Intentionally Interprofessional Palliative Care

Intentionally Interprofessional Palliative Care

Synergy in Education and Practice

Edited by

DorAnne Donesky

Michelle M. Milic

Naomi Tzril Saks

Cara L. Wallace

Editorial Consultant

Barbara A. Head

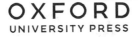

OXFORD
UNIVERSITY PRESS

OXFORD
UNIVERSITY PRESS

Oxford University Press is a department of the University of Oxford. It furthers the University's objective of excellence in research, scholarship, and education by publishing worldwide. Oxford is a registered trade mark of Oxford University Press in the UK and certain other countries.

Published in the United States of America by Oxford University Press
198 Madison Avenue, New York, NY 10016, United States of America.

© Oxford University Press 2024

Library of Congress Cataloging-in-Publication Data
Names: Donesky, DorAnne, editor. | Milic, Michelle M., editor. |
Saks, Naomi Tzril, editor. | Wallace, Cara L., editor.
Title: Intentionally Interprofessional Palliative Care /
[edited by] DorAnne Donesky, Michelle M. Milic, Naomi Tzril Saks, and Cara L. Wallace.
Description: New York, NY : Oxford University Press, [2024] |
Includes bibliographical references and index.
Identifiers: LCCN 2023036685 (print) | LCCN 2023036686 (ebook) |
ISBN 9780197542958 (hardback) | ISBN 9780197542972 (epub) | ISBN 9780197542989
Subjects: MESH: Palliative Care—methods | Interprofessional Relations | Interprofessional Education
Classification: LCC RT87.T45 (print) | LCC RT87.T45 (ebook) | NLM WB 310 |
DDC 616.02/9—dc23/eng/20231004
LC record available at https://lccn.loc.gov/2023036685
LC ebook record available at https://lccn.loc.gov/2023036686

DOI: 10.1093/med/9780197542958.001.0001

Printed by Integrated Books International, United States of America

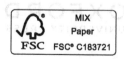

To Barbara—

This book is dedicated to the life's work and legacy of Dr. Barbara Head, who over the course of this text provided input as a nurse, social worker, mentor, mediator, friend . . . you exemplify what it means to serve passionately on and with a transdisciplinary team. This textbook is only a piece of the gifts you leave to the field of hospice and palliative care; we are forever grateful to have worked with you on it. Thank you.

Contents

Contributors

Terry Altilio, LCSW, APHSW-C
Palliative Social Work Consultant

Susan Barbour, MS, FNP
Palliative Care Advanced Practice Nurse
(retired)
University of California
San Francisco, CA, USA

Melanie Bien, LCSW
Department of Public Health
Whole Person Integrated Care: Street
Medicine, Shelter Health, and Maria
X. Martinez Health Resource Center
San Francisco, CA, USA

Rabbi Amy Ruth Bolton, BCC
Manager of Spiritual Care
NYU Langone Health
New York, NY, USA

Stephanie W. Chow, MD, MPH
Director, ALIGN (Aging, Life Innovations,
Goals & Needs) Program
Department of Geriatrics and Palliative
Medicine
Icahn School of Medicine, Mount Sinai
Hospital
New York, NY, USA
Assistant Professor
Brookdale Department of Geriatrics and
Palliative Medicine
Mount Sinai Hospital
New York, NY, USA

Lawrence Chyall, MS
Clinical Nurse Specialist
San Francisco General Hospital
San Francisco, CA, USA

Kathryn W. Coccia, MM, MT-BC
BJC Hospice
St. Louis, MO, USA

Tara M. Coles, MD, FACEP
Assistant Professor of Medicine
Department of Medicine, Division of
Palliative Care
MedStar Georgetown University Hospital
Georgetown University School of Medicine
Washington, DC, USA

Christine Corbett, DNP, APRN, FNP-BC,
CNN-NP, FNKF
Associate Chief Nursing Officer for Advanced
Practice Providers
Nurse Practitioner, Kidney Palliative Care
University Health
Kansas City, MO, USA

Jana Craig, PhD
Regional Director, NCAL Ethics Department
Kaiser Permanente
Oakland, CA, USA

Dulce M. Cruz-Oliver, MD, FAAHPM, AGSF*
Assistant Professor
Palliative Care Section, General Internal
Medicine Division
Department of Medicine
Johns Hopkins University School of Medicine
Baltimore, MD, USA

Jennifer Currin-McCulloch, PhD, LMSW
Assistant Professor
Colorado State University
School of Social Work
Fort Collins, CO, USA

Constance Dahlin, MSN, ANP-BC, ACHPN,
FPCN, FAAN*
Palliative Nurse Practitioner
Salem Hospital
Salem, MA, USA
Consultant
Center to Advance Palliative Care
New York, NY, USA

Erin M. Denney-Koelsch, MD, FAAHPM
Associate Professor of Medicine & Pediatrics
Division of Palliative Care
University of Rochester Medical Center
Rochester, NY, USA

DorAnne Donesky, PhD, ANP-BC, ACHPN,
ATSF, FHPN*,†
Professor of Clinical Nursing, Emeritus
University of California
San Francisco, CA, USA

Cathy Dundas, LCSW, APHSW-C
Norcal Regional Clinical Manager Palliative Care
Providence, Queen of the Valley Medical Center
Napa, CA, USA

Susan Enguídanos, PhD, MPH
Leonard Davis School of Gerontology
University of Southern California
Los Angeles, CA, USA

Leslie Montes Ferris, LCSW
Clinical Social Worker
IUPUI Indiana University School of Medicine
Indianapolis, IN, USA

Regina M. Fink, PhD, APRN, AOCN,
CHPN, FAAN
Professor Emeritus
School of Medicine and College of Nursing
Faculty
Interprofessional Master of Science
Palliative Care & Palliative Care Certificate
Programs University of Colorado Anschutz
Medical Campus
Aurora, CO, USA

Paul Galchutt, MPH, MDiv, BCC*
Research Staff Chaplain
M Health Fairview
University of Minnesota Medical Center
Minneapolis, MN, USA

Myra Glajchen, DSW, MSW, BSW, ACSW,
APHSW-C
Director of Education and Training
MJHS Institute for Innovation in
Palliative Care
New York, NY, USA
Assistant Professor
Department of Family and Social Medicine
Albert Einstein School of Medicine
Bronx, NY, USA

Jaime Goldberg, PhD, MSW, LCSW
Research Specialist
University of Wisconsin-Madison School of
Medicine and Public Health
Madison, WI, USA

Barbara A. Head, PhD, CHPN, ACSW, FPCN,
APHSW-C
Emeritus Professor
University of Louisville School
of Medicine
Affiliated Faculty
Kent School of Social Work
Louisville, KY, USA

Julie J. Howard, RRT, NCTTP, CCM
RT COPD Case Manager
Adventist Health + Rideout
Marysville, CA, USA

Amy W. Johnson, DO
Indiana University Health Palliative
Medicine
Ambulatory Medical Director IU Health
Palliative Care
Indiana University School of Medicine
Indianapolis, IN, USA

Barbara L. Jones, PhD, MSW, FNAP, FAOSW**
Dean and Professor
Boston University School of Social Work
Boston, MA, USA

Allison Kestenbaum, MA, MPA, BCC-PCHAC,
ACPE Certified Educator*
Supervisor of Spiritual Care and Clinical
Pastoral Education
University of California, San Diego Health
San Diego, CA, USA

Lisa Kitko, RN, PhD, FAHA, FAAN†
Dean of the School of Nursing
University of Rochester
Rochester, NY, USA

Amanda J. Kirkpatrick, PhD, RN, FAAN †
Professor, College of Nursing
Creighton University
Omaha, NE, USA

Jennifer Ku, PharmD, BCPS
Neurology and Palliative Care Pharmacist
Providence St. Peter Hospital
Olympia, WA, USA

Jennie Kung*
Director of International Partnerships and
Corporate Development
Mayo Clinic
Rochester, MN, USA

Ian B. Kwok, MD
Assistant Professor of Clinical Medicine
Weill Cornell Medical College
New York, NY, USA

Joshua R. Lakin, MD*
Senior Physician
Dana-Farber Cancer Institute
Assistant Professor of Medicine
Harvard Medical School
Boston, MA, USA

Daniel Lam, MD*
Clinical Associate Professor of Medicine
University of Washington
Seattle, WA, USA

Elizabeth Lindenberger, MD*
Professor
Brookdale Department of Geriatrics and
Palliative Medicine
Icahn School of Medicine at Mount Sinai
New York, NY, USA

Gayla Maze, MSG
Hospice Volunteer Coordinator
Lutheran Senior Services
Home & Community Based Services
St. Louis, MO, USA

Tanya Majumder, MD, MS
San Francisco Department of Public Health,
Whole Person Integrated Care: Street
Medicine, Shelter Health, and Maria
X. Martinez Health Resource Center
San Francisco, CA, USA

Mary Lynn McPherson, PharmD, PhD, BCPS,
FAAHPM
Professor and Executive Director
Advanced Post-Graduate Education in
Palliative Care
University of Maryland School of Pharmacy
Baltimore, MD, USA

Michelle M. Milic, MD, FCCP*
Associate Professor of Clinical Medicine
Division of Pulmonary, Critical Care and
Sleep Medicine
Division of Palliative Medicine
MedStar Georgetown University Hospital
Washington, DC, USA

Kafunyi Mwamba, PhD Candidate, DVM,
DMin, BCC
Volunteer Coordinator and Palliative
Medicine Chaplain Spiritual Care Service,
Stanford Health Care
Stanford University
Stanford, CA, USA

Michelle A. Neveu, AGACNP-BC, ACHPN
Lieutenant Colonel, United States Air Force
Reserve
Palliative Care Nurse Practitioner
Providence Queen of the Valley
Medical Center
Napa, CA, USA

Mark P. Pfeifer, MD, FACP
Professor of Medicine
V.V. Cooke Chair of Medicine
University of Louisville
Louisville, KY, USA

Andrea L. Pfeifle, EdD, PT, FNAP
Associate Vice Chancellor for
Interprofessional Practice and Education
Professor
Family and Community Medicine
The Ohio State University and The Wexner
Medical Center
Columbus, OH, USA

Susan R. Pollesel, MA, CCC-SLP
Speech Pathologist
Adventist Health
Ukiah, CA, USA

Jennifer D. Portz, PhD, MSW
Assistant Professor
Division of General Internal Medicine,
Department of Medicine
University of Colorado School of Medicine
Aurora, CO, USA

Dona J. Reese, PhD, MSW
Professor
Social Work Department
Southern Illinois University
Carbondale, IL, USA

Thomas Reid, MD, MA
Clinical Professor of Medicine
Division of Palliative Medicine
Department of Medicine
University of California
San Francisco, CA, USA

Karen Richards, PhD, EdS, MS
Director of Instructional Design, Media, and
Technology
MJHS Institute for Innovation in
Palliative Care
New York, NY, USA
Adjunct Assistant Professor/Instructional
Designer
School of Health Professions
Department of Psychiatric Rehabilitation &
Counseling Professions
Rutgers, the State University of New Jersey
Piscataway, NJ, USA

Masha Rand Rosenthal, MD
Assistant Professor of Clinical Emergency
Medicine
Director of Palliative Emergency Care
Medstar Emergency Physicians
Georgetown University School of Medicine
Washington, DC, USA
Department of Emergency Medicine
Medstar Union Memorial Hospital
Baltimore, MD, USA

Mateo Rutherford-Rojas, MA, MATI, CHI
Interpreting Services
UCSF Health
San Francisco, CA, USA

Naomi Tzril Saks, MA, MDiv, BCC
Clinical Health Care Chaplain
Assistant Adjunct Professor
Division of Palliative Medicine
Department of Medicine
University of California
San Francisco, CA, USA

Tara J. Schapmire, PhD, MSSW, OSW-C, FAOSW
Associate Professor of Medicine
Associate Professor of Social Work
University of Louisville
Louisville, KY, USA

Deborah Schwing, LMFT, LPCC
By the Bay Health
San Francisco, Marin, and Sonoma Counties,
CA, USA

Jennifer Seaman, PhD, RN, CHPN*
Assistant Professor
University of Pittsburgh, School of Nursing
Department of Acute and Tertiary Care
Pittsburgh, PA, USA

Deborah Witt Sherman, PhD, APRN, ANP-
BC, ACHPN, FAAN
Professor, Graduate Nursing
Soros Foundation Faculty Scholar
Faculty Senate Chair of the Interprofessional
Cross-Disciplinary Committee-
Chair of the Interprofessional Committee
Nicole Wertheim College of Nursing and
Health Sciences
Florida International University
Miami, FL, USA

Bridget Sumser, MSW, LCSW, APHSW-C
Assistant Adjunct Professor
Division of Palliative Medicine
University of California San Francisco
San Francisco, CA, USA

Niamh van Meines, PhD, ANP-BC, ACHPN
CEO
Madrone Care Network
Moraga, CA, USA

Michelle Voyer, OTD, OTR/L, C/NDT
Occupational Therapy Fieldwork Coordinator
Inpatient Occupational Therapist
MedStar Georgetown University Hospital
Washington, DC, USA

Marcie Wagner, RDH, MS
Assistant Professor
University of the Pacific
San Francisco, CA, USA
Private Practice
Marin County, CA, USA

Cara L. Wallace, PhD, LMSW, APHSW-C*
Dorothy A. Votsmier Endowed Chair, Professor
Trudy Busch Valentine School of Nursing
School of Social Work, Affiliated Faculty
Saint Louis University
Saint Louis, MO, USA

Helen Ye, MS, LAc
University of California, San Francisco
Osher Center for Integrative Health
San Francisco, CA, USA

*designates Cambia Sojourns Scholar, Cambia Health Foundation, Portland, OR, USA
**designates mentor for the Cambia Sojourns Scholar Leadership Program, Cambia Health Foundation, Portland, OR, USA
† designates Macy Faculty Scholar, Josiah Macy Jr. Foundation, New York, NY, USA

Introduction

Barbara A. Head*

As a dual professional (registered nurse and social worker), I was drawn to hospice and palliative care because of the focus on interprofessional collaboration and teamwork. The World Health Organization's definition of palliative care, one of the oldest and most accepted meanings, claims that palliative care uses a team approach to address the needs of clients and their families.[1] Teamwork is the core from which our success with clients and families emanates. We are experts in interprofessional teamwork. However, most of the publications guiding our work approach it from a single profession's viewpoint, be it medicine, nursing, social work, spiritual care, or other professions involved in the work.

When approached about helping with a textbook focused on interprofessional palliative care, it immediately appealed to me. The past 10 years of my career have been focused on interprofessional education in palliative care whereby our institutions and faculties prepare students from different professions and disciplines to work together to improve the quality of life for patients and families experiencing serious illness. This textbook would augment the profession-specific palliative care textbooks already published by Oxford University Press by focusing on the unique synergy and perspective created when professionals join and work toward one common purpose—person-centered care for the seriously ill. Such teams have learned that more is accomplished by cooperation than by working individually. The identity of the team overrides individual personal identities; leadership is shared as work is focused on mutually determined goals and accountability.

Interprofessional palliative care is modeled in the selection of authors and editors for this textbook: two individuals from different professions were selected to coauthor each chapter, and two editors, also from different professions, edited the chapter. This was an intentional means to include the perspectives of the dominant professions on each topic. Such shared leadership and mutual accountability presented challenges. We could observe the teams of two going through the forming, storming, norming, and performing stages of teambuilding[2] as they developed their chapters. Adding two editors to the mix assured that at least four professional perspectives contributed to each chapter, but also required consensus building through a series of communication efforts. In the end, we hope that the work models the teamwork we are encouraging.

---

* Final edits of Dr. Head's introduction were done by the editorial team following her death.

Some reflections on the team process experienced by the editors as this book took shape: It was fascinating to observe and experience the multiple styles of interprofessional collaboration within the author teams and within our editorial team. These teams were microcosms of the interprofessional team collaboration that we advocate, and the teams exhibited similar challenges to those experienced by clinical teams. Some authors were reluctant to collaborate with someone they did not know, while others welcomed the challenge and the new connections. Some author teams wrote their chapters together, while others were led by one author with the other serving in more of a supporting role. Some authors requested more direction from editors, while others were less enthusiastic in considering the multiple interprofessional perspectives of the editorial team. The process of writing many of the chapters became a dialogue of curiosity between authors and editors with the common goal of exploring the topic in a truly transdisciplinary manner.

Often in palliative care, we take our interprofessional practice for granted, when we are actually functioning more in parallel than truly interprofessionally or transdisciplinarily. Ideally, each team member is grounded in their own profession with a strong profession-specific voice. As they bring their ideas generated from within their perspective, those ideas are shaped by the interprofessional alchemy and transformed into a unique perspective that benefits our patients but would not be possible without the interprofessional interaction. Through the process of working on this book, we have found that the interprofessional perspective is not intuitive and must be developed over time. We found that we continue to identify areas where we are still learning about each other's perceptions. As authors and editors, we experienced each other's intersectionality—we each have a strong profession-specific voice, but many other perspectives also became evident, based on our personal backgrounds and positionality, clinical experiences, regional variation, political perspectives, educational foundation, interests, experience with COVID, individual strengths—these and more influenced thinking and discussions throughout the text. This was not always an easy process—at times we found ourselves frustrated, confused, and at odds over the topic or terminology at hand. Our deep respect for one another and our commitment to truly listening to one another's perspectives eventually allowed us to find alignment and common ground.

We have a well-publicized and ongoing challenge with language in palliative care. We are still struggling for acceptance and public understanding of the difference between palliative care and hospice. In this book, we have included some notes with standardized comments/definitions about certain words that we found used differently by different authors. Even as we were completing the manuscript, we learned that the term "providers" has fallen out of favor, with good reason related to its origin.[3] As we recognize that language is constantly changing, we decided not to reopen previously completed chapters. However, we have been careful about our word choices in this book, also recognizing that some words may sound dated in a few years. Language is often accompanied by strong emotions or polarization, and we attempt to invite discussion across professions and the wider population we serve. We welcome ongoing curiosity, graciousness, humility, and dialogue as the language of our discipline develops.

It has been said that if you want to go fast, go alone, but if you want to go far, go with a team. Our coauthors needed time to come together, focus, and divide the work. Interprofessional collaboration requires a certain mindset and willingness to focus on the task rather than on who gets credit. Some struggled while others embraced the assignment. We did not go fast, but by giving authors and editors the time needed to overcome obstacles and speak as a team, we have a more in-depth product reflective of the team's voice rather than one authority.

References

1. World Health Organization. Palliative Care Fact Sheet. https://www.who.int/news-room/fact-sheets/detail/palliative-care, 2020. Accessed 1/3/2024.
2. Tuckman BW, Jensen MAC. Stages of small-group development revisited. *Group Organiz Studies* 1977;2(4):419–427.
3. Scarff JR. What's in a Name? The Problematic Term "Provider." *Federal Practitioner.* 2021;38(10):446.

Glossary Terms

Accreditation independent, third-party evaluation of a program or institution by an assessment body, and measured against recognized standards.

Adult learning components of education directed toward mature learners. Characteristics include learner-centered, self-directed, active learning (learning by doing), reflection/drawing from past experiences, multisensory, focused on personal development of the learner, and learner engagement through feedback and consultation.

Advance care planning discussion and preparation for future decisions about medical care in advance, in case the person becomes seriously ill or unable to communicate their own wishes.

Advance care planning documents forms which document an individual's preferences for care should they become unable to communicate for themselves. Some are legal documents (living wills, designation of healthcare surrogate, advance directive); others are medical orders such as do not resuscitate orders or physician's/medical orders for life-sustaining treatment (POLST/MOLST).

Advanced practice providers (APP) physician assistants/associates and advanced practice registered nurses, including nurse practitioners and clinical nurse specialists, who are educated, licensed, and credentialed to perform basic medical activities typically performed by a physician, including physical exams, ordering diagnostic tests, and prescribing medication.

Assessment an in-depth, ongoing process of evaluating a patient's needs and resources. It includes interventions, outcomes, and evaluation and is completed by the domain expert(s) or other members of the team.

Care plan in palliative care, the plan is based upon the patient's and/or family's goals of care, input from the referring and collaborating clinicians, and the interprofessional team members' assessments. The plan is adjusted during the course of care based upon the trajectory of the illness and ongoing assessments.

Caregiver someone responsible for attending to the daily care needs of another person, either as a volunteer or as a paid employee. Caregivers provide physical, emotional, and financial support to a person who is unable to care for him/herself due to illness, injury, or disability.

Certificate designation of completion of a continuing education course or program; does not signify competence or advanced expertise (designated with lower case "c").

Certification a voluntary process whereby an individual's advanced expertise in a specialty field of practice is verified, usually on a national level. Candidates must meet defined eligibility requirements and pass a competency test. In many fields, board certification is required for practice (designated with upper case "C").

Clinician any health professional providing direct patient care to individuals and their families, whether primary care practitioners, specialist consultants, or specialist-level palliative care team members.

Collaborative practice the goal of interprofessional education, when health professionals from multiple backgrounds work together at the top of their scopes of practice in a synergistic way that benefits patients and caregivers.

Comfort care care directed at maintaining or improving the quality of life of persons with a serious illness. The goal is to prevent or treat symptoms and side effects, and address psychosocial and spiritual problems related to the disease. Although the goal of all palliative care is comfort, the term "comfort care" is often used synonymously with outpatient hospice care or the decision to forgo disease-directed therapy while hospitalized.

Comfort measures only (CMO) care in which only those interventions that relieve or prevent suffering are provided; a regional term to designate comfort care status.

Competency a combination of skills, job attitudes, and knowledge which is reflected in job behavior that can be observed, measured, and evaluated

Continuing education education beyond that which is required for an academic degree or licensure. Often required for license renewal of healthcare professionals, it is specific to each profession and each state.

Core palliative care team the four foundational palliative care professions that are named as part of the interprofessional palliative care team for both the Medicare hospice guidelines and the NCP guidelines—chaplain, nurse, physician, and social worker. Teams may include many professions in addition to the core members, and this designation does not minimize the importance of other team members who contribute to the palliative care of patients and families

Cultural competence the processes by which individuals and systems respond respectfully and effectively to people across all diversity factors in a manner that recognizes, affirms, and values the worth of individuals, families, and communities, and protects and preserves the dignity of each.[1]

Cultural humility a lifelong process of self-reflection and self-critique whereby an individual first examines and understands his or her own beliefs and cultural identities before learning about another's culture.[2]

Discipline a field of study; refers to a branch of knowledge either in healthcare (i.e., oncology, radiology, pediatrics, palliative care) or elsewhere (i.e., history, music, science, design).

Domain a sphere of knowledge, influence, or activity

End-of-life care care provided when death is imminent based on the diagnosis and prognosis.

Family significant others as defined by the patient, including blood relatives, life partners, or friends.

Familiness a term that emphasizes the unique community of caregivers who provide holistic care for the patient.[3]

Fellowship a postgraduate program in an area of specialization, ranging from one-three years.

Generalist palliative care see *Primary palliative care*

Goals of care patient-determined desired outcomes of the care provided, based on personal beliefs and values and consideration of the patient's current health situation; if the patient is unable to communicate, goals of care are developed, based on the healthcare proxy's understanding of the patient's beliefs and values.

Health professions education education for students who plan to enter a field such as medicine, nursing, chaplaincy, social work, psychology, music therapy, physical therapy. Such education is often preparatory to obtaining licensure for practice.

Hidden curriculum lessons learned that are not part of the formal curriculum. This often refers to professionalism, interpersonal interactions, coping skills, emotional responses, and communication. May have a negative connotation when referring to unintended signals that reinforce negative behaviors or interactions.

Hospice a team-oriented approach to expert medical care, pain management, and emotional and spiritual support expressly tailored to the patient's needs and wishes; support is also provided to the patient's loved ones. In the United States, hospice is an insurance benefit for people with a prognosis of 6 months or less to live.

Immersion programs intensive clinical opportunities which may offer potential for brief clinical observation and mentoring over days to weeks.

Interdisciplinary various fields of expertise or specialties (i.e., medical oncologist, radiologist, surgical oncologist, pathologist). Although Medicare policy and the NCP Guidelines use the term "interdisciplinary" when referring to teams composed of clinicians representing multiple professions, in this book we have standardized the language to use the term "interprofessional" when referring to the core members of the palliative care team and reserve the term "interdisciplinary" for referring to collaboration across specialties or with non-healthcare disciplines.

Interprofessional team team composed of members of different professions (i.e., physician, nurse, chaplain, social worker).

Interprofessional education (IPE) involves educators and learners from two or more health professions and their foundational disciplines, who jointly create and foster a collaborative learning environment. The goal of these efforts is to develop knowledge, skills, and attitudes that result in interprofessional team behaviors and competence. Ideally, IPE is incorporated throughout the entire curriculum in a vertically and horizontally integrated fashion. In palliative care, ideally IPE includes learners and faculty from all four of the core professions.[4]

Licensure granting of a permit or license, typically from a state board, which allows one to practice a certain profession within a scope of practice or care.

Multidisciplinary draws on knowledge from different disciplines but stays within the boundaries of those fields

Palliative care care provided by interprofessional team members and focused on expert assessment and management of pain and other symptoms, assessment and support of caregiver needs, and coordination of care for seriously ill patients. Palliative care attends to the physical, functional, psychological, practical, and spiritual consequences of a serious illness. It is a person- and family-centered approach to care, providing seriously ill people relief from the symptoms and stress of an illness. Through early integration into the care plan of seriously ill people, palliative care improves quality of life for both the patients and the family.

Palliative medicine subspecialty of palliative care practiced specifically by physicians.

Pimping a slang term used for quizzing learners, especially in the medical field where a more experienced physician asks questions of learners (residents or medical students). Although this is often justified as a means to test knowledge and think quickly ("good pimping"), it traditionally invokes a hierarchy, questions a learner in a public or operating room setting, and may be "malignant" and induce shame or humiliation. Some have suggested an end to the term and the practice and a renewed pedagogy in medical education.[5,6]

Postgraduate relating to or pursuing advanced study after graduating from college or professional school.

Primary (or generalist) palliative care palliative care provided by healthcare professionals who practice the foundational principles of palliative care but are not currently employed with a specialist palliative care team. This includes primary care clinicians, disease-oriented specialists, nurses, social workers, pharmacists, chaplains, and others who care for the seriously ill but have not specialized in palliative care.

Profession an occupation that requires special education and/or prolonged training and a formal qualification (i.e., medicine, nursing, social work, chaplaincy).

Provider often refers to a person or organization that provides medical care and services. Providers may include physicians, doctors of osteopathic medicine, nurse practitioners and other advanced practice registered nurses (APRNs), physician assistants/associates, and licensed medical social workers. Concerns have been raised about the use of the term "provider" in healthcare as it suggests a commercial transaction rather than a relationship between clinician and patient, and it obscures the specific role and credentials of individual clinicians. The terms "clinician," "practitioner," or "healthcare professional" are suggested as preferable when an overarching term is necessary. For this edition, the decision was made to keep the term "provider" when it was used by chapter authors, while recognizing that this change may be necessary for future editions.[7]

Residency enhanced clinical training for entry to practice.

Role blurring a characteristic of the Generalist-Specialist Model of Interprofessional Palliative Care where expert palliative care specialists learn from their interprofessional colleagues and overlap functions with specialists from other professional backgrounds. This characteristic can also be considered from a negative perspective when clear boundaries and communication are missing and lead to misunderstandings and resentment among team members.

Screening (domain-specific) a brief instrument or process, completed by all members of the palliative care team, that evaluates the presence or absence of domain-specific needs and/or distress with the goal of identifying those in need of further assessment and care to be performed by the palliative care domain expert and in collaboration with other members as indicated.

Specialist palliative care the active, total palliative care of patients with serious illness and their families, provided by an interprofessional team whose members have undergone recognized specialist palliative care training and/or certification.

Specialty Palliative care is considered to be a subspecialty within medicine and nursing, but a specialty in spiritual care and social work. For this book, we standardize the language by referring to palliative care as a specialty when referring to the team as a whole. We use the term "subspecialty" when referring specifically to nursing or medicine.

Subspecialty see *specialty*

Supportive care a term sometimes used synonymously with either comfort care or palliative care.

Synerdisciplinary care Each team member approaches patient and family encounters through their own lens, education, and experience, and recognizes different cues from the patient/family and nuances of the interaction. Palliative care team members confer about their observations, which can lead to care that far surpasses what any one person can offer on their own and better addresses the scope of patient/family needs. When a profession's perspective is absent from a team, those nuances are lost.

Team-based care the provision of comprehensive health services to individuals, families, and/or their communities by at least 2 health professionals who work collaboratively with patients, family caregivers, and community service providers on shared goals within and across settings to achieve care that is safe, effective, patient-centered, timely, efficient, and equitable. In palliative care, best practice for team-based care includes all four core professions.[8]

Tertiary palliative care In academic medical centers, specialist knowledge for the most complex cases is practiced, researched, and taught by academicians or researchers. Competence in education and research is achieved by significant advanced training and experience. Tertiary palliative care includes the complex care provided at centers with advanced clinical services such as cardiopulmonary life support (ECMO) and transplant, in addition to academic research and education.

Thanatology the study of death and dying.

Transdisciplinary an ideal model of team collaboration in which all professions on the team work as equals; shared information, communication, compassion, knowledge, and decision-making are used to co-create a unified care plan; responsibility for outcomes is shared; turf issues are minimized because each member is viewed as essential and can assume leadership at any given time. In addition, the natural, social, and health sciences are integrated in a humanities context, and in so doing transcend each of their traditional boundaries. Team members share information with each other so that the boundaries of each discipline begin to be removed and professionals gain skills in other practice areas, yet the authority for each profession remains with its respective specialist. Palliative care teams should strive to practice in this manner.

References

1. National Association of Social Workers. (2015). Standards and indicators for cultural competence in social work practice. Washington, DC: NASW. Retrieved from https://www.social workers.org/LinkClick.aspx?fileticket=7dVckZAYUmk%3D&portalid=0
2. Tervalon, M., & Murray-Garcia, J. (1998). Cultural humility versus cultural competence: A critical distinction in defining physician training outcomes in multicultural education. Journal of Health Care for the Poor and Underserved, 9, 117–125. doi:10.1353/hpu. 2010.0233
3. Schriver, J.M. (2010). Human behavior and the social environment: Shifting paradigms in essential knowledge for social work practice. (5th ed.). Needham Heights, MA: Allyn & Bacon.
4. Buring SM, Bhushan A, Broeseker A, Conway S, Duncan-Hewitt W, Hansen L, Westberg S: Interprofessional education: definitions, student competencies, and guidelines for implementation. Am J Pharm Educ 2009;73:59.
5. Chen, D.R., Priest, K. Pimping: a tradition of gendered disempowerment. BMC Med Educ 19, 345 (2019). https://doi.org/10.1186/s12909-019-1761-1
6. Kost A, Chen FM. Socrates was not a pimp: changing the paradigm of questioning in medical education. Acad Med. 2015;90(1):20–4.
7. Scarff, J. R. (2021). What's in a Name? The Problematic Term "Provider". Federal Practitioner, 38(10), 446.
8. Naylor MD, Coburn KD, Kurtzman ET, et al. Team-Based Primary Care for Chronically Ill Adults: State of the Science. Advancing Team-Based Care. Philadelphia, PA: American Board of Internal Medicine Foundation; 2010.

1

Interprofessional Teamwork in Palliative Care

Jennifer D. Portz and Joshua R. Lakin

Key Points

- While there is limited evidence directly linking interprofessional practice to domain-specific outcomes, interprofessional teams are foundational to the provision of excellent palliative care.
- Healthcare providers, patients, and caregivers highlight the importance of interprofessional work in palliative care.
- Strong theoretical foundations and growing appreciation for interprofessional education models ensure the successful future of interprofessional palliative care practice.

Introduction

A Case Study

Consider the illustrative fictional case of Ms. Smith, a 47-year-old who identifies as a Black woman with a history of sickle cell disease and who has recently been diagnosed with stage 3 breast cancer. She is being referred to the palliative care team for a painful lymph node in her left axilla as she prepares for her initial cancer treatment. As a result of her sickle cell disease, she has relapsing and remitting chronic pain, slowly worsening chronic kidney disease, and has infrequent hospitalizations for sickle disease crises. Ms. Smith has a history of anxiety and depression, now stable with treatment through a therapist with whom she has a wonderful relationship. She has 2 children, is recently divorced from her partner, and is currently enmeshed in the legal system due to custody challenges from her partner as part of divorce proceedings. She has recently joined a Jehovah's Witness Kingdom Hall at her family's encouragement.

Why an Interprofessional Team?

Palliative care is a comprehensive approach to caring for people like Ms. Smith, those with serious illness, along with supporting their families, friends, and caregivers. The focus of palliative care is on improving quality of life while addressing physical, psychological, spiritual, cultural, and social concerns of both the patient and their loved ones. Considering the many complexities of this case, no single professional could serve Ms. Smith and her family adequately; they would benefit from the synergy of an interprofessional palliative care team. Managing serious illness presents many intertwined challenges, from achieving symptom control, easing patient-family conflict, and navigating complex care systems, to tending to the dying process. As such, the interprofessional team is pivotal to addressing the multidimensional aspects of caring for people with serious illness.

Before we consider the benefits of interprofessional work, it is important to note the difference between *interprofessional* and *interdisciplinary* teams, though they frequently exist together. Much of the research in palliative care uses the terms interchangeably.[1] As you will read in Chapter 3, interdisciplinary teams incorporate various disciplines or expertise on the team, often used interchangeably with "specialties" such as pulmonology, neurology, or palliative care. While this is an important element to interprofessional palliative care work, the term *interprofessional* is additive because it calls upon individuals with diverse professional training (for example, nursing, medicine, social work, or spiritual care) to collectively muster and intentionally manage their multiple and overlapping disciplines in team-based care of vulnerable populations, such as those people with serious illness seeking care from the medical system.[1] Interprofessional teamwork is founded on collaboration to achieve a common goal. When interprofessional teamwork is successful, the unique skills and expertise of each profession synergize to create a novel and integrated care experience.

The evidence base for supporting interprofessional teams is developing. At this time there is little direct evidence verifying that interprofessional teamwork improves patient and family outcomes or quality of care. However, early indicators suggest that interprofessional teams are associated with improved patient satisfaction, reduced lengths of hospitalization, adherence to recommended practices, and better use of healthcare resources. Patients, caregivers, and palliative care providers alike all document that an interprofessional approach improves patient and family experience of palliative care.[2-6]

Interprofessional palliative care offers an opportunity to care for people and their families at a comprehensive and multidimensional level; however, the process is not without difficulties. While the benefits are clear to those who approach their work in an interprofessional manner, challenges include communication barriers, role ambiguity, team power-dynamics, professional friction, and financial resources. While these challenges are noted in the literature, the catalysts and best practices for establishing and managing high-quality interprofessional teams are well documented by team leaders, clinicians, and educators. Much of this book will highlight these facilitators for successful interprofessional work, including theoretical frameworks, education and training, and best practices across a variety of palliative care settings.

Interprofessional Teamwork by Domain of Palliative Care Practice

In 2018, the updated National Consensus Project Clinical Practice Guidelines for Quality Palliative Care (NCP Guidelines) were published. They assess, delineate, and describe the impact of interprofessional palliative care on 8 key domains of care[7] (Table 1.1). The NCP's findings highlight that palliative care, when delivered as a specialty team, can enhance quality in each of the key domains of care. Importantly, while there is a significant volume of research discoverable through

Table 1.1 The 8 Domains of Palliative Care Delivery from the National Consensus Project Clinical Practice Guidelines for Quality Palliative Care

Domain	Description
1	*Structure and Process of Care* The composition of an interdisciplinary team is outlined, including the professional qualifications, education, training, and support needed to deliver optimal patient- and family-centered care. Defines the elements of the palliative care assessment and care plan, as well as systems and processes specific to palliative care.
2	*Physical Aspects of Care* The palliative care assessment, care planning, and treatment of physical symptoms are described, emphasizing patient- and family-directed holistic care.
3	*Psychological Aspects of Care* The processes for systematically assessing and addressing the psychological and psychiatric aspects of care in the context of serious illness.
4	*Social Aspects of Care* Assessing and addressing patient and family social support needs.
5	*Spiritual, Religious, and Existential Aspects of Care* The spiritual, religious, and existential aspects of care are described, including the importance of screening for unmet needs.
6	*Cultural Aspects of Care* The ways in which culture influences both palliative care delivery and the experience of that care by the patient and family, from the time of diagnosis through death and bereavement.
7	*End-of-Life Care* The symptoms and situations that are common in the final days and weeks of life.
8	*Ethical and Legal Aspects of Care* Advance care planning, surrogate decision-making, regulatory and legal considerations, and related palliative care issues, focusing on ethical imperatives and processes to support patient autonomy.

Domains and definitions used with permission.

systematic review, the description of palliative care interventions and teamwork is varied and, overall, the quality of evidence is limited. As such, a paucity of evidence exists on how interprofessional teams drive higher quality palliative care and specifically in which domains. However, strong foundational conceptual reasons support the value of teams as best poised to affect each of the key palliative care domains.

Primary and specialty palliative care leaders, in both Europe and the United States, are calling for increased interprofessional teamwork to improve patient- and family-centered outcomes in the care of patients with serious illness.[8-11] Healthcare providers in particular care settings, such as intensive care units,[12] rural communities,[13] those caring for patients and families preparing for left ventricular assist devices,[14] and those managing advanced kidney disease[15] identify a need for interprofessional palliative care. In this chapter, we delve deeper into the impact of interprofessional work in each NCP Guideline domain.

Domain 1: Structure and Process of Care

Our team worked with a veteran in his 50s over 2 weeks while he was hospitalized for advanced cirrhosis. We determined he was at high risk of dying at the initial visit. We worked to identify his values and hopes, which was challenging as the severity of his hepatic encephalopathy changed day to day.
—David Bekelman, MD, MPH, physician, Veteran Affairs Eastern
Colorado Health Care System, Aurora, Colorado
At the request of the primary medical team, I brought our facility dog, Tootsie, who was a source of support and comfort. Later, the patient and I worked on life review and processing of childhood trauma.
—Elizabeth Holman, PsyD, psychologist, Veteran Affairs Eastern
Colorado Health Care System, Aurora, Colorado
The veteran said he would be surprised if there is a God and was not afraid of death. We discussed his lifelong experiences of trauma, abandonment, culture of violence, and complex family dynamics. Being an accomplished artist supported his spiritual sense of meaning and purpose.
—Lydia Buttner, M.Div., BCC, chaplain, Veteran Affairs Eastern
Colorado Health Care System, Aurora, Colorado
I worked on hospice placement options for him and his service dog, Milo, whom he cared about deeply. In the end, I was unsuccessful in placing them together; however, we were able to advocate for his friend and caregiver to bring Milo to the hospital to say goodbye to the veteran.
—Sarah Osani, LCSW, social worker, Veteran Affairs Eastern
Colorado Health Care System, Aurora, Colorado

As illustrated in this example of a veteran and his caregivers from the VA Eastern Colorado Health Care System, Aurora, Colorado, the domain of structure and process of care covers a wide array of palliative care activities, ranging from team-work addressing quality of life to care coordination and communication. We have rich research in this domain, and moderate-quality evidence demonstrates that a specialty palliative care team impacts patient and family quality of life, advance care planning, and patient and family satisfaction.[7] However, studies have not employed consistent team structure, and many studies are missing what would be considered a full cohort of palliative care team members and interventions.[16] While one re-view found an association between the number of professions involved and effect of intervention, the effect was limited to particular professions, such as physicians and physical therapists, and nearly half of interventions were delivered by only 1 or 2 clinicians.[16] Multiple recent studies have shown inconsistent team structures, making it difficult to tie particular aspects of interprofessional work directly to im-pact on structures or processes of care;[17-20] however, some ongoing studies are pro-spectively designed with detailed and comprehensive interprofessional components that will help to further assess the impact of teamwork in palliative care,[21-23] and some look more specifically at the impact of one role in the team.[24,25]

Conceptually, interprofessional work is foundational to the domain of struc-ture and processes of care. Working to improve the complex space that patients and families consider as good quality living, a goal that is central to the practice of palliative care and embodies all other domains of care, requires the palliative care team to assess and treat an individual from many dimensions. Activities such as advance care planning, early and late goals of care conversations, and care coordi-nation require a nuanced and interwoven knowledge of the person and their family, cultural, physical, and existential values, beliefs, and constructs. For example, Ms. Smith, who has experience with chronic serious illness and the healthcare system, is now faced with a new life-threatening illness in the context of shifting family and spiritual dynamics. Assessing the different paths to maximizing her quality of life through her possible future courses of treatment will depend upon a cohesive, well-trained, and synchronized interprofessional palliative care team. However, we know that the coordination and integration of interprofessional palliative care work, while linked to quality of life and other process outcomes in our work, requires hard work, thoughtful systems, and clear intentions; consequently, attention to this do-main of interprofessional palliative care work is critical.[26]

A key aspect to the processes of care domain is the interprofessional team itself, including team education and emotional support. Although true interprofessional work is complex and difficult to research, the effort is worthwhile for the patient, the family, and the care team. Burnout rates among palliative care providers is estimated to be 62%, with the highest rates seen among non-physicians, younger providers, and those with smaller teams.[27] With this in mind, interprofessional teams improve both provider self-care and team support, as detailed below. Palliative care providers have indicated that authentic team-member relationships and a supportive belief in an interprofessional care model foster creativity, improved energy, and emotional well-being across the team.[28] Providers have also found that networking within and across their own professions is helpful for improving their own unique skill set and managing stress when caring for the seriously ill.[29] However, providers also call for specific mechanisms and institutional support to improve self-care and team support.[30] Based on studies exploring provider experiences, training in mindfulness and stress reduction, professional workshopping, and narrative approaches show promise in fostering positive team dynamics, improved coping skills, and stress reduction among palliative care providers.[31-33] In coping with the challenges of providing palliative care, interprofessional teams are the best mechanism for supporting team members and developing coping skills.

Due to a growing appreciation and focus on interprofessional care, interprofessional education is rapidly expanding. As you will see in later chapters of this book, curricula have been developed for early medical and health professions education, advanced palliative care training, and continuing education. Interprofessional education offers new opportunities to advance participation and leadership, particularly among social workers, nurses, and chaplains.[34] Successful interprofessional education requires engaged support from professionals who traditionally have more power, such as physicians and administrative leaders. Interprofessional education and training programs are shown to improve clinician confidence in providing palliative care, enhancing understanding and promoting therapeutic changes in psychosocial care, practice knowledge, and continuity of care, and show promise when held online.[35-37] One exemplar practice of exploring the shared responsibility of all team members, and the unique contributions of each, improved the team's appreciation of the full scope of palliative care practice.[38] Importantly, all professions on the palliative care team have roles in each key domain of practice, as will be highlighted throughout this chapter. For example, the NCP Guidelines recommend that all members of the interprofessional palliative care team must be able to screen for unmet needs in all domains of care. In addition, all team members should be proficient in general palliative care functions, such as facilitating goals of care conversations, serious illness communication, and end-of-life care. Interprofessional education and ongoing training may be key to developing and maintaining successful interprofessional structures of care.

Domain 2: Physical Aspects of Care

I work on an interprofessional team providing palliative care to patients with advanced kidney disease. Symptom management in these patients is complex and non-traditional, as so many of the patients have Cicely Saunders' "total pain." Working with an interprofessional team is essential. For example, we cared for one patient with end-stage renal disease on dialysis who had chronic, non-malignant neck pain. The pain was severe and had not responded to escalating doses of opioids and other adjuvant therapies. Working closely with our nurse practitioner and social worker, we were able to discover that the patient's pain was psychosocial and existential in nature. She had deep-seated fears about her own mortality as she was the guardian for her daughter, who had disabilities and relied on her for housing and financial support. By addressing these issues and expanding our focus out from the physical aspects of her pain, we were able to titrate down her opioids and, perhaps counterintuitively, provide her with more pain relief.

—Richard E. Leiter, MD, palliative care physician,
Dana-Farber Cancer Institute, Boston, Massachusetts

To address the physical aspects of serious illness, healthcare providers indicate that the interprofessional palliative care team is essential for delivering person-centered medication regimens,[39] complex symptom-cluster management,[40] and multidimensional pain treatment.[41] We have moderate-quality evidence that comprehensive specialty palliative care impacts symptom management, though most of the evidence on specific therapeutics and interventions is quite limited.[7,42]

According to healthcare providers, facilitators influencing interprofessional collaboration for physical symptom management include several personal and team characteristics.[39-41] First, all of the providers on the team must be interested and willing to collaborate with other interprofessional members. Pharmacists, nurses, chaplains, and social workers all report that a genuine interest in teamwork results in improved identification and management of complex symptoms. A lack of interest by the team results in hierarchical decision-making, reduced team participation, and diminished creativity to address complex and multidimensional symptoms. Second, this interest in and willingness for interprofessional team engagement often depend on individual professions legitimizing the value they bring to patient care. For example, in a qualitative study of 15 pharmacists, participants indicated that if the pharmacist could demonstrate to the team that their questions, ideas, and follow-up were helpful, the team, and physicians in particular, were more likely to actively engage in medication review and incorporate pharmacist recommendations into care plans.[39]

In terms of team characteristics, role flexibility across the team is reported to improve physical outcomes. Interprofessional providers all report their ability to assess pain. This confidence in assessing pain across the team is an excellent example of flexing outside one's stereotypical role on the team. However, perceived flexibility in the treatment of physical aspects of care is less apparent. For example, in an ethnographic study of 2 hospice and palliative care teams consisting of 15 members, physicians and nurses expressed more willingness to treat pain symptoms than other professions.[41] Social workers, chaplains, and aides indicated that pain treatment was beyond their scope of practice. Yet, in this same study, physicians and nurses highlighted other professionals' abilities to treat pain. In a specific case, a nurse participant noted that the team social worker provided a stress-reducing intervention which in turn improved the patient's pain. Providers suggest that improving team logistics by incorporating diverse professional leadership roles, using a shared common language, maximizing knowledge exchange, and sharing management responsibility will lead to superior role flexibility and interprofessional practice addressing physical aspects of care.[40,41] Consider all of this in the example of Ms. Smith above. She has a history of chronic pain and is now presenting with acute pain in the context of a breast cancer diagnosed in close temporal proximity to a divorce and during a custody dispute over her children. She also has anxiety and depression and is almost certainly experiencing a complex "total pain" syndrome that must be assessed and treated through an interprofessional lens.

Domain 3: Psychological Aspects of Care

When working as a pediatric palliative care social worker, I always worked along with the physician as she would have conversations about diagnosis or transitions of care. As a team, we thought it was important that we go together and support the child and family. Sometimes I could remain with the family after the physician left and sit with their emotions, help them sort out what they heard, identify what questions they still had, or just be present as a witness. Meeting with the family together also provided support to the team. Regardless of how the conversation unfolded, it was always easier to go together and to share the emotional weight of the discussion. Being a team meant that we could help each other hold the emotions and be present for the child and family and for each other. It made us better together and helped us continue in our roles knowing we were never alone.

—Barbara L. Jones, PhD, MSW, FNAP, The University of Texas at Austin

The prevalence of psychological symptoms, such as anxiety and depression, are high in serious illness and impose a significant burden upon patients and families.[43] The evidence base for the impact of interprofessional palliative care on anxiety and depression is mixed;[7] however, a number of well-done studies demonstrate an impact of early palliative care and communication interventions on anxiety, fatigue, and depression.[44-47] As in other domains, the evidence for how the interprofessional team addresses psychological aspects of care is limited, with early evidence demonstrating the impact from music and art therapy on depression and anxiety.[7]

In terms of conceptual constructs in which interprofessional palliative care teams address the psychological burden of serious illness, one retrospective analysis of an early palliative care intervention suggests that attention to symptom management, patient and family coping, and prognostic awareness are key.[48,49] Accomplishing improved symptom management through medications and counseling, while helping patients and families to have a deeper understanding of the possible future with their illness in the context of bolstered coping resources, is the kind of task that requires the multiple inputs and the diverse expertise of an interprofessional team. Importantly, in the realm of psychological care, many individual professions have demonstrated interventions that can be effective in improving mental health, so this particular domain is one where collaboration is critical for finding synergy and providing maximum benefit. In the care of patients like Ms. Smith, who has a stable non-prescribing mental health provider but now enters a new realm where her psychological care will become more complex, one critical function of the interprofessional palliative care team is managing constructs such as the interplay of possible end-of-life planning and new cancer-directed or pain medications that could interact with antidepressant therapy.

Domain 4: Social Aspects of Care

Caregivers play a vital role in cancer care; yet, their contribution and the impact of cancer on their well-being is often overlooked. An interprofessional palliative care team sees the importance of both the patient and the context in which the patient lives, of which caregivers are a core component. Further, an interprofessional palliative care team has the expertise to care for the physical and emotional impact of illness on the caregiver, thereby improving the health of both patients and their vital support networks.
—Kelly M. Trevino, clinical psychologist, Memorial Sloan
Kettering Cancer Center, New York, New York

A paucity of research exists on the impact of interprofessional specialty palliative care in the realm of meeting social needs and providing access to relevant services for patients and families. The existing evidence points less to interprofessional work and more toward single-profession interventions.[7] An intentional, well-designed interprofessional palliative care model for addressing opiod use disorder in cancer patients sets an excellent example for how studies can more clearly demonstrate interprofessional work.[50] Social aspects of care are a key area for future research given the known significant burden of caregiving in serious illness. Informal caregiving represents a significant and unaddressed burden in the United States, and the impact on those caring for people living and dying from serious illness includes complicated bereavement, morbidity, and mortality (see Chapter 17).[51] As such, since specialty palliative care charges itself with the well-being of patients and their families, integrated and thoughtful team-based care of social networks is critical.

While further evidence directly linking interprofessional practice to improved social health outcomes is imperative, relying on the expertise of various professions to address specific social concerns cannot be underestimated. Based on the NCP Guidelines, some of the major social concerns include: home modification and transportation, family communication and experience, health insurance, medication access, and home and personal safety.[7] In respect to these concerns, interprofessional palliative care providers find that clinical pharmacists are particularly helpful in addressing medication access concerns.[52] In a study of occupational therapists' role in palliative care, they voiced their expertise in adapting patients' environments to improve the safety and function of patients.[53] Home health aides provide personal care to patients and families, and therefore have a valuable role on the interprofessional team in establishing family connections and improving communication.[54] Physical therapists indicate that they are devoted to connecting patients and families to community resources during the end of life.[55] Each team member has a role to play in identifying and addressing social concerns.

Our example case highlights why social care by an interprofessional team is so critical for palliative care interventions. Ms. Smith is at incredibly high risk of traumatic experiences in multiple dynamic social roles in her life, for example as a mother and as a wife, and her newly diagnosed and chronic illnesses further weakens her ability to manage her life in all of its facets. An interprofessional palliative care team can help to integrate the multiple roles and social aspects of her life to create a comprehensive plan for her to be able to maintain and maximize her social network and supports.

Domain 5: Spiritual, Religious, and Existential Aspects of Care

Working on an interprofessional team is a continuous reminder to all of us to attend to patients and their loved ones as whole people. Patients benefit from knowing there are skilled professionals working together for them in all kinds of ways. Simply through the presence of a chaplain who can make a spiritual assessment, patients are more likely to divulge spiritual pain and resources they may have kept hidden otherwise. It is as if a previously imperceptible frequency is tuned into and adding this knowledge about the patient can offer insight to the interprofessional team so they may collectively and more deeply overcome obstacles to achieving patients' goals of care.

—Allison Kestenbaum, MA, MPA, BCC, ACPE certified
educator, palliative care chaplain, University of California
San Diego Health, San Diego, California

There is moderate-quality evidence that therapies such as dignity therapy improve spiritual well-being, enhance interpersonal spirituality, and decrease existential distress. However, as in other domains of palliative care, the evidence base does not address how interprofessional teams affect the spiritual well-being of patients and their caregivers.[7,56] Yet we do know that spiritual concerns often go unaddressed without an interprofessional team.[57] According to interprofessional providers, there is often a lack of support at a systems level, and therefore, with busy schedules, spirituality is commonly not assessed.[57]

In a survey of interprofessional practice and palliative care, chaplains reported various roles and responsibilities across their teams. Despite differences in interprofessional practice, chaplains felt they were able to deliver high-quality spiritual care and provide personalized spiritual rituals.[58] However, just as social workers and chaplains note that treating physical symptoms is outside their scope of practice, nurses and physicians feel similarly in relation to spiritual aspects of care. For example, in a study of 19 palliative care providers, non-spiritual providers felt more comfortable assessing spiritual history but were not always clear about best practices regarding questions and language.[57] Providers were often unwilling to assess for spiritual distress if there was no spiritual specialist on the team because they were assessing for a concern they felt they could not address. Although having a spiritual provider on the team is key to improving training and support, awareness of spiritual assessments and interventions are needed across professions.

An interprofessional team is opportune for supporting Ms. Smith in this domain. Her new religious community may serve as a key social support for her during this difficult time. Her religious perceptions of illness and medical treatment are likely to influence her symptom experience and care decisions, particularly related to the use of blood products. Therefore, each team member is needed to not only identify her spiritual experience in her transition into the Jehovah's Witness religious tradition, but also the influence her former and new religious beliefs may have on all other domains of care.

Domain 6: Cultural Aspects of Care

It's every interprofessional team provider's social responsibility to approach those that we care for with a sense of cultural humility; an openness, curiosity, and sensitivity to learn the cultural nuance of the patients and families that we serve. Music, as an expressive art, can be a gateway for the team into this deeper humanistic understanding, acting as a guide to help us learn from our patients through their unique musical preferences and/or story. We meet people where they are and do not necessarily need words, but rather use music as a tool, to express or foster a connection to one another while also honoring the roles that music has played in the context of the person's life. Providing culturally affirming and relevant music interventions can take many forms including musical improvisation, songwriting, receptive music, or music-facilitated relaxation, while helping the interprofessional team respect a person's cultural identity.

—Angela Wibben, MM, MT-BC, board-certified music therapist,
University of Colorado Hospital, Aurora, Colorado

Some evidence addresses the impact of culturally sensitive care on palliative measures, with low-quality evidence showing possible positive impacts to care decisions at the end of life, depression, quality of death, and coping skills. Low-quality evidence implies that interpreters may have an impact on the quality of communication and care.[7] However, despite the lack of evidence, careful attention to cultural currents is foundational to palliative care and fundamentally requires differing disciplines, worldviews, and experiences, mustered together in an interprofessional way. As Ms. Wibben so thoughtfully highlights above, good palliative care requires approaching the care of complex, seriously ill patients in a way that demonstrates that we are thoughtfully sensitive and curious about their background and cultural factors that affect their quality of life, choices about therapies, and conceptualization of illness.

Although limited evidence exists within the cultural domain, provider experiences corroborate the value of interprofessional practice for improving patient and family experiences of care. According to intensive care unit (ICU) physicians, nurses, and interpreters, limited English proficiency creates barriers to culturally appropriate end-of-life communication with patients and families.[59] Facilitators for achieving high-quality end-of-life conversations included pre-meetings with the entire team, interpretation that emulates empathy for the patient and family while improving messaging, bidirectional provider-patient cultural communication, and cultural humility.[60,61] However, language is only one aspect of cultural care. Collecting all culturally relevant information would simply be impossible by one individual provider. Therefore, culturally relevant information should be collected across team members and shared among the team.[62]

Considering the case of Ms. Smith, in the little we know about her, we see that she presently identifies as a Black woman, a mother, and someone whom we observe as making a religious change based on input from her family. We also can see that she has lived with an inherited chronic illness that disproportionately affects non-White populations. She is someone who is highly likely to have experienced systemic and interpersonal, individualized racism. In addition, there is so much about where she is from and who she is that we still have yet to learn. We also do not know anything about the cultural views of her care team that will, in turn, affect the way she receives and perceives her cancer care (the reason why the palliative care team is involved at this moment of her care). A structured assessment, aimed at delving into attitudes, beliefs, context, decision-making style, and environment,[63,64] completed by a self-aware and coordinated interprofessional team, is the best way to thoughtfully navigate the multifaceted inputs defining an individual's underlying culture in its collision with the complex overlapping cultures in our evolving medical system.

Domain 7: End-of-Life Care

Our interprofessional team (social worker, nurse practitioner, physician) recently cared for a hospitalized gentleman who was actively dying. It became clear that dying at home was of the utmost importance to the patient and family. The patient was experiencing a high level of symptoms, making transition to home challenging and potentially traumatizing. By being able to view the case from 3 different professional angles, we were able to provide comprehensive care planning to the patient and family. The social worker helped to prepare the patient and family for the possible heavy emotional burden of the transfer, as well as address their anticipatory grief and anxiety. The physician coordinated with the medical team and collaborated with the nurse practitioner to develop a symptom management plan. The nurse practitioner provided logistical support to the outpatient team. We were able to provide comprehensive palliative care to this patient and family through the ability to see the case from different perspectives and collaborate closely with one another on our team.

—Kate Sciacca, NP, palliative care nurse practitioner,
Brigham & Women's Hospital, Boston, Massachusetts

Care for patients at the end of life is a core role for palliative care teams and often represents a period when each of the other 7 domains of care reach their peak complexity. Moderate-quality evidence demonstrates that interprofessional care improves dying at home, family bereavement, and grief outcomes, and low-quality evidence supports the value of the team for symptom and medication management at the end of life.[7] However, as with previous studies, the teamwork portion of this literature is largely insufficient to be able to directly connect interprofessional interaction to patient and family outcomes.

The specific role of the interprofessional team during end-of-life care varies based on the setting of care (e.g., home vs. inpatient) and family and caregiver involvement.[65] From the provider perspective, interprofessional teamwork during the provision of end-of-life care offers several benefits. First, due to the complexity of illness trajectories and care-specific characteristics, the identification of dying patients is challenging.[66,67] Healthcare providers indicate that collaboration among the interprofessional team allows for improved identification of patients nearing the end of life.[68] In a study of 28 interviewed nurses and physicians, the informants stated that, in addition to other clinical practices, team collaboration facilitated the identification of dying patients across a variety of primary care and hospital settings.[69] As one cardiologist in the study noted: "And of course consultation with a colleague, like: 'Well, this is what I see. Do you see that as well?'" Similarly, in the United Kingdom, a qualitative study noted that general practitioners relied on the interprofessional team to identify patients in need of palliative and end-of-life care.[70]

Second, healthcare providers confirm that interprofessional teams are necessary to facilitate high-quality end-of-life care decisions. Analysis of 40 interviews with interprofessional care providers, including physicians, nurses, social workers, therapists, and spiritual clinicians, revealed that interprofessional teamwork was a key facilitator to initiating, strategizing, and completing end-of-life conversations with patients and their families.[71] Among these providers, they highlighted the importance of team cohesion and early clinical planning to achieve successful end-of-life planning discussions. Providers also stated that ambiguous roles among the team around responsibility for leading these conversations often hindered the process, suggesting a need for effective team awareness, communication, and leadership.

The need for interprofessional end-of-life care planning has also been emphasized specifically for the pediatric population. In a study of focus groups with 36 interprofessional palliative care providers, participants described a process for providing high-quality end-of-life care planning for youth and their families.[72] This study reported that using the process of (1) team pre-briefing, (2) collaborative work across settings, and (3) providing essential information was successful for preparing and conducting end-of-life care discussions in this population.

End-of-life decision-making can be particularly difficult when discussing do-not-resuscitate orders or the removal of life-sustaining treatment. In these incidences, the multiple professions present on the team are able to contribute their unique perspectives and work together to address the complex and difficult decisions with respect to patient and family wishes.[73] Physicians and nurses highlight the need for interprofessional practice in making end-of-life decisions, stating that collaborative team decision-making and communication with the patient and family improve compliance with the established plan of treatment and emotional burden among team members.[74]

Patient and family perspectives also confirm the benefits of interprofessional palliative care during the end of life. A qualitative study of 23 interviews with a diverse sample of family caregivers explored the impact of inpatient palliative care consults on family members' understanding of the patient's condition, knowledge of available care options, and decision-making ability.[75] The authors found that caregivers reported positive aspects of interprofessional palliative care on communication, access to providers, and increased time to discuss prognosis. As one study participant noted, "If I learned anything new [from the interprofessional palliative care consult] . . . I suppose I learned about my mom's attitude towards her care and . . . allowing her to have more of a say of what she wanted."

Domain 8: Ethical and Legal Aspects of Care

Since ethical issues arise at the end of life, collaboration with palliative care colleagues is essential. This is particularly true in situations of complexity, where disagreements about the goals of care or uncertainty about prognosis necessitate teamwork. The interprofessional team works to elucidate the multidimensional core values of patients and families, which provides critical information when brainstorming about the ethically possible, and preferable, paths forward.

—Aimee Milliken, PhD, RN, HEC-C, clinical ethicist, nurse,
researcher, Brigham & Women's Hospital, Boston, Massachusetts

Ethical and legal aspects of the delivery of specialty palliative care covers a broad range of topics and challenges, from surrogate decision-making and legal documents to constructs of futility and clinician-assisted death. Evidence for the impact of interprofessional palliative care in the ethical and legal realm is sparse and focuses on utilization outcomes, such as changes in code status orders or hospitalizations, rather than assessing the impact of interprofessional palliative care teamwork on patients, families, or clinicians.[7,76] One study, a social work–led structured debriefing for ICU nurses, suggests that interprofessional work can decrease clinician distress around providing nonbeneficial care in the ICU.[77]

Conceptually, several realms related to the ethical and legal aspects of palliative care may be considered within the context of an interprofessional team. In each realm, the interprofessional teamwork aims to mitigate patient, family, and medical team distress and trauma in complex and charged clinical situations. First, in the selection and preparation of surrogate decision-makers,[78] an interprofessional team can help to identify and prepare chosen proxies to make the myriad of healthcare choices that arise when seriously ill patients are incapacitated. Interprofessional palliative care teams can infuse cultural and religious views into the choice, activation, and empowerment of surrogates at the appropriate time. Consider the case of Ms. Smith, someone who is recently divorced and still involved in legal proceedings around her children; this is a case where a team-based approach to preparation for surrogate decision-making is critical.

Second, interprofessional palliative care teams, as highlighted by the example from Dr. Milliken above, are a critical contributor to ethics consultation, which has been demonstrated to help find consensus around decisions and to affect medical care in the ICU.[79,80] Adding multiple coordinated professional views to a comprehensive ethics consultation strengthens the depth of exploration and decision-making. In a similar vein, interprofessional teamwork is foundational in addressing the construct of medical futility when it arises in the specialty palliative care realm. A team, with its varied worldviews and professional training, is essential when teasing out the differential diagnoses for disagreements around whether and how a treatment is "futile." For example, when a family presses for artificial nutrition and hydration in advancing dementia, an interprofessional team is the only way to tease out that the pressure comes from the family's attempt to honor the patient's religious wishes and trauma experienced while nearly starving to death in a concentration camp—highlighting that the feeding tube may not extend life but is certainly not futile in the care of the whole patient and family, when considering their religious, cultural, bereavement, and psychosocial well-being.

Last, an interprofessional team and the multiple expertise and points of view are central to comprehensive evaluations before applying advanced palliative care therapies such as palliative sedation or, where legal, clinician aid in dying. The need for team input in such situations is both legally required and protective for patients, families, and clinicians to help ensure broad and complete assessment of all factors weighing into treatment decisions.

Conclusion

In conclusion, interprofessional collaboration and teamwork are a foundational element of good palliative care and weave deeply through the 8 key domains of palliative care work. However, we lack direct evidence linking interprofessional teams to specific outcomes in palliative care, though some studies do shed light on the teamwork that can drive outcomes. Providers, patients, and caregivers highlight the importance of interprofessional teamwork in palliative care and how teamwork is conceptually critical to all domains of care. This book will discuss the theoretical foundations of successful interprofessional education, structure, and work needed to deliver high-quality palliative care.

Discussion Questions

1. Although the direct evidence for the efficacy of interprofessional practice is limited, in your opinion, what are the benefits of having an interprofessional team in palliative care?
2. How can interprofessional clinicians and researchers work together to build the evidence base exploring how interprofessional palliative care teams affect our key outcomes?
3. In your practice, how confident are you in the assessment and treatment of each domain? How can the interprofessional team support you in fostering new skills?
4. Why do you think interprofessional teams promote positive practice skills, provider self-care, and team support among palliative care clinicians? Why are these skills and support important in palliative care?

References

1. Parse RR. Interdisciplinary and interprofessional: what are the differences? *Nurs Sci Q.* 2015;28(1):5–6.
2. Klarare A, Rasmussen BH, Fossum B, Fürst CJ, Hansson J, Hagelin CL. Experiences of security and continuity of care: patients' and families' narratives about the work of specialized palliative home care teams. *Palliat Support Care.* 2017;15(2):181–189.
3. Sagin A, Kirkpatrick JN, Pisani BA, Fahlberg BB, Sundlof AL, O'Connor NR. Emerging collaboration between palliative care specialists and mechanical circulatory support teams: a qualitative study. *J Pain Symptom Manage.* 2016;52(4):491–497.e491.
4. Svensson G, Wåhlin I. Patient perceptions of specialised hospital-based palliative home care: a qualitative study using a phenomenographical approach. *Int J Palliat Nurs.* 2018;24(1):22–32.
5. Brooks LA, Manias E, Nicholson P. Communication and decision-making about end-of-life care in the intensive care unit. *Am J Crit Care.* 2017;26(4):336–341.
6. Brooks LA, Manias E, Nicholson P. Barriers, enablers and challenges to initiating end-of-life care in an Australian intensive care unit context. *Aust Crit Care.* 2017;30(3):161–166.

7. Ahluwalia SC, Chen C, Raaen L, et al. A systematic review in support of the National Consensus Project Clinical Practice Guidelines for Quality Palliative Care, fourth edition. *J Pain Symptom Manage*. 2018;56(6):831–870.

8. Albers G, Froggatt K, Van den Block L, et al. A qualitative exploration of the collaborative working between palliative care and geriatric medicine: barriers and facilitators from a European perspective. *BMC Palliat Care*. 2016;15:47.

9. Bergman J, Lorenz KA, Acquah-Asare S, et al. Urologist attitudes toward end-of-life care. *Urology*. 2013;82(1):48–52.

10. Gidwani R, Nevedal A, Patel M, et al. The appropriate provision of primary versus specialist palliative care to cancer patients: oncologists' perspectives. *J Palliat Med*. 2017;20(4):395–403.

11. Geiger K, Schneider N, Bleidorn J, Klindtworth K, Jünger S, Müller-Mundt G. Caring for frail older people in the last phase of life: the general practitioners' view. *BMC Palliat Care*. 2016;15:52.

12. Nelson JE, Puntillo KA, Pronovost PJ, et al. In their own words: patients and families define high-quality palliative care in the intensive care unit. *Crit Care Med*. 2010;38(3):808–818.

13. Wallerstedt B, Benzein E, Schildmeijer K, Sandgren A. What is palliative care? Perceptions of healthcare professionals. *Scand J Caring Sci*. 2019;33(1):77–84.

14. Brush S, Budge D, Alharethi R, et al. End-of-life decision making and implementation in recipients of a destination left ventricular assist device. *J Heart Lung Transplant*. 2010;29(12):1337–1341.

15. O'Hare AM, Szarka J, McFarland LV, et al. Provider perspectives on advance care planning for patients with kidney disease: whose job is it anyway? *Clin J Am Soc Nephrol*. 2016;11(5):855–866.

16. Phongtankuel V, Meador L, Adelman RD, et al. Multicomponent palliative care interventions in advanced chronic diseases: a systematic review. *Am J Hosp Palliat Care*. 2018;35(1):173–183.

17. Beasley A, Bakitas MA, Edwards R, Kavalieratos D. Models of non-hospice palliative care: a review. *Ann Palliat Med*. 2019;8(Suppl 1):S15–s21.

18. Fulton JJ, LeBlanc TW, Cutson TM, et al. Integrated outpatient palliative care for patients with advanced cancer: a systematic review and meta-analysis. *Palliat Med*. 2019;33(2):123–134.

19. Kaasa S, Loge JH, Aapro M, et al. Integration of oncology and palliative care: a Lancet Oncology Commission. *Lancet Oncol*. 2018;19(11):e588–e653.

20. Norton SA, Ladwig S, Caprio TV, Quill TE, Temkin-Greener H. Staff experiences forming and sustaining palliative care teams in nursing homes. *Gerontologist*. 2018;58(4):e218–e225.

21. Fukui S, Fujita J, Ikezaki S, Nakatani E, Tsujimura M. Effect of a multidisciplinary end-of-life educational intervention on health and social care professionals: a cluster randomized controlled trial. *PLoS ONE*. 2019;14(8):e0219589.

22. Graney BA, Au DH, Barón AE, et al. Advancing Symptom Alleviation with Palliative Treatment (ADAPT) trial to improve quality of life: a study protocol for a randomized clinical trial. *Trials*. 2019;20(1):355.

23. Siegle A, Villalobos M, Bossert J, et al. The Heidelberg Milestones Communication Approach (MCA) for patients with prognosis <12 months: protocol for a mixed-methods study including a randomized controlled trial. *Trials*. 2018;19(1):438.

24. Nasu K, Konno R, Fukahori H. End-of-life nursing care practice in long-term care settings for older adults: a qualitative systematic review. *Int J Nurs Pract*. 2020;26(2):e12771.

25. Wilson CM, Briggs R. Physical therapy's role in opioid use and management during palliative and hospice care. *Phys Ther*. 2018;98(2):83–85.

26. Head BA, Furman CD, Lally AM, Leake K, Pfeifer M. Medicine as it should be: teaching team and teamwork during a palliative care clerkship. *J Palliat Med*. 2018;21(5):638–644.

27. Kamal AH, Bull JH, Wolf SP, et al. Prevalence and predictors of burnout among hospice and palliative care clinicians in the U.S. *J Pain Symptom Manage*. 2020;59(5):e6–e13.

28. Cain CL, Taborda-Whitt C, Frazer M, et al. A mixed methods study of emotional exhaustion: energizing and depleting work within an innovative healthcare team. *J Interprof Care*. 2017;31(6):714–724.

29. Bam NE, Naidoo JR. Nurses experiences in palliative care of terminally-ill HIV patients in a level 1 district hospital. *Curationis*. 2014;37(1):1238.
30. Riotte CO, Kukora SK, Keefer PM, Firn JI. Identifying the types of support needed by interprofessional teams providing pediatric end-of-life care: a thematic analysis. *J Palliat Med*. 2018;21(4):422–427.
31. Orellana-Rios CL, Radbruch L, Kern M, et al. Mindfulness and compassion-oriented practices at work reduce distress and enhance self-care of palliative care teams: a mixed-method evaluation of an "on the job" program. *BMC Palliat Care*. 2017;17(1):3.
32. Perez GK, Haime V, Jackson V, Chittenden E, Mehta DH, Park ER. Promoting resiliency among palliative care clinicians: stressors, coping strategies, and training needs. *J Palliat Med*. 2015;18(4):332–337.
33. Goldsmith J, Wittenberg-Lyles E, Rodriguez D, Sanchez-Reilly S. Interdisciplinary geriatric and palliative care team narratives: collaboration practices and barriers. *Qual Health Res*. 2010;20(1):93–104.
34. Forrest C, Derrick C. Interdisciplinary education in end-of-life care: creating new opportunities for social work, nursing, and clinical pastoral education students. *J Soc Work End Life Palliat Care*. 2010;6(1–2):91–116.
35. Lansdell J, Beech N. Evaluating the impact of education on knowledge and confidence in delivering psychosocial end-of-life care. *Int J Palliat Nurs*. 2010;16(8):371–376.
36. van der Plas AG, Hagens M, Pasman HR, Schweitzer B, Duijsters M, Onwuteaka-Philipsen BD. PaTz groups for primary palliative care: reinventing cooperation between general practitioners and district nurses in palliative care: an evaluation study combining data from focus groups and a questionnaire. *BMC Fam Pract*. 2014;15:14.
37. Graham R, Lepage C, Boitor M, Petizian S, Fillion L, Gélinas C. Acceptability and feasibility of an interprofessional end-of-life/palliative care educational intervention in the intensive care unit: a mixed-methods study. *Intensive Crit Care Nurs*. 2018;48:75–84.
38. Lippe M, Linton B, Jones B. Utilizing a collaborative learning activity to sensitize interprofessional students to palliative care scopes of practice with adolescent and young adults. *J Interprof Care*. 2019;33(2):267–269.
39. Disalvo D, Luckett T, Bennett A, Davidson P, Agar M. Pharmacists' perspectives on medication reviews for long-term care residents with advanced dementia: a qualitative study. *Int J Clin Pharm*. 2019;41(4):950–962.
40. Dong ST, Butow PN, Agar M, et al. Clinicians' perspectives on managing symptom clusters in advanced cancer: a semistructured interview study. *J Pain Symptom Manage*. 2016;51(4):706–717.e705.
41. Dugan Day M. Interdisciplinary hospice team processes and multidimensional pain: a qualitative study. *J Soc Work End Life Palliat Care*. 2012;8(1):53–76.
42. Bausewein C, Schunk M, Schumacher P, Dittmer J, Bolzani A, Booth S. Breathlessness services as a new model of support for patients with respiratory disease. *Chron Respir Dis*. 2018;15(1):48–59.
43. Rosenstein DL. Depression and end-of-life care for patients with cancer. *Dialogues Clin Neurosci*. 2011;13(1):101–108.
44. Temkin-Greener H, Mukamel DB, Ladd H, et al. Impact of nursing home palliative care teams on end-of-life outcomes: a randomized controlled trial. *Med Care*. 2018;56(1):11–18.
45. Bekelman DB, Allen LA, McBryde CF, et al. Effect of a collaborative care intervention vs usual care on health status of patients with chronic heart failure: the CASA randomized clinical trial. *JAMA Intern Med*. 2018;178(4):511–519.
46. Temel JS, Greer JA, Muzikansky A, et al. Early palliative care for patients with metastatic non-small-cell lung cancer. *N Engl J Med*. 2010;363(8):733–742.
47. Paladino J, Bernacki R, Neville BA, et al. Evaluating an intervention to improve communication between oncology clinicians and patients with life-limiting cancer: a cluster randomized clinical trial of the Serious Illness Care Program. *JAMA Oncol*. 2019;5(6):801–809.
48. Jacobsen J, Jackson V, Dahlin C, et al. Components of early outpatient palliative care consultation in patients with metastatic nonsmall cell lung cancer. *J Palliat Med*. 2011;14(4):459–464.

49. Hoerger M, Greer JA, Jackson VA, et al. Defining the elements of early palliative care that are associated with patient-reported outcomes and the delivery of end-of-life care. *J Clin Oncol.* 2018;36(11):1096–1102.

50. Arthur J, Edwards T, Reddy S, et al. Outcomes of a specialized interdisciplinary approach for patients with cancer with aberrant opioid-related behavior. *Oncologist.* 2018;23(2):263–270.

51. https://www.caregiving.org/wp-content/uploads/2020/06/AARP1316_RPT_Caregivinginthe eUS_WEB.pdf.

52. Kuruvilla L, Weeks G, Eastman P, George J. Medication management for community palliative care patients and the role of a specialist palliative care pharmacist: a qualitative exploration of consumer and health care professional perspectives. *Palliat Med.* 2018;32(8):1369–1377.

53. Tavemark S, Hermansson LN, Blomberg K. Enabling activity in palliative care: focus groups among occupational therapists. *BMC Palliat Care.* 2019;18(1):17.

54. Fryer S, Bellamy G, Morgan T, Gott M. "Sometimes I've gone home feeling that my voice hasn't been heard": a focus group study exploring the views and experiences of health care assistants when caring for dying residents. *BMC Palliat Care.* 2016;15(1):78.

55. Wilson CM, Stiller CH, Doherty DJ, Thompson KA. The role of physical therapists within hospice and palliative care in the United States and Canada. *Am J Hosp Palliat Care.* 2017;34(1):34–41.

56. van de Geer J, Veeger N, Groot M, et al. Multidisciplinary training on spiritual care for patients in palliative care trajectories improves the attitudes and competencies of hospital medical staff: results of a quasi-experimental study. *Am J Hosp Palliat Care.* 2018;35(2):218–228.

57. Siler S, Mamier I, Winslow BW, Ferrell BR. Interprofessional perspectives on providing spiritual care for patients with lung cancer in outpatient settings. *Oncol Nurs Forum.* 2019;46(1):49–58.

58. Fitchett G, Lyndes KA, Cadge W, Berlinger N, Flanagan E, Misasi J. The role of professional chaplains on pediatric palliative care teams: perspectives from physicians and chaplains. *J Palliat Med.* 2011;14(6):704–707.

59. Barwise AK, Nyquist CA, Espinoza Suarez NR, et al. End-of-life decision-making for ICU patients with limited English proficiency: a qualitative study of healthcare team insights. *Crit Care Med.* 2019;47(10):1380–1387.

60. Murray-García J, Tervalon M. The concept of cultural humility. *Health Aff (Project Hope).* 2014;33(7):1303.

61. Tervalon M, Murray-García J. Cultural humility versus cultural competence: a critical distinction in defining physician training outcomes in multicultural education. *J Health Care Poor Underserved.* 1998;9(2):117–125.

62. Boucher NA. Direct engagement with communities and interprofessional learning to factor culture into end-of-life health care delivery. *Am J Public Health.* 2016;106(6):996–1001.

63. Koenig BA, Gates-Williams J. Understanding cultural difference in caring for dying patients. *WJM.* 1995;163(3):244–249.

64. Kagawa-Singer M, Blackhall LJ. Negotiating cross-cultural issues at the end of life: "You got to go where he lives." *JAMA.* 2001;286(23):2993–3001.

65. Lysaght Hurley S, Barg FK, Strumpf N, Ersek M. Same agency, different teams: perspectives from home and inpatient hospice care. *Qual Health Res.* 2015;25(7):923–931.

66. Abarshi EA, Echteld MA, Van den Block L, Donker GA, Deliens L, Onwuteaka-Philipsen BD. Recognising patients who will die in the near future: a nationwide study via the Dutch Sentinel Network of GPs. *Br J Gen Pract.* 2011;61(587):e371–e378.

67. Kennedy C, Brooks-Young P, Brunton Gray C, et al. Diagnosing dying: an integrative literature review. *BMJ Support Palliat Care.* 2014;4(3):263–270.

68. Åvik Persson H, Sandgren A, Fürst CJ, Ahlström G, Behm L. Early and late signs that precede dying among older persons in nursing homes: the multidisciplinary team's perspective. *BMC Geriatr.* 2018;18(1):134.

69. Flierman I, Nugteren IC, van Seben R, Buurman BM, Willems DL. How do hospital-based nurses and physicians identify the palliative phase in their patients and what difficulties exist? A qualitative interview study. *BMC Palliat Care.* 2019;18(1):54.

70. Mitchell H, Noble S, Finlay I, Nelson A. Defining the palliative care patient: its challenges and implications for service delivery. *BMJ Support Palliat Care*. 2013;3(1):46–52.
71. Ho A, Jameson K, Pavlish C. An exploratory study of interprofessional collaboration in end-of-life decision-making beyond palliative care settings. *J Interprof Care*. 2016;30(6):795–803.
72. Henderson A, Young J, Herbert A, Bradford N, Pedersen LA. Preparing pediatric healthcare professionals for end-of-life care discussions: an exploratory study. *J Palliat Med*. 2017;20(6):662–666.
73. Imhof L, Mahrer-Imhof R, Janisch C, Kesselring A, Zuercher Zenklusend R. Do not attempt resuscitation: the importance of consensual decisions. *Swiss Med Wkly*. 2011;141:w13157.
74. Kryworuchko J, Strachan PH, Nouvet E, Downar J, You JJ. Factors influencing communication and decision-making about life-sustaining technology during serious illness: a qualitative study. *BMJ Open*. 2016;6(5):e010451.
75. Enguidanos S, Housen P, Penido M, Mejia B, Miller JA. Family members' perceptions of inpatient palliative care consult services: a qualitative study. *Palliat Med*. 2014;28(1):42–48.
76. Ma J, Chi S, Buettner B, et al. Early palliative care consultation in the medical ICU: a cluster randomized crossover trial. *Crit Care Med*. 2019;47(12):1707–1715.
77. Browning ED, Cruz JS. Reflective debriefing: a social work intervention addressing moral distress among ICU nurses. *J Soc Work End Life Palliat Care*. 2018;14(1):44–72.
78. Sudore RL, Fried TR. Redefining the "planning" in advance care planning: preparing for end-of-life decision making. *Ann Intern Med*. 2010;153(4):256–261.
79. Au SS, Couillard P, Roze des Ordons A, Fiest KM, Lorenzetti DL, Jette N. Outcomes of ethics consultations in adult ICUs: a systematic review and meta-analysis. *Crit Care Med*. 2018;46(5):799–808.
80. Kryworuchko J, Hill E, Murray MA, Stacey D, Fergusson DA. Interventions for shared decision-making about life support in the intensive care unit: a systematic review. *Worldviews Evid Based Nurs*. 2013;10(1):3–16.

2

Palliative Care

History, Terminology, and Definitions

Terry Altilio and Jennifer Seaman

Key Points

- Palliative care as a specialty, over 4 decades, has moved from the siloed setting of oncology across diagnoses and settings and has built a research base and demand for service.
- A specialty that engages the multidimensional aspects of living with serious illness and the universal experience of death presents challenges in terms of definition and scope.
- The discourse, written and spoken, surrounding the specialty, its scope and practice and the process of team that is foundational to the work, invites reflection and intention in order to build coherence of meaning and purpose as the specialty continues to build its culture and identity.
- Exploring the origins and current dialogue related to palliative and team-based care as well as the argots, or specialized jargon, that have grown up within the practice world, is essential to cohering a path forward with attention to language that grounds the practice for colleagues, patients, and families, and informs policy.

Introduction

Authoring this chapter has brought together 2 palliative care clinicians with an interest in language and word choice—one who wanders in the macro and micro landscapes where palliative care continues to be defined and words and phrases have become the jargon of the specialty* and another who writes at the group level, the meso landscape of team terminology and process. The intention of this chapter

---

* Palliative care is considered to be a subspecialty within medicine and nursing, but a specialty in spiritual care and social work. For this book, we standardize the language by referring to palliative care as a specialty when referring to the team as a whole. We use the term "subspecialty" when referring specifically to nursing or medicine.

is to explore the macro, meso, and micro[1] landscapes, the history of terminology within palliative care, and to give voice to some of the challenges that continue to percolate around the most basic question of what we call this specialty after almost 5 decades in development. We will provide definitions and ponder the unique histories of professions that may influence our worldviews and how we cohere around the work and the language we use to describe its process. As this chapter is written by a nurse and a social worker, with editors representing medicine and spiritual care, readers might sense the shifting and blend of the unique frames which construct our disciplines[†] and ways of seeing the world—perhaps a metaphor for what we might achieve in our teams and an invitation for readers to consider alternate frames and narratives.[2]

We are writing in an exceptional time, when the unprecedented impact of COVID-19, with inequities laid bare, and the killings of Black and Brown people by police have placed social justice and equity center stage.[3-6] Attention to history, authenticity, activism, and intention is at the center of dialogues about these painful realities, and in some way attending to the language of palliative care may not seem to be related. Yet how we see and describe our work and purpose relates to the culture and values of those who have built a largely White specialty. As we explore history, the work, and related language, we will invite reflection about values and terminology that infuse the specialty and may or may not be shared across cultures and ethnicities—language that bridges and affirms and that which assumes and distances. We will look at how teams are a microcosm of society and how, as a collective, as professionals and individuals, we may struggle with identity, power, and hierarchy within and beyond the actual practice of palliative care.

Reflections on the Macro Landscape: An Origin Story

In 1974, Balfour Mount, a Canadian surgeon, proposed the term "palliative care" to describe a model of care informed by the work of Dame Cicely Saunders. Dame Saunders, the founder of the modern hospice movement, trained as a physician, nurse, and social worker and enriched the care of dying patients beyond a mind–body dualism to a "Total Pain" construct, integrating the physical, social, psychological, and spiritual aspects of personhood.[7] Dr. Mount had observed Dame Saunders at St. Christopher's Hospice in 1973, and as he considered establishing a pilot project at Royal Victoria Hospital, he chose to call it "palliative care." This choice was influenced by "my francophone colleagues (who) said that we could not use the term 'hospice' because in France the word had a pejorative connotation

---

[†] Although often used interchangeably, "discipline" refers to a branch of knowledge, while "profession" refers to an occupation that requires special education and/or prolonged training and a formal qualification. In this book, we have attempted to standardize the use of the term "profession" when referring to occupations such as spiritual care, medicine, nursing, and social work, but occasionally the term "discipline" is used, especially when focused on the theory and knowledge development of the professions.

that suggested a dumping ground of mediocrity of care, signifying the worst of nursing homes."[8] Dr. Mount believed the term "palliative care" answered the question: "What are our goals and how can they be conveyed?" The etymology of the word was perfect. It means "to improve the quality of."[8] The "palliative care" program focused on research and teaching, and services included a home care program that cared for about 100 patients in the community, an inpatient unit, a consultative service to the active treatment programs, and a bereavement team to follow families assessed to be at higher risk for complicated bereavement.[8] While a search of relevant sources defines palliate as "to cloak," definitions also include that which mitigates or alleviates and, depending on the source, often integrates what many would think is the intention of palliative care as it has evolved since 1975—"to reduce in violence; to lessen or abate; to mitigate; to ease without curing; as, to palliate a disease."[9]

As one looks at this sketch of an origin story, it is interesting to observe that "palliative" was in some way chosen to disassociate from the French meaning of the word "hospice," even as the intention was to replicate the compassionate, competent, and integrated care for the dying provided at St. Christopher's.[8] This effort to craft acceptable language for different settings, countries, and colleagues continues and extends to fashioning our specialty for patients, families, and funding and referral sources, challenging palliative care to frame the scope of our practice and make it "palatable" to others.

Palliative Care—What's in a Name?

As recently as September 2020, the discussion about the name of our specialty reached the public press in the United States with an article in the *Washington Post* titled "In Pandemic Era, the Term Palliative Care Is Even More Scary for Some. So, Specialists Want to Rename It." As palliative care teams worked intensively during an unprecedented time of suffering and death, questions about what to call our specialty arose again.[10] What is it about the origin story and evolution of palliative care that keeps us defining what we do and who we are, at the same time that research related to our specialty grows and our work continues to integrate and enrich care across countries, settings, and diagnoses?

The deliberations over decades about the acceptability of the term "palliative care" has led to alternate descriptors, including supportive care, often favored in the oncology setting, symptom management, and comfort care. Table 2.1 includes a sampling of terms used by varied organizations to define "palliative care" and related terms. Language related to pain and symptoms, holistic care, serious illness, quality of life, and the patient/family as the unit of care is common to most of the definitions. Reference to suffering, the clinical setting, life-threatening illness, early intervention, continuum of illness, and the interprofessional team is less consistent across the definitions. These definitions are found in the virtual world, accessible

Table 2.1 Definitions of Palliative Care: Palliative Care Defined across Organizations

Organization	Terms	Definitions
National Consensus Project (NCP) for Quality Palliative Care	Palliative Care	Palliative care focuses on expert assessment and management of pain and other symptoms, assessment and support of caregiver needs, and coordination of care. Palliative care attends to the physical, functional, psychological, practical, and spiritual consequences of a serious illness. It is a person- and family-centered approach to care, providing seriously ill people relief from the symptoms and stress of an illness. Through early integration into the care plan of seriously ill people, palliative care improves quality of life for both the patient and the family.[11]
World Health Organization	Palliative Care	Palliative care is an approach that improves the quality of life of patients (adults and children) and their families who are facing problems associated with life-threatening illness. It prevents and relieves suffering through the early identification, correct assessment, and treatment of pain and other problems, whether physical, psychosocial, or spiritual.[12]
International Association for Hospice and Palliative Care	Palliative Care	Palliative care is the active holistic care of individuals across all ages with serious health-related suffering due to severe illness and especially of those near the end of life. It aims to improve the quality of life of patients, their families. and their caregivers. Definition endorsed by 1180 clinicians and 188 organizations.[13]
National Cancer Institute	Palliative Care Comfort Care Supportive Care Symptom Management	Care given to improve the quality of life of patients who have a serious or life-threatening disease such as cancer . . . an approach that addresses the person as a whole, not just their disease . . . goal is to prevent or treat as early as possible the symptoms and side effects of the disease and its treatment in addition to related psychological, social and spiritual problems . . . *also called comfort care, supportive care and symptom management* . . . may be received in hospital, outpatient clinics, long-term care facilities, or at home under the direction of a physician.[14]
National Hospice & Palliative Care Organization	Palliative Care	Integrates the NCP definition: Palliative care is patient and family-centered care that optimizes quality of life by anticipating, preventing, and treating suffering. Palliative care throughout the continuum of illness involves addressing physical, intellectual, emotional, social, and spiritual needs; facilitating patient autonomy, access to information, and choice.[15]
	Hospice	Hospice is considered the model for quality compassionate care for people facing a life-limiting illness. Hospice provides expert medical care, pain management, and emotional and spiritual support expressly tailored to the patient's needs and wishes. Support is provided to the patient's family as well.[16]

Table 2.1 Continued

Organization	Terms	Definitions
Center to Advance Palliative Care (CAPC)	Palliative Care	Specialized medical care for people living with a serious illness. This type of care is focused on providing relief from the symptoms and stress of a serious illness. The goal is to improve quality of life for both the patient and the family. Palliative care is provided by a specially trained team of doctors, nurses, and other specialists who work together with a patient's other doctors to provide an extra layer of support. Palliative care is based on the needs of the patient, not on the patient's prognosis. This care is appropriate at any age and at any stage in a serious illness, and it can be provided along with curative treatment.[17]
Institute of Medicine	Basic—also called primary palliative care	Palliative care that is delivered by healthcare professionals who are not palliative care specialists, such as primary care clinicians; physicians who are disease-oriented specialists (such as oncologists and cardiologists); and nurses, social workers, pharmacists, chaplains, and others who care for this population but are not certified in palliative care.[18]

to the public, colleagues, funders, and policymakers, and thus have the potential to confuse or clarify.

Complicating the effort to harmonize definition and practice is the reality that in the United States, for example, the ideals of scope and practice put forth in the National Consensus Project's Domains of Palliative Care might be quite achievable in educational settings and/or well-resourced hospitals and communities, yet are unattainable in many other settings.[19] In the real world of inequitable resources and workforce challenges, services are often maximized through creative networks of community resources. Most recently, as a consequence of the pandemic, in some areas the use of virtual care has proliferated. Services actually provided may or may not fully reflect the expectations established in the formal definitions and guidelines.

In addition to palliative care being framed within parameters of what is possible in underserved and under-resourced settings and in a continuing process of self-definition, the scope of palliative care lacks clarity among stakeholders. Referring clinicians may describe the specialty according to well- or ill-informed perceptions, or according to their hopes for what the service might bring to their patients and families. Phrases that have infused the world of palliative care, such as "goals of care," "comfort care," or "support," may differ in meaning for referring sources, patients and families, and palliative clinicians themselves. A referral for "goals of care" may not have unified meaning, and goals may range from a hope to align on a decision to forgo an attempt at resuscitation to a discussion of values and goals that guide treatment decisions that are much broader than singular issues such as resuscitation decisions. [20] "Comfort measures only (CMO)" has evolved as a code or shorthand communication for a care plan focused on interventions designed to alleviate symptoms, enhance quality of life, and relieve suffering for patients when disease-directed therapy is no longer deemed beneficial and the sole objective is comfort. While the intention in our fast-paced system is to develop argots or specialized jargon that serves to save time and can be abbreviated to check boxes in an electronic medical record, the unintended consequences of our word choice as heard by patients, families, and colleagues in each situation are essential to consider. These unintended consequences, as they relate to the language which informs the culture of palliative care, will be explored and are exemplified in Table 2.3 as micro elements of practice that inform communication within the team and beyond.

The Search for Definition: The Macro World of the United States

Perhaps the privilege we possess to ponder definitions and terms is both an asset and a liability as we try to remain centered on the shared mission of returning to the goals of providing humane care and the relief of pain and suffering. The World Health Organization (WHO) identifies 40 million persons in need of palliative care in a world where vast numbers experience profound inequity.[12] In the setting of devastating inequities and reimbursement structures that are often not driven by the needs of patients and families, nor by clinical expertise, engaging in ongoing defense of the name of our specialty seems like a diversion from the shared work of joining with primary teams and patients and families as they negotiate illness, uncertainty, and eventual death. Using the power of our collective voice to define and defend the name of the specialty when payment and reimbursement drive priorities, amidst heavily regulated, inadequately funded, and inequitable systems of care, may be viewed as a priority of the privileged.

Yet many concur about the need to forge a universal, global definition of palliative care to set a standard for what care, expertise, and compassion require of us, to inform the public, and to be able to speak to funders and governments with one voice.[21] While many palliative care pioneers are engaged in this enduring effort to define palliative care on an international level with intention and focus, we begin by shining a light on the United States and its efforts to enhance how the specialty is understood and received by the public and referring colleagues. A survey undertaken in 2011 by the Center To Advance of Palliative Care (CAPC) and repeated in 2019 used a telephone survey to sample 800 adults aged 25 and over with an oversampling in order to reach 347 persons aged 65 and over. In 2019 they added an online survey to reach 252 patients with serious illness, 262 family caregivers, and 317 physicians. The definition of palliative care used in these surveys was as follows:

Palliative care is specialized medical care for people living with a serious illness. This type of care is focused on providing relief from the symptoms and stress of a serious illness. The goal is to improve quality of life for both the patient and the family. Palliative care is provided by a specially trained team of doctors, nurses and other specialists who work together with a patient's other doctors to provide an extra layer of support. Palliative care is based on the needs of the patient, not on the patient's prognosis. This care is appropriate at any age and at any stage in a serious illness, and it can be provided along with curative treatment.[17]

Of the 800 adults surveyed, there was no significant change in public awareness of palliative care between the survey of 2011 and 2019. A second online Harris poll of 2029 adults conducted with the University of Rochester Medical Center reported that 71% had never heard of palliative care or had limited knowledge, a figure very similar to the 2011 CAPC results when 70% were "not at all knowledgeable."[22] While public awareness essentially remained the same, awareness among patients and families improved. Those with palliative care experience for self or others were more likely than those without experience to report being very or somewhat knowledgeable (76% vs. 43%). There is an implication that personal involvement with palliative care may be a pathway to gradually changing public opinion, along with data that support the essential importance of definition and messaging aligned across providers.[17]

Distinguishing palliative care from hospice and end-of-life care continues to inform efforts to educate the public, clinicians, funders, and policymakers. In the United States, a secondary analysis, published in 2020, looked at self-reported data from the 2018 Health Information National Trends Survey to examine the association between palliative care knowledge and misconceptions of palliative care. This analysis found that 12.6% who reported knowing about palliative care and held no misconceptions were female, caregivers, college educated with higher income, and served by a primary care provider. Others who believed they knew about palliative care often had misconceptions: 44.4% automatically thought of death; 38% equated palliative care with hospice; 17.8% believed you must stop other treatments; and 15.9% saw palliative care as giving up.[23] The connection made by many that links palliative care to end of life brings back the origin story where the word "palliative" was chosen to mitigate the connection to "hospice," even though the pilot project was focused on care for those coming to the end of life.[8] The following summary statement links the macro work of defining the specialty to the micro work of the words we choose to describe that work: "Language and definition and messaging make a big difference in public attitude toward palliative care."[17] The desire to promote and accurately represent palliative care to the public is juxtaposed with an awareness that the demand for services cannot be met with the current workforce and the inequitable access to care, even with the expansion of telehealth across this country and the world. The evolving attention to primary palliative care, while a recognition of the values and skills that all clinicians do or might integrate, is also a response to workforce issues and the desire to bring palliative care to all seriously ill patients through the care of their primary teams.

The Macro World of International Practice

Palliative care specialists around the world contribute expertise, endless commitment, and passion to patients, families, colleagues, and communities. It is both instructive and humbling to move beyond a U.S.-centric discussion and explore the global definitions and adaptations in parts of the world where deliberations about the meaning and structure of a team may be framed differently—as cultures, politics, economics, and the absence or presence of will or resources influence scope and definition.

In 2014, the WHO passed a comprehensive resolution welcoming the inclusion of palliative care in the definition of universal health coverage and emphasizing the need for health services to provide integrated palliative care in an equitable manner to address the needs of patients in the context of universal health coverage.[12]

At the same time, the WHO resolution recognized the limited availability of palliative care services in much of the world, which leads to avoidable suffering for millions of patients and their families, and emphasized the need to create or strengthen health systems to include palliative care as an integral component of the treatment of people within the continuum of care.[12] While an important milestone and affirmation of a shared humanity, as well as the value of palliative care at the primary and specialist level, the documentation of need and the passing of resolutions are far removed from actually touching the lives of patients and families.

In 2017, the Lancet Commission produced a report titled "Alleviating the Access Abyss in Palliative Care and Pain Relief: An Imperative of Universal Health Coverage."[24] Moving beyond an affirmation of need, the Lancet report broadened the conversation to include practical issues such as cost, budgeting, and strategies for expanding access. The report identified the lack of access to pain relief and palliative care throughout the life cycle as a global crisis, and consequent action to close this divide between rich and poor as a moral, health, and ethical imperative.[25] The emphasis on cost and budget calls attention to the absence of analyses that attach value to the services of professions such as social work, nursing, and spiritual care, making it more difficult to advocate for funding within a budget.

In 2018 a Vatican initiative, "Pal-Life," was launched, reflecting the words of Pope Francis and describing palliative care as an

> [e]xpression of our uniquely human need to take care of each another, particularly
> to care for persons who are suffering. Palliative care is a witness to the fact that
> the human person is always precious, even if old, even if sick. The human person,

whatever his circumstances, is always a good, for himself and for others, and is loved by God.[25]

Concurrent with documented evidence of the need for palliative care has been the recent international effort to create a consensus process to "define" palliative care, launched by the International Association of Hospice and Palliative Care (IAHPC). The consensus process built the following definition:

> Palliative care is the active holistic care of individuals across all ages with serious health-related suffering due to severe illness, and especially of those near the end of life. It aims to improve quality of life of patients, their families and their caregivers.[26(p 761)]

This process engaged 38 participants, primarily physicians, across 22 countries and surveyed over 400 IAHPC members from 88 countries. The definition includes bullet points and qualifiers designed to clarify the definition, as well as recommendations for government.[26] This mammoth consensus process also set off controversy and commentary within and between other organizations such as the Worldwide Hospice and Palliative Care Alliance, with a central area of difference relating to whether palliative care encompasses all suffering or only provides care to those with limited life expectancy.[27] David Clark, a professor of medical sociology at the University of Glasgow's School of Interdisciplinary Studies, reflected on this controversy, pondering whether it is possible and/or desirable to have a universal definition for a specialty that is multifaceted, global, and continuing to evolve.[28] Is it possible to agree on a definition and scope that might apply in intersectional contexts where the variation in values, policies, resources and beyond might be almost endless?[27] Yet, the need for definition is essential for identity and advocacy. Thus Dr. Clark proposed the following definition for comment:

> Most people who have a life-threatening condition can benefit from palliative care, whether or not they are having active treatment. Palliative care helps with personal, social and medical problems associated with potentially mortal illness, especially pain and other distressing symptoms. It assists families and cares and supports them in bereavement. It uses skilled approaches from a trained team, but often involves friends, family members and the wider community. Palliative care improves wellbeing and, in some instances, has even been shown to extend life.[27]

These processes, designed to define and support the work of palliative care around the world and create relevance to varied cultures and countries, relate to the macro environment of the specialty. Moving to the meso level of practice brings us to craft an understanding of the models of traditional and non-traditional teams and related processes, which will be followed by a walk through the micro level, the weeds and wildflowers—an invitation to consider the argots and jargon that have infused the work of palliative care in the United States.

The Whole Is Greater than the Sum of Us: The Meso Perspective

When considering palliative care either as a philosophy of care or as a specialty, its single unifying feature is care delivery by a group of individuals, working in concert, with the patient and family as the unit of care. The multidimensional nature of serious illness, suffering, and death demands care from a group of diverse clinicians individually skilled in physical, psychological, social, spiritual, or practical support—a team. Across the United States and internationally, the team model may be operationalized in different ways. Large academic medical centers often have a full complement of clinicians—physicians, nurses, psychologists, pharmacists, social workers, and chaplains—all dedicated members of the palliative care service. In many inpatient and outpatient settings in the United States, palliative care rests in a singular clinician who creatively joins with colleagues across specialties and community resources, often virtually, to create a team to serve the needs of specific patients. In rural communities, the team care expected from a hospice program may be influenced by distance and staffing with "teams" organized by honoring and accessing community resources, such as neighbor, church member, storekeeper— perhaps linked to a healthcare provider through technology. Regardless of its composition, the defining element is the team.

Team-Based Care: The Origin Story

Until the early twentieth century, clinicians in England practiced almost universally within rigid, vertical, hierarchical structures, with consultants at the top, followed by physicians, surgeons, dentists, apothecaries, matrons, ward sisters, and nurses. Communication between the ranks was also highly structured, and deviation from accepted protocol, even to convey lifesaving information, would result in disciplinary action.[28] The rapid industrial expansion and waves of immigration experienced in the United States in the late 19th and early 20th centuries, along with advances in medical science, brought new challenges to the healthcare infrastructure. During this time, a "team approach" to care was first implemented.[29]

Richard Cabot, a young physician influenced by the ideas of philosopher and social reformer John Dewey and social worker Jane Addams, chose to work in the outpatient department of the prestigious Massachusetts General Hospital. The department served a patient population that was unable to afford inpatient care and suffered from chronic conditions such as tuberculosis. Cabot quickly realized that regardless of the interventions that medicine could offer, the conditions in which patients lived, and to which they returned after treatment, would preclude any substantive recovery. In 1905, he proposed an unprecedented arrangement—a program in which he partnered physicians, social workers, and nurses to address the multidimensional needs of patients and their families and thereby improve the effectiveness of medical care.[30] While this model would serve as the template for hospital-based social work programs throughout the country, at the time it was considered so radical that Cabot was required to pay for the team members from his own funds.[30]

As medical care in hospitals expanded in scope and complexity, it became ever apparent that a single profession could not singlehandedly direct such complex organizations.[31] Instead, a team of interdependent members could better ensure the efficient management of departments *and* the patients they served. Dorothy Rogers, a nurse, proposed this idea in a 1932 editorial, very diplomatically noting that the "game depends" upon each member playing their assigned role and no members seeing themselves as "solo performers."[31]

Another early example of team-based care is the work of the Montefiore Hospital Home Care Program, which sought to understand patients as whole persons and provide care that met their physical, social, and spiritual needs. This comprehensive home-based program, led by physician Martin Cherkasky in the mid-1940s, included physician visits, nursing care, medication, housekeeping services, physical and occupational therapy, and transportation assistance. According to Cherkasky, this program achieved positive outcomes, at a lower cost; and more importantly, it allowed patients to recover in the comfort of their homes, as opposed to the regimented environment of the hospital.[32] This home-based model of whole-person care predated modern home hospice care by nearly a quarter of a century, but bore many of the attributes that would come to be embodied in the modern hospice movement in America.

During the 1940s and 1950s, we begin to see editorials and position papers calling for health professionals to work collaboratively, as opposed to hierarchically, in care delivery.[31,32] But it was the impact of World War II that solidified the shift to a team-based model of care. The war brought home millions of injured service personnel who required the multifaceted care of interprofessional teams specializing in burns, rehabilitation, and mental health.[28] Beyond the practical need for care from a range of professionals, healthcare was being influenced by the novel work of behavioral and social scientists. Theories from fields such as group dynamics and organizational development promoted the concept of synergy—the idea that the impact of a team is greater than the contributions of its individual members.[28]

In 1974, the first U.S. hospice was founded by Florence Wald (then dean of the Yale School of Nursing), along with 2 pediatricians and a chaplain, creating a path for what would become the first categorically interprofessional specialty.[33] Throughout the arc of the 20th century we see a shift from a vertical chain of command to a spoke and wheel structure that places the patient and family at the center of care and a coordinated team of clinicians working together to support them.

Unintended Consequences of Developing a Specialty

The specialty of palliative care which followed the modern hospice movement eventually received official recognition and gained widespread, if somewhat reluctant acceptance into the acute care setting. As life expectancy continues to rise and there is ever-increasing development *and* use of technological advances to sustain life, there arises the need to address the burden of serious illness and the impact of its treatment. Specialty palliative care has come forward and has made great strides toward addressing this gap. However, 2 main problems emerged—one philosophical and one practical. First, by creating a specialty whose raison d'être is to manage pain, suffering, and difficult decisions, primary providers can offload the responsibility of addressing these needs for their patients. Second, the demands of an aging population and trends toward greater use of acute and intensive care at end of life will far outstrip the supply of palliative care clinicians in practice and in the training pipeline.[34] To address both these issues, a hybrid model using both primary and specialty palliative care has been introduced[35-39] and supported across professions. Primary palliative care equips clinicians at the bedside with basic skills to assess and address pain and symptoms, to communicate effectively, and to provide practical and emotional support to patients and their families (see Chapter 11 for the concept of "familiness"), enabling them to navigate the serious illness.

Another unintended consequence of the establishment of a palliative care specialty in the setting of our current fee-for-service model is the medico-centricity of the specialty. In the current model, only physicians and advanced practice providers (APPs) can bill for specialty consultative services, including palliative care. Thus, a palliative care service must have physicians and/or APPs to be revenue-generating and must creatively manage the costs of other team members, who function as critical members of the team but cannot bill for their services. Hospice operates under a different payment model, which may allow its members to function in a more team-like fashion. Yet, the current payment structure literally defines and circumscribes what hospice can provide. No matter how great the burden of a person's unmet palliative care needs and no matter how willing they are to forgo curative or life-extending treatment, if they are not "terminally ill"—as defined by a life expectancy of less than 6 months—they do not qualify for hospice care.

Teaching Individuals to Be a Team

Although evidence grew for the value of team-based models of care delivery during the mid-20th century, the education of the team's members remained firmly rooted in traditional disciplinary silos.[28] Teams function best when there is shared knowledge about other members' skills and roles, but there were no opportunities beyond "on-the-job learning" for clinicians to acquire this information.

The first report of interprofessional education was published by Szasz in 1969 and described an experiment conducted at the University of British Columbia, wherein selected didactic classes were "interprofessionalized" to include students from more than one of the health professions—medicine, dentistry, nursing, physical therapy.[40] The experiment demonstrated that this model was feasible to implement but did not measure any outcomes related to team performance among participants.

In 1972, the Institute of Medicine (IOM) delivered the results of their report, *Education for the Health Team*, at their conference on interprofessional education, recommending that a concerted effort be made to integrate the education of diverse healthcare team members in classroom and clinical settings.[41] From that point forward, there was an exponential increase in programs providing interprofessional education opportunities for those in healthcare and grant funding to support these efforts.[28] However, Baldwin notes that in the 1980s much of the federal funding for these programs ceased, though select foundations have continued to fund programs committed to interprofessional education for healthcare professionals in academic-community partnerships.[28] In 2009, the Interprofessional Education Consortium (IPEC) was founded by 6 national education associations of schools of the health professions to promote the value of interprofessional education, to set educational standards across institutions, and to develop core competencies for the education of health professionals.[42] In 2012, the National Center for Interprofessional Practice and Education, a public-private partnership, was established to serve as a resource for interprofessional education and collaboration in healthcare.[43] Recognizing that palliative care is an inherently interprofessional specialty, numerous training programs have been developed and tested to educate members of the palliative care team in a manner that reflects their practice model[44-47] (see Chapters 8–10 for discussion of academic, clinical, and continuing education in interprofessional palliative care).

Throughout the evolution of team-based care and education, we see the terms "interdisciplinary" and "interprofessional" used intermittently, and often inconsistently. "Discipline" refers to knowledge, and "profession" refers to praxis or practice. The label "profession" emerged in medieval times and was first applied to physicians, lawyers, and clergy. Those who wished to be in these roles were required not only to acquire distinct knowledge, but also to publicly *profess* to safeguard the interests of vulnerable persons. Thus, being a professional implied responsibility beyond the transacting of services; and each profession operated autonomously, under a code of professional ethics. Since that time, multiple healthcare professions have emerged, each with their unique disciplinary knowledge *and* professional rules and ethics. The label "interdisciplinary" when referring to various professionals on a healthcare team can lead to confusion, as the term is also used to describe those with different specialties (e.g., oncology, cardiology, and pulmonology). Some in the field of palliative care would argue for reclaiming the term "interprofessional" because it is additive (implying richer meaning) and inclusive (recognizing equal status among members of the team).[48] However, this proposed shift in nomenclature is not without challenges. The term "interdisciplinary"‡ has been incorporated into federal regulations for the provision and reimbursement of hospice and palliative care, and change would require extensive revision. See Table 2.2 for a summary of team terms.

Table 2.2 Teamwork Terminology

Term	Definition	Caveats
Interdisciplinary	"Of or pertaining to two or more disciplines or branches of learning; contributing to or benefiting from two or more disciplines."[50]	In terms of healthcare, this refers only to knowledge and does not take aspects of practice into account.
Interprofessional	"Occurring between or involving two or more professions or professionals."[51]	Refers to both knowledge and practice, ascribing full membership to all professions within the team.
Transprofessional	"Transprofessionalism is defined as a process of collaboration between two or more professionals across and beyond professional and disciplinary boundaries, such that boundaries blur and new synergies flourish."[52]	The ability of diverse professionals on a team to practice across and beyond their traditional disciplinary and professional boundaries has tremendous potential to maximize benefits to care recipients. However, there is also considerable potential for role ambiguity and role confusion, potentially resulting in missed care or duplicative care.
Interdisciplinary team	Members with diverse knowledge and skills work together proactively.[53]	May not have shared leadership or decision-making authority. The term may introduce confusion among medical colleagues.
Interprofessional team	Professionally diverse team with knowledge and skills working together proactively.[53]	The term offers clarity as to members comprising the team.
Transprofessional team	Members with diverse knowledge and skills who "create a shared mission, have role overlap, and have integrated responsibilities, leadership and training."[53]	This model is ideally suited to stable teams in non-teaching settings, but may be difficult to implement in teaching organizations that have rotating staff and waves of learners. In the palliative care context, the term "transprofessional team" is most appropriate.

‡ Although Medicare policy and the NCP Guidelines use the term "interdisciplinary," in this book we have standardized the language to use the term "interprofessional" when referring to the core members of the palliative care team.

Beyond the debate around the root terms, "discipline" and "profession," there is also the issue of prefix: *multi-*, *inter-*, or *trans-*. Most would argue that the terms "interdisciplinary" or "interprofessional"—in reference to a team—suggest a level of coordination beyond merely multidisciplinary or multiprofessional. However, transdisciplinary§ or transprofessional teamwork implies that members of the team can work interchangeably, with overlapping skill sets. Team members in settings with a stable, enduring staff describe this fluid and adaptive team model as the apex of evolutionary development. However, those in large teaching organizations with rotating students see this as potentially chaotic and virtually unattainable.

A Hike through the Wildflowers and Weeds of Terminology: The Micro Perspective

Beyond the ongoing quandary of defining and branding of palliative care in the national and international landscape, and the essential importance of team as a foundational construct, are the words we choose, the silence we observe, and the argots, or jargon, we integrate—all within our personal power to control. Word choice may serve many purposes. For some, adopting the language of hierarchy and of those in power is a path to acceptance—this process serves to protect and mitigate the discomfort that might evolve from questioning or disagreement. While palliative care seeks to be egalitarian, it can never be purely so, as the risk and responsibility are not equal, nor are the sheer numbers within each profession (see Chapter 3). Social workers and chaplains are minority disciplines in medical settings, and negotiating this positionality may involve adopting the vernacular of the majority.[54] Social work and spiritual care identify not only with the legacy of their profession, but also with a history of each profession's relationship to the other and to healthcare institutions. Physicians and nurses have unique professional histories of relationship not shared by social workers and chaplains. Each profession is perceived differently by patients and families and brings unique training that enriches listening and informs practice. Added to the rich complexity of what each profession brings to the work and what patients and families expect is healthcare financing, which may infuse relationships and hierarchy within teams and yet never be discussed. Some team members carry the responsibility for billing, generating income, and contributing to the financial viability of the service, and others depend on departments or institutions to support their work. Unique responsibilities, such as the writing of orders and the prescribing role of physicians and nurse practitioners, engage a process of discernment, decision-making, and risk that differs from that of other team members. No

---

§ The term "transdisciplinary" is more accurately described as transprofessional, since it illustrates the collaboration and synergy between professions rather than disciplines. However, in this chapter and throughout the book, the term "transdisciplinary" is used since it is currently the word most commonly used in the literature to signify this form of team collaboration.

When we refer to "interprofessional," it is within this framework of working at the transdisciplinary collaborative level. It is referring to an advanced level of professional synergy.

matter the structure of the team and the terms used to describe it, each member by their choice to participate as a team member has a shared responsibility to evolve voice, to contribute, challenge, and question. To that end, we move to a micro level to bring attention and intention to the terms and phrases that inform the voice of palliative care in many settings.

This process of creating a specialty and a language with which to talk about our purpose and intentions has, over time, integrated words and phrases that have become ubiquitous. Words and phrases such as "suffering," "dignity," "goals of care," "comfort care," and "quality of life" have become automatic—argots which may or may not have shared understanding among clinicians, patients, and families. The intention of this section is to draw attention to a micro level of practice that may have become useful in teaching, serves to mask our discomfort or aid in negotiating the demands of fast-paced health systems, yet may leave behind the critical discernment and rich narrative discovery that enriches the mind and soul of many who chose this work. The purpose of this exploration, which is reflected in Table 2.3,

Table 2.3 Micro Terminology

Argots	Descriptor	Caveats
Suffering	Distress brought about by the actual or perceived impending threat to the integrity or continued existence of the whole person.[55] . . . any aspect of person; comparable to "Total Pain" construct.[56]	A ubiquitous term often engaged before or without any awareness of the historical "suffering" that infuses a families' life and legacy. Patients may be described as suffering at the same time we are assisting families to integrate, cognitively and emotionally, an absence of consciousness and brain function.
Loved ones	An assumed relationship of love	The automatic assumption that a patient is "loved" is a bias, perhaps a hope or a wish, and can impact another's willingness to share the authenticity of the relationship.
Caregiver/care partner	Caregiver: someone who provides care; one gives and the other receives—a one-way relationship. Care partner: a partnership with opportunity to give and receive; more inclusive and egalitarian.[57]	The concept of burden floods the caregiver literature. Caregiver implies a dependence, yet patient goals may include enhancing autonomy, control, and agency. The distinction in this word choice creates opportunity to join and adapt language as the trajectory of illness evolves and needs change. It is important to recognize that dependence does not obviate the ability to give as well as receive.
Withhold/forgo care/treatment	Care is constant, treatments are withdrawn and withheld. To withhold means to refuse to give or hold back; forgo includes to give up or do without—a subtle difference in tone.	To withhold, for some, may be heard as a profound responsibility and assertion of power . . . to forgo may be heard as a message of deliberative weighing and a consequent informed choice. The patient becomes the "object" of withholding; the patient or surrogate is the "agent" of forgoing.
Goals of care	Explored within the landscape of intersecting variables and values and goals extending beyond medical decisions.	For example, in many settings referrals for "goals of care" are a metaphor reflecting clinician distress when patients and families do not accept a recommendation, such as agreeing to a "do not attempt resuscitation" order.

Table 2.3 Continued

Argots	Descriptor	Caveats
Comfort care	May be used as a simplified descriptor of a specialty or a transition in a plan of care. Implies a binary about the humane goal of comfort which rests in a continuum.[59]	Often used by referral sources to abbreviate and protect self, patient, and family from the work and distress of linking history, treatment outcomes, goals, and hopes to a changing focus. Implies that the universal ethical mandate to maximize comfort was not a concurrent focus of all who provided care.
Death with dignity	A term which may assume rather than discover the unique meaning of dignity in the histories and legacies of patients and families; used to promote and name laws that support aid in dying.	Equating dignity with the freedom to end one's life implies that other care may not be dignified. A clinician's view of dignity may combine a subjective, cultural, and spiritual lens with data—a self-awareness that can lead to an authentic discovery of the values that inform "dignity" for the other.
End of life, dying	In a culture that assumes death denial, the work of discovering how others view the end of biologic "life" may help to bridge cultural and ethnic divides.	Palliative care in a multiethnic society requires humility and acceptance that even death may be viewed and described from unique histories and belief systems that create such descriptors as "crossing over" and "traveling." Death may be seen as a "transition" rather than an "end."

is not to achieve agreement, but rather to encourage attention and intention in word choice. This table is organized around 3 aspects of practice: words and phrases often central to palliative care communication; descriptors or definitions; and lastly, questions and comments to broaden and enrich the frames within which we understand the intention and unintended messages that some may receive from the language we have evolved.

At the heart of palliative care practice is joining across teams, with patients and families. This joining is hindered or enriched by word choice, by the process of discovery to create "intersubjective understanding." Attention to culture, spirituality, and history requires moving beyond the assumption that we have shared understanding about such individual concepts as suffering and dignity. It is at this micro discussion of terminology that we end this chapter, as it is the choice of words, spoken or written, or the choice to be silent, that pervades all aspects of interprofessional practice—no matter the setting.

Reflection questions

1. How can your team limit argots, or specialized jargon, to enhance the messaging of palliative care?
2. In what way does your team practice in a transdisciplinary/transprofessional manner?
3. How can you increase this level of teamwork?

4. In your current practice setting, what terminology at the micro- meso- and macro- levels might interfere with advocating for palliative care among stakeholders, including administration, patients, families, clinicians, payment sources, or advocacy groups?

Acknowledgments

Jennifer Seaman wishes to acknowledge the contributions of the Cambia Sojourns Scholar Interprofessional Special Interest Group (IP SIG), whose thoughtful questions and grappling with the topics of history and team terminology were foundational to the development of this chapter.

References

1. Krawczyk M, Sawatzky R, Schick-Makaroff K, Stajduhar K, Öhlen J, Reimer-Kirkham S, Mercedes Laforest E, Cohen R. Micro-meso-macro practice tensions in using patient-reported outcome and experience measures in hospital palliative care. *Qual Health Res.* 2019 Mar;29(4):510–521. doi: 10.1177/1049732318761366. Epub 2018 Mar 15. PMID: 29542400.
2. McKee M. Excavating our frames of mind: the key to dialogue and collaboration. *Soc Work.* 2003;48:401–408.
3. Thakur N, Lovinsky-Desir S, Bime C, Wisnivesky JP, Celedón JC. The structural and social determinants of the racial/ethnic disparities in the U.S. COVID-19 pandemic: what's our role? *Am J Resp Crit Care Med.* 2020;202:943–949.
4. Bailey ZD, Krieger N, Agénor M, Graves J, Linos N, Bassett MT. Structural racism and health inequities in the USA: evidence and interventions. *Lancet (London)* 2017;389:1453–1463.
5. Seervai S. It's harder for people living in poverty to get health care. *The Commonwealth Fund*; 2019. https://www.commonwealthfund.org/publications/podcast/2019/apr/its-harder-peo ple-living-poverty-get-health-care
6. Farmer B. Long-standing racial and income disparities seen creeping into COVID-19 care. *Kaiser Health News*; 2020. https://kffhealthnews.org/news/covid-19-treatment-racial-inc ome-health-disparities/
7. Saunders C. The management of terminal malignant disease. In: Saunders C, ed. *The Management of Terminal Malignant Disease.* Hodder and Stoughton; 1993:1–14.
8. Balfour Mount. Accessed December 12, 2020. https://www.mcgill.ca/palliativecare/portra its-0/balfour-mount.
9. Palliative care. http://www.finedictionary.com/palliate.html.
10. Warraich HJ. In pandemic era, the term palliative care is even more scary for some. So specialists want to rename it. *Washington Post*, September 7, 2020. https://www.washingtonp ost.com/health/palliative-care-supportive-hospice/2020/09/04/07bf5236-e6d8-11ea-97e0-94d2e46e759b_story.html
11. Clinical Practice Guidelines for Quality Palliative Care, 4th edition. National Coalition for Hospice and Palliative Care, 2018. https://www. nationalcoalitionhpc.org/ncp/.
12. Palliative Care Key Facts, WHO, 2020. https://www.who.int/news-room/fact-sheets/detail/ palliative-care.
13. International Association for Hospice and Palliative Care. 2019. https://hospicecare.com/ what-we-do/projects/consensus-based-definition-of-palliative-care/definition/.
14. NCI Dictionary of Terms. https://www.cancer.gov/publications/dictionaries/cancer-terms/ expand/P.

15. Explanation of Palliative Care. 2018. https://www.nhpco.org/palliative-care-overview/expl anation-of-palliative-care/.
16. Hospice Facts and Figures. August 20, 2020. https://www.nhpco.org/factsfigures/.
17. Meier DE. Key Findings on the Perceptions of Palliative Care; 2019. https://media.capc.org/ recorded-webinars/slides/1lessAudience_Research_Webinar_Aug_8-2019_FINAL.pdf.
18. Institute of Medicine. *Dying in America: Improving Quality and Honoring Individual Preferences Near the End of Life*. National Academies Press; 2015:ii.
19. Clark D. From margins to centre: a review of the history of palliative care in cancer. *Lancet Oncol*. 2007;8:430–438.
20. Klement A, Marks S. The pitfalls of utilizing "goals of care" as a clinical buzz phrase: a case study and proposed solution. *Palliat Med Rep*. 2020;1:216–220.
21. Xiao J, Brenneis C, Ibrahim N, Bryan A, Fassbender K. Definitions of palliative care terms: a consensus-oriented decision-making process. *J Palliat Med*. 2021;24:1342–1350.
22. Ladwig S, Quill T, Horowitz R, Weibel A, Dickson RB. Public opinion about palliative care in 2019: the needle hasn't moved. 2019. https://media.capc.org/posters/2019/717019.pdf.
23. Flieger SP, Chui K, Koch-Weser S. Lack of awareness and common misconceptions about palliative care among adults: insights from a national survey. *J Gen Intern Med*. 2020;35:2059–2064.
24. Knaul FM, Farmer PE, Krakauer EL, et al. Alleviating the access abyss in palliative care and pain relief-an imperative of universal health coverage: the Lancet Commission report. *Lancet (London)* 2018;391:1391–1454.
25. Discourse of Pope Francis to the participants in the Plenary Assembly of the Pontifical Academy for Life, March 5, 2015. http://www.academyforlife.va/content/pav/en/projects/ pallife/pallife-project.html.
26. Radbruch L, De Lima L, Knaul F, et al. Redefining palliative care: a new consensus-based definition. *J Pain Symptom Manage*. 2020;60:754–764.
27. Controversies in palliative care: A matter of definition. January 18, 2019. http://endoflifestud ies.academicblogs.co.uk/controversies-in-palliative-care-a-matter-of-definition/.
28. Walton MM. Hierarchies: The Berlin Wall of patient safety. *Qual Saf Health Care*. 2006;15:229–230.
29. Baldwin DC, Jr. Some historical notes on interdisciplinary and interprofessional education and practice in health care in the USA, 1996. *J Interprof Care* 2007;21(Suppl 1):23–37.
30. History of Social Service Massachusetts General Hospital. https://www.massgeneral.org/soc ial-service/about/history.
31. Rogers D. Teamwork within hospitals. *Am J Nursing*. 1932;32:657–659.
32. Cherkasky M. The Montefiore Hospital Home Care Program. *Am J Public Health*. 1949;39:163–166.
33. Adams C. Dying with dignity in America: the transformational leadership of Florence Wald. *J Prof Nurs*. 2010;26:125–132.
34. Hua MS, Li G, Blinderman CD, Wunsch H. Estimates of the need for palliative care consultation across United States intensive care units using a trigger-based model. *Am J Resp Crit Care Med*. 2014;189:428–436.
35. Quill TE, Abernethy AP. Generalist plus specialist palliative care: creating a more sustainable model. *N Engl J Med*. 2013;368:1173–1175.
36. Murray SA, Boyd K, Sheikh A, Thomas K, Higginson IJ. Developing primary palliative care. *Br Med J*. 2004;329:1056–1057.
37. Sumser B, Altilio T. *Palliative Care: A Guide for Health Social Workers*. Oxford University Press; 2019.
38. Wheeler MS. Primary palliative care for every nurse practitioner. *J Nurse Pract*. 2016;12:647–653.
39. Paice JA, Battista V, Drick CA, Schreiner E. Palliative nursing summit: Nurses leading change and transforming primary palliative care: nursing's role in providing pain and symptom management. *JHPN*. 2018;20:30–35.
40. Szasz G. Interprofessional education in the health sciences: a project conducted at the University of British Columbia. *Milbank Q*. 1969;47:449–475.
41. Institute of Medicine. *Education for the Health Team*. National Academies Press; 1972.

42. Interprofessional Education Collaborative (IPEC). Accessed December 14, 2020. https://www.ipecollaborative.org/about-us.

43. National Center for Interprofessional Practice and Education. Accessed December 14, 2020. https://nexusipe.org/informing/about-national-center.

44. Gadoud A, Lu W-H, Strano-Paul L, Lane S, Boland JW. A pilot study of interprofessional palliative care education of medical students in the UK and USA. *BMJ Support Palliat Care.* 2018;8:67–72.

45. Head BA, Schapmire T, Hermann C, et al. The Interdisciplinary Curriculum for Oncology Palliative Care Education (iCOPE): meeting the challenge of interprofessional education. *J Palliat Med.* 2014;17:1107–1114.

46. Hall P, Weaver L, Fothergill-Bourbonnais F, et al. Interprofessional education in palliative care: a pilot project using popular literature. *J Interprof Care.* 2006;20:51–59.

47. Gellis ZD, Kim E, Hadley D, et al. Evaluation of interprofessional health care team communication simulation in geriatric palliative care. *Gerontol Geriatr Educ.* 2019;40:30–42.

48. Seaman JB, Lakin JR, Anderson E, et al. Interdisciplinary or interprofessional: why terminology in teamwork matters to hospice and palliative care. *J Palliat Med.* 2020;23:1157–1158.

49. Merriam-Webster Dictionary. https://www.merriam-webster.com

50. Oxford English Dictionary online. www.oed.com

51. Chiocchio F, Richer M-C. From multi-professional to trans-professional healthcare teams: the critical role of innovation projects. In Gurtner S, Soyez K, eds. *Challenges & Opportunities in Health Care Management.* Springer; 2015:127.

52. Otis-Green S, Ferrell B, Spolum M, et al. An overview of the ACE Project—advocating for clinical excellence: transdisciplinary palliative care education. *J Cancer Educ.* 2009;24(2):120–126.

53. Higgins PC. Guess who's coming to dinner? The evolving identity of palliative social workers. In Altilio T, Otis-Green S, Cagle J, eds. *Oxford Textbook of Palliative Social Work.* Oxford University Press; 2022:65–76.

54. Cassel EJ. *The Nature of Suffering.* Oxford University Press; 1991.

55. Saunders C. The symptomatic treatment of incurable malignant disease. *Prescrib J.* Oct 1964;4(4):68–73.

56. Care Partner's Guide: Care Partner versus Caregiver. Huntington's Outreach Project for Education, at Stanford. 2018. https://hopes.stanford.edu/care-partners-guide-care-partner-versus-caregiver/.

57. Patek BK. Liberation from mechanical ventilation. Merck Manual Professional Version, 2020. https://www.merckmanuals.com/professional/critical-care-medicine/respiratory-failure-and-mechanical-ventilation/liberation-from-mechanical-ventilation.

58. Kelemen AM, Groninger H. Ambiguity in end-of-life care terminology: what do we mean by "comfort care?". *JAMA Intern Med.* 2018;178(11):1442–1443.

59. Wailoo K. *Whose Pain Matters: Reflections on Race, Social Justice and Covid 19's Revealed Inequities* [Video]. 2020.

3

Profession-Specific Roles in Palliative Care

Naomi Tzril Saks, Cara L. Wallace, DorAnne Donesky, and Michelle M. Milic

Key Points

- The transdisciplinary team collaboration framework in palliative care is distinguished from other approaches to teamwork in that it involves a shared team vision for both the inclusion and transcendence of professional boundaries.
- Interprofessional roles are synergistic rather than interchangeable or working side by side. Optimal interprofessional practice requires team members who are confident and mature in their own discipline and respectful of their own and others' roles.
- The proposed Generalist-Specialist Model of Interprofessional Practice in Palliative Care, founded on the transdisciplinary framework for collaboration, allows members to function as an integrated, supportive team.
- Each profession defines their own scope of practice and values.
- Despite evolving national standards for profession-specific roles in palliative care, specialized education, credentialing, responsibilities, and general practice vary across professions, teams, services, and institutions.
- While experiential understanding of profession-specific roles in palliative care is supported by some empirical evidence, role definitions and responsibilities are often poorly communicated or understood.
- Many palliative care teams do not include core professions in full-time positions, such as chaplain, social worker, nurse, and physician. A priority of palliative care leadership is developing the financial models and clinical efficiencies that support the hiring of the full, nationally endorsed, interprofessional team.

Introduction

The demand for palliative care continues to grow rapidly, with a limited workforce scrambling to meet the need and to expand palliative care training[1] across

---

Box 3.1. Administrator

Jennie Kung

One of my most rewarding experiences has been serving as a hospital administrator at a large academic medical center for advance care planning, palliative care, and hospice, among other areas. In that role, I led the co-creation of the service strategy with the clinical team. Importantly, it required guiding and nurturing the strategy to fruition by navigating the financials, staffing, policies and procedures, human resources, and a whole bevy of responsibilities so that the clinicians could focus on taking care of the patients and their families. An administrator responsible for the end-of-life care continuum requires breaking down silos to create pathways that may not currently exist. Imagine a network of bridges in a highly matrixed organization, enabling everyone in the continuum to communicate and deliver thoughtful, goal-concordant care.

Success in this role means that the administrator needs to have an array of tools in their toolbox to drive efficiency and effectiveness, thus ensuring that the organization can deliver high-quality care in a financially sustainable manner. One important tool I utilize time and time again is human-centered design (HCD) to spark engagement and buy-in from stakeholders. Widely used in technology and product development, HCD is often overlooked in healthcare as an effective method to uncover the needs of our patients and their families, as well as perspectives of our care teams and teammates. HCD builds empathy into the solutions we create. As champions across the system are trained in HCD, they are armed with tools to solve problems in an empathetic manner. Administrators who embrace HCD are able to inject innovative, human-centered solutions so that we can all be empowered to make improvements for everyone involved.

---

professions. Ideally, palliative care is practiced by an interprofessional* team minimally staffed by the core members† (chaplain, nurse, physician, and social worker). As each profession grapples with growing and training its workforce, in systems challenged by chronic workplace stress2 and healthcare disparities, how team members individually function and successfully collaborate deserves focused attention.

Collaboration between the professionals on a team in the context of family-centered models for care is associated with positive outcomes that address the quadruple aim of improving patient and clinician experience of care, improving the health of populations, and reducing per capita costs of healthcare.[3,4] In addition, palliative care facilitates safer care, better communication, and improved adherence to treatment.[5-7] However, in practice, interprofessional collaboration is a work-in-progress, and success is dependent on the sincere commitment of each team member and the institutions and cultures that support the specialty. Successful palliative care and the sustainability of each team member depends on functioning teams built on team-reflective practice, and awareness of individual and systemic power dynamics and sources of well-being. How do we move beyond good intentions and general core competencies for collaboration to co-create teams where the focus on collaborative practice results in higher-quality care?

In this chapter, the authors introduce a road map they created which conceives interprofessional cooperation rooted in the framework of transdisciplinary[‡] team collaboration and operationalized in the Generalist-Specialist Model of Interprofessional Practice in Palliative Care (GSM) (see Figure 3.1). For teams to function at their best, understanding others' roles is key. Included in the chapter is a brief description of the professional background of each core team member with a summary of profession-specific education, licensure, and certification for professional practice, specialization, and certification in palliative care, and a description of each professions' roles and responsibilities (see Table 3.1). Contributions of a broad range of essential team members are included in separate boxes (see Boxes 3.1–3.12). The chapter concludes with a brief discussion of challenges to role identity and development that impact synergy and recommendations for the growth of sustainable models of interprofessional teamwork.

Theoretical Framework for Interprofessional Collaborative Practice

While palliative care prides itself on an interprofessional approach, minimal guidance exists on best practices for the *implementation* of this approach. Transdisciplinary team collaboration serves as a theoretical foundation alongside the GSM to provide a framework for discussion of roles and contributions of each core profession.

---

‡ The process this framework is pointing to is more accurately described as transprofessional, since it illustrates the collaboration and synergy between professions rather than disciplines. However, in this chapter and throughout the book, the term *transdisciplinary* is used since it is currently the word most commonly used in the literature to signify this form of team collaboration. When we refer to interprofessional it is within this framework of working at the transdisciplinary collaborative level. It is referring to an advanced level of professional synergy.

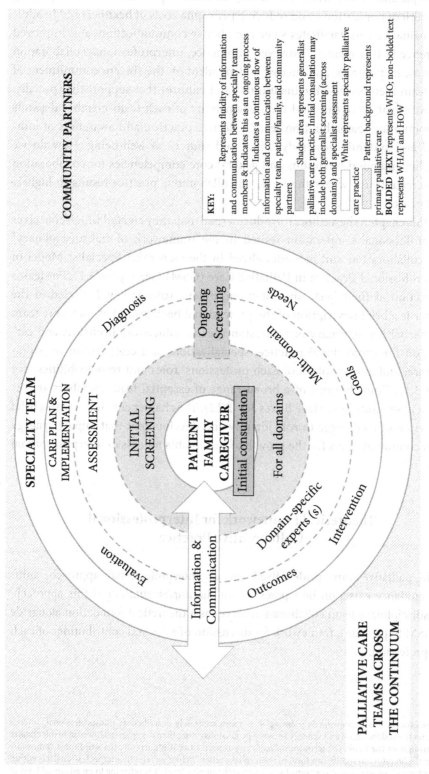

Figure 3.1 Generalist-Specialist Model of Interprofessional Practice in Palliative Care

Definitions & Additional Information

Circular Format: Indicates there is a continuous cycle of interprofessional screening, assessment, and rounding resulting in an ongoing process of identification of needs/diagnosis, care planning, interventions and outcomes.

Generalist-Specialist Palliative Care: Screening and foundational palliative care interventions provided by palliative care specialist team members focused on areas outside of their primary domains

Primary Palliative Care: Screening and foundational palliative care interventions provided by any health care team member across practice settings and specialties that do not specialize in palliative care

Specialty Palliative Care: Collective assessment and advanced palliative care interventions provided by the palliative care specialist team within team members' primary domains.

Palliative Care Specialist: A professional with additional certification, training, and experience in palliative care who provides generalist palliative care outside their domain and specialty palliative care within their domain.

Screening: A few sentence instrument, completed by all members of the team, that evaluates the presence or absence of domain specific needs and/or distress with the goal of identifying those in need of further assessment and care to be performed by the palliative care domain expert and in collaboration with other members as indicated.

Assessment: An in-depth, on-going process of evaluating a patient's needs and resources. It includes interventions, outcomes and evaluation and is completed by the domain expert(s) or other members of the team

Foundational Palliative Care Interventions: Interventions that all palliative care specialists on the team, regardless of professional background, provide including (not exhaustive): facilitating family meetings, serious illness communication, and anticipatory guidance at end of life

Domains: Per NCP guidelines, palliative care domains include structure and processes, physical, psychological/psychiatric, social, spiritual/religious/existential, cultural, end of life, ethical/legal.

Multi-domain refers to the fact that all members of the team may contribute to assessment and intervention in all domains of care per their expertise and training.

Initial Consultation: Multi-domain comprehensive evaluation to capture a patient's characteristics, resources, and needs in all key palliative care domains. May be done with multiple team members present and labeled as H&P in inpatient setting or admission visit in hospice setting.

Palliative Care Teams Across the Continuum: Includes teams that perform specialty palliative care ex. outpatient, home-based, hospice, consulting teams etc.

Community Partners: Individuals and organizations that contribute to the ongoing care and support of the seriously ill and their caregivers and provide primary palliative care (i.e. primary care providers, home health, psycho-social professionals, religious/spiritual leaders, etc)

Figure 3.1 Continued

Table 3.1 Education, Licensure, Certification

	Education and Licensure (state-specific)	Certification for Professional Practice (met minimum criteria to practice)	Certification for Palliative Care
Chaplain			
Clinical Healthcare Chaplain	Master's degree in related field and at least 2 units of Clinical Pastoral Education (CPE); no state licensure	Board Certification available from multiple organizations. Requires master of divinity (or equivalent), 1600 total hours CPE and 2,000 hours of employment as a chaplain, endorsement by a spiritual or philosophical tradition, and demonstration of competencies in front of a certifying committee.	Each of the following is available after prior general board certification status Palliative Care and Hospice Advanced Certification (BCC-PCHAC) Hospice and Palliative Care Specialty Certification (APBCC-HPC)
Nurse			
Aide (HHA/MA/CNA)	No degree; requirements vary by state but commonly 60 hours of classroom; 100 hours of clinical practice; no licensure exam	Optional National Nurse Aide Assessment Program (NNAAP) certification	Certified Hospice and Palliative Nursing Assistant (CHPNA®)
LVN/LPN	No degree; 12–20 months after high school; 1530 hours of education (576 theory hours; 954 clinical hours); National Council Licensure Examination (NCLEX)	Not available	Certified Hospice and Palliative Licensed Nurse – CHPLN®
RN	Associate degree, minimum; 600 hours of didactic courses and 270 hours in clinical practice; NCLEX exam	Optional American Nurses Credentialing Center (ANCC) certification	Certified Hospice and Palliative Nurse (CHPN®)
APRN	Master's degree and 1000 clinical hours; no licensure exam	ANCC or American Association of Nurse Practitioners (AANP) certification exam required to bill for services	Advanced Certified Hospice and Palliative Nurse (ACHPN®)

Table 3.1 Continued

	Education and Licensure (state-specific)	Certification for Professional Practice (met minimum criteria to practice)	Certification for Palliative Care
Physician			
MD/DO	Bachelor's degree, then 4-year doctoral program 3 exams for MD license spaced during and after medical school by US Medical License Exams (USMLE)	Minimum residency training is 3 years. Requires 40–80 hours/week for 3–5 years American Board of Internal Medicine (ABIM) or other primary board certification for specialty (surgery, emergency med, etc.) exam	One additional year of fellowship training in subspecialty of palliative medicine and an additional exam Subspecialty certified by the ABIM in Hospice and Palliative Medicine
Social Worker			
Bachelor's level social worker (LBSW)	Bachelor's degree; minimum of 400 hours field education; licensure exam by state (titles vary by state across all levels)	National Association for Social Work (NASW) offers certification across specialized areas of practice. No additional certification needed following licensure	Both available across levels based on a combination of years of experience and education.
Master's level social worker (LMSW)	Master's degree; minimum of 900 hours field education; licensure exam by state		Advanced Palliative Hospice and Social Work Certification (APHSW-C), endorsed by Social Work Hospice & Palliative Network
Independent clinical social worker (LCSW; can bill insurance independently)	3000 hours of supervised clinical experience after MSW; licensure exam by state		NASW offers (Advanced) Certified Hospice and Palliative Social Worker (CHP-SW or ACHP-SW)

Abbreviations: APRN: Advanced Practice Registered Nurse; BCC: Board Certified Chaplain; BSN: Bachelor of Science in Nursing; CNA: Certified Nursing Assistant; DO: Doctor of Osteopathic Medicine; HHA: Home Health Aide; LCSW: Licensed Clinical Social Worker; LPN: Licensed Practical Nurse; LVN: Licensed Vocational Nurse; MA: Medical Assistant; RN: Registered Nurse.

Transdisciplinary Team Collaboration

Historically, palliative care team culture is distinguished by high levels of autonomy, a flattened hierarchy, a focus on sustainable workload, and members who possess an openness to personal feedback from colleagues, patients, and caregivers.[8] More recently, this collaborative culture has been described with the term "transdisciplinary," as opposed to multidisciplinary or interdisciplinary. The distinctions between the prefixes are defined in Table 3.2. Teams are more

Table 3.2 Disciplinary* Approaches to Care

Uni/intra-disciplinary	Professionals from a single discipline working together toward a common goal
Multidisciplinary	A "parallel play" approach to care; clinicians from different professions working independently and from a profession-specific perspective; goals include combining efforts to address a shared problem.
Interdisciplinary	An interactive model where professionals work jointly each from their profession-specific perspective to address a common problem
Transdisciplinary	A synergistic framework blurring professional role boundaries and with overlapping functions. Where all professions on the team work as equals; shared information, communication, compassion, knowledge, and decision-making are used to co-create a unified care plan.

* Although often used interchangeably, "discipline" refers to a branch of knowledge, while "profession" refers to an occupation that requires special education and/or prolonged training and a formal qualification. In this book, we have attempted to standardize the use of the term "profession" when referring to occupations such as spiritual care, medicine, nursing, and social work, but occasionally the term "discipline" is used, especially when focused on the theory and knowledge development of the professions.

Source: Adapted from Rosa WE, Anderson E, Applebaum AJ, Ferrell BR, Kestenbaum A, Nelson JE. Coronavirus disease 2019 as an opportunity to move toward transdisciplinary palliative care. *J Palliat Med.* 2020;23(10):1290–1291; Institute of Medicine. *Establishing Transdisciplinary Professionalism for Improving Health Outcomes: Workshop Summary.* National Academy Press; 2014.

successful in moving toward a professionally inclusive, egalitarian practice, free of stereotyped professional images that previously resulted in siloed care, when they aim to practice transdisciplinary collaboration.[9] Transdisciplinary team collaboration in palliative care is distinguished from other approaches to teamwork in that it includes both the inclusion and transcendence of professional boundaries in the evolution of holistic care. All professions work as equals at the height of their abilities. All members of the team assist in creating transdisciplinarity by clarifying roles and responsibilities, improving communication, addressing conflict, and developing shared policy and practices. Limiting boundaries recede, healthy differentiation develops, and a new alchemy arises as shared decision-making, team support, and professional growth[9] result in quality services.

With transdisciplinarity, all healthcare clinicians work collaboratively, yet authority and scope of service for each profession remain with its respective specialist.[10] Palliative team cooperation is dependent upon formal and informal communication, shared team philosophy, smooth work flow, and team commitment.[11] These key variables for cooperation are continually evaluated and improved within the framework of transdisciplinary team collaboration. When this approach works, a high-level interchange of knowledge develops. Team members understand the clinical methods and competencies of one's own and others' professions, leading the outsider to observe seamless joint care planning.

Box 3.2. Healthcare Interpreter

Mateo Rutherford-Rojas
"Holding the Emotional Charge"

As medical interpreters, our primary purpose is to be a conduit, allowing clinicians and patients to effortlessly communicate with each other as if speaking the same language. In palliative care, goals-of-care, and end-of-life discussions, the emotional charge can significantly complicate our success. The professional interpreter must employ every technique possible to dissipate the emotional charge until it has flowed through them to avoid a communication breakdown. Once the intended ears, minds, and hearts of the message receive it and react to it, the interpreter is free to release their emotions.

Interpreting for a young couple (both under 20) whose first-born son was dying, the parents were challenged to accept the fact that the best hospital in the state could not save their baby, holding to the belief that hope would bring the miracle they needed. I was interpreting the turning point when they finally realized they had to choose between watching their baby die in pain, hooked up to machines and tubes, or to let him go painlessly held in their arms and feeling their warmth and love. When asked what they most wished for, their response was immediate and determined, "We want other people to never experience this." Their sincerity and concern for others at a time when most people would be focused on their own pain and suffering was so overwhelming that everyone burst into tears; nurse, surgeon, social worker, interpreter. It was a very appropriate response for a culture with a collectivist perspective where suffering is shared. Later that night, the team removed the machines and tubes so the parents could hold their son in loving arms while he passed away. Over the months, every Spanish interpreter had worked with this family and care team. To help us bring closure, we sent a card to the family expressing how they had touched our lives and the honor we felt to serve them and their baby.

As an interpreter, our emotional response would be completely out of context until the message is transmitted into the listener's language. Then, and only then, can we share the emotional impact of the words and feelings. This is perhaps the biggest challenge for the healthcare interpreter in palliative care.

Though team members share many tasks and responsibilities, actualizing this concept does not simply refer to the conflating of or dissolution of roles; rather, when the collaborative process is effective, it underlines the commitment to individual expertise and scope of service within shared goal setting, a common reference framework, and the interplay between team members.[12] The transdisciplinary approach to collaboration is the philosophical and functional foundation that supports individual clinicians and teams to function successfully within the GSM.

Generalist-Specialist Model (GSM) of Interprofessional Practice in Palliative Care

The GSM operationalizes the transdisciplinary framework for implementation of interprofessional and multi-domain screening, assessment, and intervention in palliative care (see Figure 3.1). The chapter authors conceptualized the GSM with inspiration from the Inpatient Spiritual Care Implementation Model[13] and the fourth edition of the National Consensus Project's Clinical Practice Guidelines for Quality Palliative Care (NCP Guidelines) recommendations for cross-domain screening by all professions.[14] The GSM includes all core professions across inpatient and outpatient palliative and hospice settings. The term *generalist-specialist* refers to a unique process of transdisciplinary collaborative practice within advanced practice palliative care teams trained in and practicing skills for managing complex and difficult cases.

The terms *generalist, primary, specialist,* and *specialty* are commonly used in healthcare to differentiate between care delivered by trained specialists in a particular healthcare area or population and care provided by clinicians who are broadly trained across practice areas or populations. However, the terms, as used in this model, do not refer to the distinction between primary and specialty care, but rather illustrate, when hyphenated together, a successful ongoing collaboration across professions among individuals within a specialist palliative care team.

The GSM is grounded in the assumption that all team members are experts in advanced practice palliative care competencies (see Chapters 6 and 17). For example, all team members lead rounds, facilitate serious illness communication and goals of care meetings, provide anticipatory guidance at end of life, and offer basic bereavement care. As *generalist*s in the ongoing practice of care planning, every member of the palliative care team screens for need in all domains of palliative care. As *specialists* within their domains of palliative care, chaplains, nurses, physicians, social workers, and other team members provide clinical assessment and care planning unique to their training and role. Each profession is the qualified expert or specialist in one or more domains of care.

At the same time, all members of the team are *generalists* in domains of care outside of their profession-specific areas of clinical expertise. For example, all physicians are *specialists* in assessing and treating the physical aspects of care, and at the same time they function as *generalists* as they regularly complete brief spiritual-existential and psychosocial screens for need and distress as part of every initial consult and follow-up visit. Similarly, chaplains complete a physical and psychosocial screen during each clinical visit in addition to their spiritual, religious, and existential assessment and care plan. Although the NCP Guidelines recommend that each profession screen in each domain, currently validated screens only exist for the spiritual/existential domain[15,16] and not for the other domains. Many teams use portions of existing validated assessment tools to screen in the physical,

---

Box 3.3. Occupational Therapist

Michelle Voyer

Occupational therapists (OT) seek to understand the life roles of their patients/clients and facilitate participation and engagement in meaningful occupations. OTs support patients receiving palliative care and hospice services by identifying barriers and creating client-centered strategies to preserve independence and enhance quality of life.

Mr. G is a 71-year-old who was diagnosed with amyotrophic lateral sclerosis (ALS). He began experiencing weakness in his dominant hand that limited his independence in self-care activities and affected his engagement in social activities. He was not comfortable sharing his diagnosis, and his deficits were becoming more noticeable when dining with his friends. He struggled with cutting his food and with clothing management when using the bathroom. The OT recommended that Mr. G research the menu ahead of time and either plan to order something that he could eat using one hand or discretely notify the waiter that he would like his food cut into bite-sized pieces. The OT suggested either wearing pants that were easy to pull up and down (elastic waistband) or use a buttoner/zipper pull small enough to fit in his pocket. Mr. G was able to employ the strategies learned in OT to plan his activities, limit anxiety when in social situations, and enhance meaningful engagement with his friends.

---

psychological, social, spiritual, religious, existential, cultural, end of life, and ethical domains of care.

All team members offer basic responses to the need in all domains during the patient encounter and then summarize the information learned from the screening and encounter to communicate to the rest of the team. Clinicians must specifically know when and what information needs to be referred to colleagues who are the domain experts[14] and what needs further assessment and intervention rooted in their own expertise and training. Often team members assess, intervene, and collaborate on multiple domains. When team members have a high level of trust and familiarity, domain and role boundaries may be blurred (see Chapters 4 and 11). Team members flow in and out of screening, assessment, and interventions in all domains, depending on the situation and the needs of the patient and caregivers.

Constant communication and information ideally flow between specialty palliative care and hospice teams in the community. This occurs in the form of regular rounds, case updates, clear and transparent handoffs, post-discharge clinical and well-being debriefs, and evaluation. A similar and simultaneous stream of information flows between the specialty palliative care team and primary teams, who are regularly reporting their primary palliative care assessment and interventions. The specialty team is in ongoing communication with the continuum of community partners, such as primary care providers, spiritual leaders, home health agencies, and psychosocial professionals, to ensure consistent care during transitions between levels of service.

For the GSM model to be successful, all core professions must be represented. Individual team members and institutional leadership must be familiar with the significance of each palliative care domain and professional role within a care plan and with the screening practices of all domains. Team members of all professions share leadership in structure and processes of care, such as improving service workflow. The transdisciplinary approach to team collaboration, coupled with training in and implementation of the GSM, sanctions and emboldens all members of the team and referring clinicians to holistically assess, identify, and address multiple aspects of the experience of serious illness.

Profession-Specific Roles and Contributions to Palliative Care

A strong sense of professional identity is related to professional competency in one's own field, which, in turn, is integral to building trust and respect as part of a team.[17] Awareness among team members and institutional leadership of the background and roles of team members is an important prerequisite to competency in interprofessional collaboration.[18] The evolving framework of transdisciplinary team collaboration in palliative care, one that is more egalitarian than traditional hierarchical models, is based upon a shared appreciation of the roles and skills that each member brings to the team.[19] However, palliative care educational backgrounds vary vastly, both between individuals of the same profession and across professions. Professionalization as a chaplain, nurse, physician, and social worker takes many hours of education and practice, licensure or certification, with wide variation in these requirements across professions.

Physicians, nurses, and social workers all require state licensure to practice in the United States, with opportunities for certification in both general practice and specialty areas. Chaplains do not receive licensure but depend upon board certification for general practice based on specific national qualifications, with opportunities for additional certification for specialized practice. Prior to palliative care specialization, each clinician receives extensive education and preparation, but only physicians have a required fellowship that leads to palliative care specialty practice and certification (see Chapter 9). The considerable personal and financial cost is a barrier to higher education, and variations exist between professions. For instance, physicians are required to take 3 exams costing over $2000 before they are licensed,[20,21] as compared to the one licensure exam costing a few hundred dollars that is required for the other licensed professions (nursing and social work) (see Table 3.1).

Box 3.4. Palliative Care Clinical Pharmacist

Jennifer Ku

As clinical specialists in medication stewardship and drug information, pharmacists are uniquely suited in helping the interprofessional palliative care team ensure safe and effective pharmacotherapy that aligns best with patients' goals of care. A pharmacist is especially helpful in assisting with medication-related decision-making, overcoming issues related to medication access and medication burden, adjusting medication regimens to account for drug interactions and altered pharmacokinetics, and problem-solving in situations with limitations in medication administration or availability.

For example, TC's cancer pain was only tolerable while on an intravenous ketamine infusion, oral long-acting morphine 100 mg every 8 hours, and an intravenous hydromorphone PCA. Her clinical picture was complicated by active polysubstance use disorder, a complex behavioral health history requiring treatment with multiple psychotropic medications, cardiac dysfunction, and a desire to not go home while tethered to any intravenous lines. The palliative care pharmacist was integral in transitioning her to an oral analgesic regimen tailored to her clinical case and goals of care.

The pharmacist helped design a 4-day cross-taper plan in collaboration with anesthesiology to safely transition TC onto an oral regimen of methadone and as needed oxycodone. The pharmacist also worked with her psychiatry team to adjust psychotropic medications to minimize drug interactions with her analgesics and the cocaine and cannabis TC intended to continue to use after discharge. The palliative care pharmacist advised TC's internal medicine team on cardiac monitoring for methadone initiation, prior authorization requirements, and opioid risk mitigation strategies to take at time of discharge. Finally, the pharmacist provided a warm handoff to the outpatient interprofessional palliative care team to ensure smooth transitions of care.

The NCP Guidelines,[14] along with current literature across professions, provides relevant information for describing the role and contributions of each profession within the hospice and palliative care field. While only the core palliative care roles are covered here in detail (presented in alphabetical order: chaplain, nurse, physician, and social worker), this chapter also includes boxes describing various other professionals often involved as part of the interprofessional team, each offering a unique perspective that enhances the effectiveness of palliative care (see Boxes 3.1–3.12). Many other healthcare professions also provide valuable primary and specialty palliative care, and their absence from this chapter does not in any way minimize their value in providing palliative care. Table 3.1 includes a comparison of education, licensure, and certification across the 4 core palliative care professions, with additional description of each professional role in the sections below.

Chaplain

Education, Licensure, and Certification for Professional Practice

The professional healthcare chaplain has master's level education in an academic field related to spiritual and existential care and has completed formal clinical training in spiritual, religious, existential, and emotional care. The chaplain is accountable to a code of ethics that includes a commitment to appropriate professional boundaries and respect for the values and beliefs of those for whom they care. A professional chaplain has a core knowledge base and array of spiritual care competencies, including the ability to support the inner life of all patients and caregivers, whatever their beliefs or understanding of life, and to advocate for the equitable and just inclusion of spiritual, religious, existential, and cultural beliefs and preferences into care.

In the practice of spiritual care, clinical healthcare chaplains are board-certified by one of the nationally recognized professional certifying bodies. Most, but not all, institutions require generalist-level board eligibility or board certification as a basic requirement for employment. Prior to board certification, one must obtain a master of divinity degree (M.Div.) or the educational equivalent. While most other master's degrees require 32–36 credit hours, or 1–2 years of full-time study, the M.Div. (or evaluation of equivalency of the M.Div.) is minimally 72 credit hours and 3 years of full-time study.[22] Board certification also commonly requires: 4 units (1600 hours) of Clinical Pastoral Education (CPE) practicum and coursework; ordination or commissioning by one's community to serve as a leader; endorsement or official recognition by that spiritual or philosophical tradition to function as a chaplain; 2000 hours as an employed chaplain; accountability for ethical conduct; and approval of written and verbal demonstration of competencies by a certifying committee.

Palliative Care Specialization and Certification

In general, most healthcare chaplains receive preliminary training in palliative care–related functions, such as caring for the seriously ill, complex communication, active listening, emotional counseling, end-of-life care, death and dying, grief and bereavement, bioethics, and well-being support for teams through their general graduate and CPE coursework. Throughout their training, chaplains may participate in palliative care rotations, internships, didactics, and primary palliative care electives. A growing number of pre- and postgraduate programs provide palliative care education for chaplains, such as the University of California, San Diego, Clinical Pastoral Education practicum with a focus on palliative care.[23] Chaplains also participate in interprofessional master's programs and academic certificates in palliative care (see Chapter 8). There are few chaplain-specific fellowships or interprofessional fellowships in palliative care that include chaplain learners. With limited protected educational or academic time and modest salaries, working chaplains often do not have access to academic fellowships or additional degrees;

Box 3.5. Music Therapist

Kathryn W. Coccia

As defined by the American Music Therapy Association, music therapy is "an established health profession in which music is used within a therapeutic relationship to address physical, emotional, cognitive, and social needs of individuals."[a] Utilizing patient-preferred music, music therapists provide musical interventions to address physical pain, isolation, anxiety, depression, and other needs that arise for patients and their families during serious illness. Music therapists utilize a variety of evidence-based interventions, including singing, instrument playing, songwriting, music-based life review, and receptive music listening, and cater interventions to each patient's strengths and needs. Music therapy increases meaningful communication between patients and their families, allows patients to create lasting legacies through song writing and recording, and provides a non-threatening space for emotional expression.

Clinical music in hospice care can include music thanatologists, who are specifically trained to utilize music at the very end of life. Music thanatologists provide a prescribed music cycle with harp and voice at the bedside of someone in their final days and moments of life. The Threshold Choir is a group of volunteer singers who seek to alleviate suffering for those in need by surrounding them with song.

Music helps hospice patients and families in many ways, big and small, while honoring the patient's individuality and spirit. Music can turn a potentially traumatic end-of-life moment into a peaceful and meaningful one. In one instance, a full-code patient was rapidly declining and the caregiver needed to decide whether to sign the DNR or have the nurse resuscitate the patient. The family gathered around the patient to sing her favorite songs, and ultimately the caregiver signed the DNR as the family continued to sing with the music therapist. Following the patient's death, her loved ones told family members that "we sang her into heaven." Music created a calm container for emotional processing, fostered a sense of community and safety, and honored the patient and her family during the final moments of her life.

https://news.stlpublicradio.org/health-science-environment/2020-03-25/heart-wrenching-joy-music-therapist-sets-hospice-patients-heartbeats-to-song.

[a] American Music Therapy Association website. https://www.musictherapy.org/#:~:text=Music%20Therapy%20is%20an%20established,and%20social%20needs%20of%20individuals. Accessed 10/19/23.

---

continuing education certificates and interprofessional continuing education courses are often more feasible (see Chapter 10).

The Board of Chaplaincy Certification, Inc., an affiliate of the Association of Professional Chaplains, together with the National Association of Catholic Chaplains, offers a palliative care and hospice advanced certification.[24,25] The Spiritual Care Association also offers a hospice and palliative care specialty certification for advanced practice board-certified chaplains.[26] These palliative care certifications require the applicant to meet written and oral competencies after completing required practice hours. Certification includes the expectation that chaplains will participate in ongoing research and quality improvement in the field. Advanced practice hospice and palliative care chaplains have specialized training and expertise in palliative care. This expertise includes: leadership, mentoring, and teaching in general palliative care practice; serious illness communication; teamwork; ethical and moral issues related to serious illness and death; the delivery of care and continuity of care; diversity, equity, and inclusion in healthcare; team well-being and resiliency.[27,28]

Role Description and Responsibilities

At the epicenter of the philosophy of palliative care is the belief that we are only successful if we are able to invite the experience of the whole person into the service of their healing. Intimately addressing the spiritual, religious, and existential realm of being human is essential to a medical specialty that is focused on improving quality of life and relief of suffering for the seriously ill.[29-32] Before the conception of the modern interprofessional team, the first formal role supporting those facing serious illness was one focused on caring for the inner life and spiritual well-being of the ill and dying. The significance of this legacy is rooted in the healing work of many traditions and communities approximately dating back to the sixth century BCE.[33-35] Today, the palliative care chaplain serves as a clinical palliative care expert on the team and is endorsed by the NCP Guidelines as the spiritual and existential expert and specialist in the field to be included in interprofessional teams in all settings. The NCP Guidelines recognize spirituality, broadly defined, "as a fundamental aspect of compassionate, patient and family-centered palliative care" and a focus on spiritual, religious, and existential respect, assessment, and coping as central to the provision of care.[14(p 32)]

Palliative care chaplains continue to endeavor to differentiate skills for a chaplain subspecialty. Few studies demonstrate how palliative care chaplains currently function in their positions.[28] Beyond the guideline to include a specially trained chaplain on palliative care teams, the field has not reached consensus on standards for the role. The palliative care chaplain is the trained spiritual, religious, and existential care specialist and expert within the GSM, functions as an advanced practice palliative care practitioner,[27] and is an equal and integrated member of the transdisciplinary palliative care team. The palliative care specialist chaplain is not an interchangeable role with other healthcare chaplains or clergy.

Within the context of the GSM, all team members complete a brief, 1- or 2-sentence screen with patients and caregivers to identify spiritual or existential distress and to assess for referral to the spiritual-existential specialist on the team, the palliative care chaplain, for timely, in-depth assessment, care plan, and intervention.[15,16,36] Palliative care nurses, physicians, and others may also perform a more comprehensive spiritual history using a tool specifically designed for non-chaplains,

---

Box 3.6. Hospice Volunteer Coordinator

Gayla Maze

Hospice volunteers improve quality of life by providing companionship and a supportive presence to hospice patients and their family members. The volunteer coordinator—a paid position required by CMS (Centers for Medicare & Medicaid Services) regulations—recruits, trains, manages, and retains volunteers while being enthusiastic about the care provided by hospice and supportive of the volunteers and staff. The volunteer coordinator monitors and assesses volunteer activities, and coaches volunteers to ensure adherence to CMS regulations.

Hospice volunteers bring a variety of talents and skills, and the volunteer coordinator taps into those talents to assign volunteers for a good fit. Volunteer Don Coles enjoys building conversation around life stories and discovering common interests to bond with patients and families. Volunteer Susan Hoffman, who is creative with shared activities, was challenged by a nonverbal dementia patient. The volunteer coordinator coached Susan to bridge that gap by teaching her to communicate through sensory stimulation. At the next visit, Susan brought chunky jewelry and a pinwheel for the patient to touch and experience, prompting smiles and laughter. Shared tips like these are continually exchanged between the interprofessional team and volunteers, allowing for the best quality of care through teamwork, a hallmark of hospice care.

Volunteers have provided written waivers to use their names/stories.

---

such as FICA Spiritual Assessment Tool.[37] During assessment, the chaplain uses evidence-based clinical tools to assess for spiritual and existential distress, illness coping, relational and community support, and evidence of suffering, well-being, and inner strengths based on standards of practice.[38,39] The team continues to re-evaluate for ongoing need and, if appropriate for the setting, the chaplain refers for community-based care near discharge or in the outpatient setting.

As with all healthcare professions in palliative care, spiritual care is evolving to focus on clinical outcomes.[40] Seminal studies point to positive outcomes related to a chaplain-performed spiritual consultation with people facing serious illness and interventions in goals-of-care discussions. Chow and colleagues[41] found that after a chart review of 11,053 oncology patients at Yale New Haven Hospital, spiritual care assessment of existential distress, complex grief, and faith-based support was positively associated with patient care and quality of life, healthcare utilization, and outcomes. Balboni and colleagues' extensive literature review and multidisciplinary assessment of the evidence related to spirituality in serious illness and positive health outcomes produced 3 top-ranked implications for spiritual care and serious illness: (1) incorporate spiritual care into care for patients with serious illness; (2) incorporate spiritual care education into training of interdisciplinary teams caring for persons with serious illness; and (3) include specialty practitioners of spiritual care in the care of patients with serious illness.[42] A growing body of positive evidence illustrates chaplains' extensive facilitation of advance care planning and goals of care conversations.[43-45] This research is especially important since end-of-life treatment decisions are known to be highly dependent on the existential, religious, cultural, moral, and ethical values of patients and caregivers.[46-48] Yet in goals-of-care discussions, patients' and surrogates' religious and spiritual beliefs are often unexamined by non-chaplain team members.[49]

Skilled interventions almost always include offering calming presence, deep listening, and compassionate emotional support. In addition to the foundational interventions related to building therapeutic relationships and supporting patients' religious, spiritual, and social rituals and practices, palliative care chaplains often counsel patients on issues of meaning, identity, personhood, dignity, and loss. They help patients and their caregivers with multifactorial spiritual and existential pain and guide people through life review and legacy planning. Common interventions also include counsel on complex ethical and moral issues in decision-making and exploration of the meaning of suffering, well-being, death, dying, the afterlife, and bereavement support.[27] The chaplain connects patients and caregivers with supportive community resources, including spiritual or philosophical leaders. The standard training and official role description for specialist palliative care chaplains include sustainability and well-being support for the palliative care and primary teams. With training in group emotional debrief, grief counseling, justice-responsive communication, and de-escalation, palliative care chaplains are positioned to intervene with team members when collaboration is in jeopardy by establishing mutual trust, psychological safety, and healthy vulnerability.

In the absence of a specialized role understood and adapted across institutions, an integral part of the palliative care chaplain's job is educating healthcare colleagues and institutions about interprofessional and transdisciplinary spiritual care as an essential component of palliative care. Chaplains benefit from the egalitarianism inherent in the transdisciplinary framework; team members and services profit as chaplains are invited to serve, teach, and model outcome-based care at the height of their credentialing and abilities.[50]

Nurse

Education, Licensure, and Certification for Professional Practice

The spectrum of nursing includes assistants or aides who have a few months of training to nurses with associates, baccalaureate, master's, or doctoral degrees. This diversity of educational preparation allows people from many different backgrounds to enter the nursing profession and work their way toward additional levels of responsibility. The home health aide (HHA), certified nursing assistant (CNA), and medical assistant (MA) in a medical practice typically provide

---

Box 3.7. Dental Hygienist

Marcie Wagner

A dental hygienist is in a position to observe oral manifestations of systemic disease, such as those seen in diabetes, as well as less obvious disease connections. As an example, a long-time patient was no longer able to take care of a particular area of her mouth. Although normally meticulous about her oral hygiene, she wasn't able to properly clean a lower left molar. When I attempted to clean the same area, I noticed her tongue was very rigid and difficult to move. I encouraged her to see her primary care provider, who eventually diagnosed early Parkinson's disease.

Hygienists should be included in the care team early. Not only can hygienists help with comfort care or prevention when a patient is bedbound; but, when we are apprised of a chronic condition in the early stages, we can mitigate side effects from medications and keep the patient's oral tissues comfortable and healthy. If patients are uncomfortable to the point of not being able to eat or reluctant to speak, it greatly impacts their quality of life.

We see patients every 3–6 months for an hour at a time and often treat multiple generations of the same family. Because of this ongoing connection, we develop trusting relationships and are often privy to very personal narratives. We recognize when a patient needs the support of a palliative care team and can direct them accordingly. Sometimes, the patient may inform us of another family member in need of help. The dental hygienist is in a distinctive position to recognize and intervene with all family members.

---

hands-on care within their setting and have completed a brief (6 months or less) training program. A licensed vocational or practical nurse (LVN/LPN; terminology differs regionally) receives a certificate after an intensive year of nursing education and often serves as the nurse in a medical practice or skilled nursing facility. A registered nurse (RN) can enter practice at the associate, baccalaureate, or master's degree educational level and typically has 1–3 years of combined clinical experiences and didactic nursing education prior to sitting for licensure examination. Once a person becomes an RN, additional opportunities exist to become an advanced practice registered nurse (APRN), which is an umbrella term that includes nurse practitioners (NP), clinical nurse specialists (CNS), certified nurse midwives (CNM), and certified registered nurse anesthetists (CRNA). Depending on the university, a master's degree in nursing can also prepare a nurse for advanced roles in nursing education, case management, health policy, informatics, integrative health, clinical nurse leader (CNL), or a wide variety of other specialty areas.

Although licensure is state specific, the standardized National Council Licensure Examination (NCLEX) is used by all states for both LVN/LPN and RN licensure. A state licensing exam is not required at the APRN level, but billing eligibility for APRNs is contingent upon board certification. After completing an approved course of study, board certification examinations are offered by the American Nurses Credentialing Center or other specialty-specific credentialing organizations. APRN board certification is specific to the type of APRN (NP, CNS, CNM, or CRNA) and population (adult/gerontology, pediatrics, family, women's health, psychiatric, etc.). Palliative care board certification is considered a subspecialty.

Palliative Care Specialization and Certification
The entrée for most nurses who specialize in palliative care is often through employment in oncology or hospice. Some nurses have been introduced to palliative care through their work in symptom management or chronic care co-ordination. Introductory palliative care content is now required for prelicensure nursing education, but graduate-level palliative care nursing education is mostly absent, beyond nurses who specifically seek it out. Most nurses specialize in pal-liative care through on-the-job training, supplemented by continuing education coursework.

In nursing, the Hospice and Palliative Credentialing Center (HPCC), affiliated with the Hospice and Palliative Nurses Association (HPNA), maintains 7 hospice and palliative nursing certification options. Specialty certification for nurses at the RN, APRN, LVN/LPN, and CNA/HHA levels requires state licensure, verification of recent clinical experience in the field of palliative care, and a passing score on a standardized examination.

Role Description and Responsibilities
Nursing's foundation is caring and respect for human dignity.[51] Nursing practice includes a professional intimacy.[52] Nurses recognize the patient's expertise in their own situation; nurses have "expert intuition," an empathetic understanding of suf-fering; and create a psychologically safe space to discuss emotionally demanding topics. Dame Cecily Saunders recognized the nursing role at end of life, related to constant presence and skill in finding peace in suffering.[51]

Nursing practice overlaps with palliative care in its focus on alleviation of suffering through attention to whole-person human responses with the goal to maximize quality of life.[51,53] Nurses partner with the patient and family (however the patient defines their family), in providing care within the context of the patient and family system's wholeness and complexity. Florence Nightingale observed that nurses can re-lieve suffering without treating disease—a foundational principle of palliative care.[51]

A position statement available to members of the Hospice and Palliative Nurses Association documents the value of the professional nurse in palliative care.[54] The statement includes the importance of vocational/practical nurses (LVN/LPN), pro-fessional nurses (RN), and advanced practice nurses (APRN). The position state-ment affirms the critical role of LVN/LPNs and RNs in supporting patients and families to meet their goals as they approach end of life and affirms APRNs as a resource to increase access to palliative care and provide primary palliative care. Palliative nursing incorporates the nursing values of assessment, diagnosis, and treatment, a focus on responses to actual and potential health problems, care for both the patient and their family as defined by the patient, and an emphasis on relief of suffering and optimizing health.[51,53] The nurses' position at the bedside gives them the opportunity to recognize the patient's response to serious illness and to support patients throughout their experience and illness trajectory.

Nurses are ubiquitous in palliative care. In fact, the scope of practice for nursing, with its emphasis on holistic care, treating the patient and family as a unit, quality of life, symptom management, and care across the continuum of illness, has a large degree of overlap with definitions of palliative care. Some have observed that hospice care is the epitome of good nursing.[51] Nurses are the

---

Box 3.8. Respiratory Therapist

Julie J. Howard

Respiratory therapists (RT) are responsible for airway management, respiratory equipment, patient education, and providing pulmonary care for patients with respiratory difficulties or chronic lung disease. They work in the hospital setting, or in outpatient pulmonary rehabilitation programs where the goal of enhanced quality of life and symptom management provided by a holistic interprofessional care team overlaps with the philosophy of palliative care.[a]

Often, patients are admitted repeatedly for acute or chronic respiratory failure associated with chronic lung disease. An RT background allows the case manager to uncover barriers and challenges with patients' home pulmonary care program that may not be evident to other team members who don't have pulmonary expertise. RTs work collaboratively with nurses, physicians, and other therapists to help optimize a patient's dyspnea and movement or rehabilitation potential. Access to maintenance medications, with education on how to use the various inhalation devices, prepares and empowers the patient to manage their pulmonary symptoms at home. Difficulties with home durable medical equipment (DME) such as a noninvasive ventilator or nebulizer can be explored and resolved, in collaboration with the DME company. Patients can be referred for specialty outpatient care at the pulmonologist's office and also with the local pulmonary rehabilitation program. RT case managers' close working relationship with patients positions them well to explore code status and assist with completion of advance directive and POLST documents. Follow-up calls once or twice a week after discharge, and an open invitation for patients to call with questions, allow the RT case manager the opportunity to develop rapport over time and journey with the patient over the trajectory of illness.

[a] Reticker AL, Nici L, ZuWallack R. Pulmonary rehabilitation and palliative care in COPD: Two sides of the same coin? *Chronic Resp Dis.* 2012 May;9(2):107–116. doi:10.1177/1479972312441379.

primary clinician to interact with patients in hospice and home-based palliative care programs. In under-resourced and rural hospitals, they are often the only clinician available to provide palliative care. Part of nursing practice includes convening and coordinating care provided by others. Even when the nurse is the lead clinician, the interprofessional team is consulted frequently, depending on the needs of the patient.

The professional nurse (RN) is trained to assess the patient with a focus on the whole person. In nursing, health is defined broadly and can include function, comfort, strength, integrity, intactness, or wholeness.[51] Nurses are trained to look for indicators of distress from a physical, psychological, social, and spiritual point of view. They are natural conveners—bringing together other members of the team to care for the patient. When considered through the lens of the GSM, nurses serve as the safety net for all of the domains, implementing other team members' care plans when they aren't available. Even before specializing in palliative care, nurses are trained to screen holistically for physical, psychosocial, spiritual, and cultural factors that might be affecting their patients' lives and to coordinate with the appropriate specialist for additional assessment and therapy. They are educated to monitor the patient over time. In the inpatient setting, nurses are present 24/7, continuing to monitor the patient and provide both nursing-specific interventions and continuation of the care plan for all team members, when others are not available.

APRNs bring all the expertise of the nursing profession to the care of the patients, and they have additional education and experience in assessment and medical management. These overlapping functions allow APRNs to play a unique role on the team—providing leadership in the medical care of patients, freeing up physicians to care for the patients who can most benefit from their expertise, and bringing the holistic assessment and therapeutic skills of nursing to patient care in a wide range of settings. The APRN is often preferred to represent nursing on the specialty palliative care team because the APRN can bill separately for services. Given the ubiquity of nursing, most patients are already well-served by nurses in the hospital, medical office, or home health setting. The exception is hospice, where the RN often serves as case manager and primary clinician on-site at the patient's home.

Nurses are part of the checks-and-balances of the healthcare system, providing medications and other treatments that are ordered by other team members. They speak up to question any medications or interventions that may not be appropriate for the patient. They also provide their own nursing interventions, and often embrace nonpharmacological interventions and integrative therapies that might be valuable for their patients. Nurses also focus on patient and family education. They are good at translating medical language to the level that the patient and family can understand. Though some of these skills overlap with the skill set of other team members, in transdisciplinarity this blurring of boundaries and roles is not a cause for concern.

Physician

Education, Licensure, and Certification for Professional Practice

The road to becoming a physician can be arduous, as it involves 8 years of formal education—an undergraduate degree and 4 years of medical education (either medical school or osteopathic medical school, MD or DO, respectively). Prospective students take the Medical College Admission Test (MCAT) to determine their eligibility for admission, which also includes an application, review of transcripts from undergraduate education, and if invited, participation in multiple interviews at each school. Physician licensure is regulated by individual states with varying requirements,[20] though each includes performance on a national license exam by US Medical License Exams (USMLE).[55] This exam is divided into 3 parts, with the first 2 parts taken during medical school and the third part following graduation. In total, the USMLE is 33 hours of written as well as practical history taking and physical exam skills testing.

During the final year of medical school, students choose a field of medicine and apply for a residency training program, which can vary in length from 3 to

---

Box 3.9. Speech Pathologist

Susan R. Pollesel

In nearly every serious illness, the ability to eat and drink or take in sufficient quantities of food is impacted. The speech pathologist may be the first clinician to recognize physical decline, when dysphagia is the presenting symptom. Speech and language pathologists (SLP) hold a master's degree, with additional certification depending on their area of expertise. Palliative care certification specific to SLP is not currently available. Because we swallow 2000–4000 times per day, dysfunction can be as life altering as organ failure. The speech pathologist has expertise in alternative feeding methods, dietary modifications, compensatory strategies, muscle strengthening and toning to protect the airway, and positioning. They also have expertise in assessment and interventions related to cognitive function.

An expert speech pathologist educates the patient and family about the physiology of airway protection, using diagrams and photos from swallow studies to communicate a unique perspective on the patient's health situation. A compassionate SLP may recognize preexisting neurological dysfunction based on historical information. The SLP's tangible data and information can support the patient and family during a very emotional time when they are called upon to make difficult decisions. Inviting the SLP to collaborate with the palliative care team, and recognition of the emotional connection between caregiving and food, can provide the SLP with opportunities to communicate compassionately with the patient and family in ways that are not available to other team members.

5 years depending on the field of study, up to 80 work hours per week with 2–4 weeks of vacation per year. For example, internal medicine and pediatrics are each 3-year training programs, a combined medicine/pediatrics residency is 4 years, and general surgery is 5 years. Physicians are then required to take a board certification exam in their primary field of study following successful completion of their training. If their residency includes 2 fields of study (medicine/pediatrics, for example), the physician is required to take a board certification for each field. Each board certification traditionally requires re-examination every 10 years in addition to continuing education on a yearly basis. A newer quarterly home study Longitudinal Knowledge Assessment for the American Board of Internal Medicine (ABIM) was launched in 2022. Physicians are required to be licensed in an individual state of practice, and this licensure involves renewal every 1 to 4 years, with additional continuing education requirements, to remain active. Following residency, some choose to complete a fellowship, which adds 1–3 years of additional training in a subspecialty[§] area. Each of these areas requires additional certification boards through the primary field of specialization, for example, within ABIM, pulmonary and critical care medicine are often combined subspecialties for training, yet have specific requirements for education and separate board examinations, each associated with an additional fee.

Palliative Care Specialization and Certification

Medicine is the only profession that has a designated path all the way to specialty training in palliative care. Physicians can choose to subspecialize in palliative medicine following residency in 1 of 10 other fields of study (anesthesiology, emergency medicine, family medicine, internal medicine, obstetrics and gynecology, pediatrics, physical medicine and rehabilitation, psychiatry and neurology, radiology, and surgery) by completing a 1-year fellowship at an accredited institution.[56] After the fellowship is completed, they are considered "board eligible" until they successfully pass the certification exam and become board certified as a hospice and palliative medicine (HPM) specialist. More than 130 HPM physician fellowships currently exist (see Chapter 9). In addition to board certification in HPM, an additional certification exists to serve as a hospice medical director. Each of these certifications requires its own ongoing maintenance, continuing education, and re-examination testing.

Role Description and Responsibilities

For centuries, physician-patient relationships have been founded on important and trusted encounters. From the earliest days, the physician was the individual with the medical knowledge and information to whom patients and families turned for

---

[§] Palliative care is considered to be a subspecialty within medicine and nursing, but a specialty in spiritual care and social work. For this book, we standardize the language by referring to palliative care as a specialty when referring to the team as a whole.

Box 3.10.   Bioethicist

Jana Craig

Although bioethicists work in a variety of settings, the role of bioethicists everywhere is to address moral problems. I consider myself a clinical ethicist because I have always worked in a clinical setting. In general, an ethics consultation is a service provided by an individual or a group to help patients, families, surrogates, healthcare providers, or other involved parties to address uncertainty or conflict regarding value-laden issues that emerge in healthcare.[a] Most clinical ethics work involves ethics consultation, but also normally includes: committee service (e.g., hospital ethics committees, institutional review boards, patient advisory boards); policy development (e.g., Withholding or Withdrawing of Life Sustaining Treatments, Futility or Non-Beneficial Care, etc.); and education (e.g., CME workshops, in-service education, grand rounds). Ethics and palliative care intersect over issues of withholding or withdrawing aggressive intervention (e.g., ventilator support, etc.), issues involving profound disability or diminishment of quality of life, and end-of-life issues, such as the provision of non-beneficial treatment.

The case of Mrs. A illustrates the clinical work of the ethicist related to the issue of non-beneficial treatment. Mrs. A is a 70-year-old woman recently diagnosed with a terminal glioblastoma, admitted to the hospital 1 month prior to this consult for altered mental status. Mrs. A remained obtunded throughout her stay and the medical team believed she was at end of life. Sadly, there were no medical or surgical options. Palliative care was consulted to maximize her comfort and also to discuss the goals of care and to optimize these in coordination with her husband and 4 adult children. The palliative care team confirmed the bedside provider's belief that Mrs. A's family would like her to continue to receive any and all treatment to extend her life, including resuscitation should her heart stop. Mrs. A continued to decline and after a "successful resuscitation," an ethics consultation was called. The interdisciplinary team (ICU, Neurology, Palliative Care, Spiritual Care, Social Work, Ethics) gathered to discuss whether Mrs. A should be resuscitated again when her heart inevitably fails and how best to support both the patient, her family, and the medical team caring for Mrs. A.

[a] Core Competencies for Health Care Ethics Consultation, *The Report of the American Society for Bioethics and Humanities*, Glenview, IL, 2006.

---

advice, counsel, and care. The physician's roles, responsibilities, and relationships with patients and families have evolved with the ever-changing landscape of our world, across cultures, and with technological advancements. Once the central person for information, coordination, and care, the physician is increasingly moving away from this focal point for an individual patient. Shifting toward putting the patient first in the patient-physician relationship, patients have become more active consumers of medical information with improved medical literacy. However, the physician still plays a critical role in this trusted and committed relationship. Since its origins, physicians have been core members of the palliative care team, with a mandate to oversee the general medical care and treatment of the patient. The physician's roles on the palliative care team may include: lead clinician for patient care; communicator with patients, families, and other providers; educator; researcher; manager of healthcare; and team lead.

Supervising the overall healthcare plan for the patient may take place in a variety of settings, including the hospital, outpatient clinics, long-term-care facilities, inpatient hospice units, and home or residential hospice. Regardless of the setting, the scope of a physician's practice is to focus first on the patient, assess for symptoms, needs, and suffering, and make recommendations to alleviate these issues and concerns.

A comprehensive H&P (history and physical) is needed to assess for both acute and chronic diagnoses. The H&P points to areas of patient physical distress and pain (primary domains of the physician), or need for emotional, psychosocial, and spiritual support—generalist areas the physician can assess, intervene, and refer to other team members as needed. Physicians must achieve a level of training and expertise to assess, synthesize, and prioritize large amounts of clinical data in terms of treatment, planning, and coordination of care. To provide holistic care and create a medical plan and recommendations, physicians need to have the general medical knowledge of the underlying chronic illness and an understanding of prognosis and treatment options for various medical conditions. With this level of involvement, the physician assumes responsibility for the patient's care from a clinical, quality and safety, and medical-legal standpoint.

Following the comprehensive H&P, the physician develops a medical and interventional plan to address each patient's specific clinical needs and coordinates consultation of additional services or care teams, advocating and communicating within the team and with other providers as outlined in the GSM. Commitment to the patient requires the physician to become an educator for the patient and family. This may include disease state education, availability of community resources, prognostication, and discussion of patient values and goals as the disease progresses. Communication is key for navigating the medical system, advocating for patients, empowering patients and families to participate in their care, revisiting disease burden, and quality of care toward the end of life. Physicians may be asked to assess decision-making capacity, and as the "attending of record" they are ultimately responsible for the patient's physical care, medical course, complications, or potential iatrogenic issues that arise.

As technology improves and medical care becomes more complex, additional challenges to implementing therapeutic interventions include communicating and incorporating goals of care and values-based decisions into the patient's care plan. Critical communication skills are taught in training and honed over time and include written and oral communication with patients, families,

---

Box 3.11. Integrative Health Practitioner

Helen Ye

Licensed acupuncturists can improve quality of life at any stage of illness. They support a patient's desire to find complementary ways to support pain management, address stress and depression, and manage a range of symptoms, including nausea and other digestive issues. An acupuncturist is required to complete more than 3000 hours of training, earning a postgraduate degree. Licensure requirements, professional title, and insurance reimbursement vary by state or region. Bethany's case exemplifies the efficacy of acupuncture in palliative care. Bethany was a 57-year-old woman with stomach cancer. She was given a 6-month prognosis after her last course of chemotherapy. She had peripheral neuropathy, multiple joint pain, fatigue, brain fog, depression, and hypertension. She was skeptical of acupuncture initially, but she found the acupuncture treatments helped ease the nausea and vomiting due to chemotherapy. It also helped ease her physical pain, neuropathy, and lightened her moods. Bethany chose to stop all curative treatments to live a better quality of life. She wanted to enjoy her family, especially her children, the outdoors, and her music. She outlived her prognosis by 6 months. Acupuncture treatments gave her peace and allowed her the transition she desired for herself and her family.

---

and other providers. Physicians follow the core bioethical principles of autonomy, beneficence, nonmaleficence, and justice, and need to have a working understanding of how this framework applies to each patient. Legal aspects of care, including Physician Orders for Life-Sustaining Treatment (POLST) Medical Orders for Life-Sustaining Treatment (MOLST) forms and shared decision-making, often fall on the physician in charge of the care. With this comes an increased level of stress and responsibility in terms of outlining and documenting a plan of care and addressing and supporting any medical-legal issues which might arise.

Social Worker

Education, Licensure, and Certification for Professional Practice

Professional titles of social workers vary, based upon the state providing the credentials. Essentially social workers are licensed following an exam at 3 different levels—completion of a baccalaureate degree (i.e., LBSW, LSW), completion of a master's degree (i.e., MSSW, LMSW, LISW), and finally licensed clinical social worker (LCSW, LICSW). These most advanced practitioners complete a minimum of 2 years of full-time clinical experience and 3000 supervised hours post-master's degree, after which they can bill insurances and practice independently. Prior to licensure and as part of degree completion, all graduate social work students are required to complete a minimum of 900 hours in partnership with an agency, guided by social work competencies.[57] At the baccalaureate level, a minimum of 400 hours is required. A bachelor's degree in social work is not required to seek and obtain a master's degree in social work (MSW). Licensure requires renewal every 2 years with adherence to the National Association of Social Workers Code of Ethics[58] and ongoing continuing education.

Palliative Care Specialization and Certification

Many social work students receive specific education in hospice, palliative care, death, dying, or grief through an elective or limited content interspersed through graduate program coursework. Rarely do social workers receive in-depth education in hospice or palliative care beyond their practicum or field education position. While a master's program in social work does prepare students in an area of specialization (i.e., by specific population, problem area, type of intervention or approach to practice),[57] few educational opportunities in hospice and palliative care exist and palliative care fellowships open to social workers are rare (see Chapter 9). More opportunities exist in broader fields such as gerontology or health. Consequently, most hospice and palliative care social workers develop their specialized and advanced practice skills on the job.

Some social workers seek additional credentials specific to hospice and palliative care, such as the National Associations for Social Worker's (NASW) Certified Hospice and Palliative Social Worker (CHP-SW or ACHP-SW), Association for Death Education and Counseling's (ADEC) Certification in Thanatology: Death, Dying and Bereavement (CT), and the more recently developed Advanced Palliative and Hospice Social Work Certification (APHSW-C). Certifications are available to social workers across educational levels; both the APHSW-C and NASW certifications require social work licensure. All 3 certifications require documentation of 2–3 years of supervised experience in hospice and palliative care within the past 5 years (1–3 years for CT) depending on education and/or professional licensure, along with previous related continuing education content for NASW and CT credentials. An evidence-based exam is required for both the APHSW and the CT. All require recertification (ranging from 2 to 4 years) and ongoing continuing education hours.

Role Description and Responsibilities

Social work is defined by the International Federation of Social Workers as "a practice-based profession and an academic discipline that promotes social change and development, social cohesion, and the empowerment and liberation of people."[59] Guided by an ecological systems approach, or person-in-environment, social work practice considers challenges through the interaction of forces (psychological, social, economic, political) and through transactions between a person and their environment. Social workers commit to abiding by a professional Code of Ethics,[58] are trained in applying ethical decision-making models to complex cases, and can be found in an array of environments, from hospitals, schools, and prisons to communities of all types.[57] Social workers provide engagement, assessment, intervention, and evaluation with individuals, families, groups, organizations, and communities, using a biopsychosocial, evidence-based approach with attention to various cultural, spiritual, ethical, professional, and political aspects related to their care.[57] Training involves gaining expertise in communication, family systems, and interpersonal dynamics, which often propel social workers to positions of leadership in their respective teams and agencies.

Palliative social workers build on these generalist-level competencies with additional focus on serious illness, death, grief, and bereavement.[60] Social workers are identified as a core component of the interprofessional team in hospice[61] and palliative care.[14] Broadly speaking, social work roles in hospice and palliative care include "medical social services" and "counseling,"[61] or attention to family dynamics, coping mechanisms, social determinants of health, access to resources, and conflict mediation.[14]

Though no standardized competencies for palliative social work yet exist in the United States, several resources serve as guidance for social workers in this area.[59,60,62-65] As supported by the GSM, and like each of their core interprofessional team members, the palliative social worker is involved across all 8 domains of the NCP Guidelines, serving as specialists in some domains (i.e., psychological, social, cultural) and generalists in others (i.e., physical, spiritual). During the first visit with a patient and family, regardless of setting, the palliative social worker provides a comprehensive assessment of relevant biopsychosocial

---

Box 3.12. Bereavement Services Manager

Deborah Schwing

Millie, a 72-year-old accomplished artist with end-stage amyotrophic lateral sclerosis (ALS), was lovingly cared for by her retired dentist husband, Stan, with the support of the palliative care team. Millie opted for hospice care when she could no longer lift a paintbrush to a tiny bedside canvas without extreme fatigue. Three months later, she died peacefully, surrounded by family.

Stan came in to see Kate for bereavement counseling 2 months after Millie's funeral. Despite weekly family dinners and occasional meetings with friends, he anguished privately, adrift in grief. Kate skillfully helped Stan name and normalize his myriad of unfamiliar feelings. She encouraged him to give voice to the tender vulnerabilities of grief: loneliness, social awkwardness, and rumination on lingering fears and regrets. For Stan, bereavement counseling provided an anchoring refuge for compassionate reflection to integrate his loss, to appreciate the loving moments he and Millie shared, and to redirect his future.

factors and needs across domains, using clinical interviewing, behavioral observation, and validated assessment tools.[60,66] They develop a detailed plan of care and communicate needed areas for follow-up with their specialty interprofessional palliative care team.

In addition to recurrent communication within the specialty team and with the patient and family, social workers provide ongoing information and communication as appropriate with clinicians providing care across other settings in the GSM (see Figure 3.1). Social workers in primary palliative care are more likely to address social work competencies related to social, spiritual, cultural, and ethical/legal aspects of care domains.[64] Open communication with referral sources and review of available case notes allow the palliative social worker to focus on unaddressed needs, including competencies best provided in specialty palliative care, such as those related to structure and process of care (i.e., conducting advance care planning or end-of-life care conversations, educating about treatment options), physical care (i.e., pain and symptom management, tailoring information about treatment and side effects, assuring patient understanding of medical language, assessing impact of physical symptoms), psychological care (i.e., providing anticipatory grief intervention, identifying and addressing complicated grief, identifying impact of illness on sexual functioning or body image, assessing psychosocial impact of symptoms, cognitive behavioral techniques), and care specific to end of life (i.e., completion of advance directives, therapeutic techniques for crisis intervention, legacy building, educating about the dying process, anticipatory guidance, and discussion of funeral and post-death arrangements).[64,67]

While many articles highlight the role and importance of a palliative care social worker across settings—with advanced cancer patients and in oncology,[68-70] heart failure patients,[71] pediatric patients,[72,73] in emergency departments,[74] and in the intensive care unit (ICU)[75,76]—little research documents standardized quality metrics for palliative social work assessments and interventions.[77] More recent research is beginning to demonstrate outcomes related to social work involvement and interventions. For example, community-based palliative care, provided by social workers and nurses, demonstrated significant reduction in costs, ICU and hospital admissions, and reduction in overall hospital days for patients compared to those engaged in traditional phone-based case management.[78] Other research evaluated involvement of the specialist palliative care social worker over a 4-year period in a tertiary academic medical center and demonstrated growth in consults over time along with greater likelihood for discussion of goals of care and improvement in dyspnea with social work involvement.[79] Finally, Lichti and Cagle[77] presented a model demonstrating ability to capture quality metrics of palliative social work assessments and interventions in inpatient electronic medical records. One goal of transdisciplinary teams must be including all members in the development of research and evaluation processes.[80]

Challenges to Role Identity and Development

As addressed in Chapter 4 of this text, institutional and systemic tension affects professional growth, identity development, and teamwork. A lack of shared vision and mission, decisions about team composition and structure, and variation in education and training can strain communication and interpersonal relations.[81] The social and cultural systems of inequality in which palliative care teams function can also create barriers to effective team collaboration. Barriers include: social hierarchy; lack of training in collaborative practice; lack of role definition or awareness; differing perceptions or values; and poor funding for inclusion of interprofessional participation.[82] Exploring each of these barriers is beyond the scope of this chapter, but considering challenges to team members' role identity and growth across professions can assist in overcoming barriers due to poor awareness and understanding of each other's roles. Though not an exhaustive list, a few challenges to role identity and development include pressure to continually advocate for one's role on the team, lack of ability to practice at the top of one's expertise, and training in limiting professional silos.

With ongoing financial pressures and minimal data related to positive outcomes associated with a fully staffed team, palliative care team leaders often experience administrative and institutional resistance to hiring a fully staffed core team. Many practitioners, especially from historically understaffed and underrepresented professions and populations in palliative care (such as chaplains and social workers), are encumbered with the obligation to continually advocate for their role while also managing their clinical load. For example, though the chaplain is the nationally recognized expert in the field in spiritual care, the only current regulating bodies that require, rather than recommend, chaplains as members of the interprofessional team are Medicare Hospice Conditions of Participation[83] and the Joint Commission palliative care certification.[84] Unfortunately, recent efforts toward greater inclusion of the spiritual domain in palliative care and recognition of the chaplain as domain specialist have not directly or immediately translated into a universal understanding of the role, a significant increase in national staffing (except for hospice mandated but not funded by Medicare) or broad integration of full-time chaplains on inpatient, outpatient, and home-based palliative care services.[29,85] Improvement in chaplains' abilities to speak the value of what they do in measureable, successful healthcare outcomes will help advance their colleagues' understanding of their contributions to care.[86] The necessity for chaplains to advocate for their role may also be due to a gap between the large percentage of patients who desire for clinicians to know and consider their religious and spiritual needs and the relatively small percentage of interprofessional providers who indicate that they discuss these topics with patients.[87]

Program and system-wide limitations impede team members' abilities to work at the height of their profession.[67,88] A team may respect a particular person in a professional role and still not value or know how to integrate that expert's profession or domain into practice.[89] At times, the medically trained members of the team may view skills and interventions that are considered "not scientifically validated" or "soft skills" as skills that anyone can perform. Social workers in health settings must regularly educate other professionals, including leadership, about the full scope of their role beyond simply offering support and community resources.[90] Chaplain experts report that they are often not consulted in the creation of their palliative care job descriptions. Without clear role delineation or acknowledged respect for a profession, tensions arise which can result in the palliative care provider "becoming engaged in a saga of struggle, where they are trying to differentiate themselves from other healthcare professionals on the team in order to promote their own professional identity and, hence, the value of their place in the team."[91(p 134)]

Perceptions of professionals needing to "protect their turf" is a barrier to nurses' ability to operate at the top of their license.[88] Some nurses report feeling like chameleons, trained as generalists to implement care plans for other team members when they are not available, and in the process they may lose focus on their unique role on the team. Unclear boundaries between professions can further this struggle. For example, though nurse practitioners are often hired because of their ability to prescribe medications and bill for medical services, tension exists between them and physicians when nurse practitioners are perceived as overstepping in a medical role or operating as "little doctors."[92]

Finally, uni-professionality and training in silos prevent development of dual identities, a culture that "[embraces] the uniqueness of each profession while cultivating interprofessional collaboration."[93(p 473)] Physicians experience a hidden curriculum[94] that informs how they interact with various team members. Physicians are also expected to "have the answers" and are legally responsible as the attending of record, causing immense pressure and forced authority.[95] Across professions, team members learn how to operate on interprofessional teams in practice, rather than within educational programs. While developing professional identities is an important aspect to contributing on interprofessional teams,[90] a lack of information about *how* interprofessional teams function or about other team members' roles hinders one's ability to function effectively, particularly early in a career.

Recommendations

Those committed to integrating a transdisciplinary framework into palliative care have few models to consider, relying mainly on lived experience of successful interprofessional collaboration and outcomes. The GSM can provide teams with a starting place for implementing a transdisciplinary approach, though it should be evaluated and validated along with other potential inclusive models. Moving beyond theoretical support for successful teams to a landscape marked by multiple sustainable models of outcome-based collaboration between palliative care practitioners and services as the standard of practice across sites will take commitment and attention. Cultivating the art and science of transdisciplinary collaboration is the next frontier in the advancement of ubiquitous, accessible, interprofessional palliative care for all. Though challenges remain and more research is needed, one systematic review of 64 studies over 20 years found that professionals can actively contribute to interprofessional practice "by *bridging* professional, social, physical, and task-related *gaps*, by *negotiating overlaps* in roles and tasks, and by *creating spaces* to be able to do so."[96(p 332)] To this end, the authors include the following comments with recommendations for future growth in developing and sustaining fully staffed teams who are supported in personally sustainable, advanced practice, holistic, and comprehensive care.

Bridging Gaps

Varying professional perspectives, diverse personalities and social preferences, geographical and working proximity, and care tasks that fall outside of defined professional roles all create common gaps that teams must navigate to operate successfully as an interprofessional team.[96] To bridge these gaps, professions can "actively [transfer] knowledge or information from one professional to another" in addition to "making oneself available to others."[96(p 336)] Successful transdisciplinarity can only occur when each team member respects the expertise and contributions of others so that bridging can occur. Advocacy for the creation and support of teams staffed with, at least, the core professions as the standard of practice is key to fulfilling the palliative care promise of whole-person care. Leaders must go beyond simply advocating for other professions with less power or influence, and use professional privilege to challenge and change existing inequitable and inadequate conditions.

Negotiating Overlaps

A team may theoretically value a transdisciplinary approach to care, but actualizing it requires great personal awareness and moments of humbly surrendering individual ego and personal recognition to the collective team and patient good. Stereotyped ideas that limit perceptions about one's own and colleagues' professions need to be released. No standards currently exist that address overlapping functions between the clinicians on the team. Movement toward GSM practice and some spontaneous blurring of roles are signs of a trusting and cooperative team culture and, at the same time, maintenance of clear professional boundaries is important to team health and harmony. Commitment to individual professional self-awareness and substantive understanding of others' vocational background, role, and clinical identity are essential. Definition and dissemination of professional roles and responsibilities improve each member's understanding of the other. Further studies validating the benefit of interprofessional practice and of each profession on the team are needed.

Creating Spaces

Transdisciplinarity requires shared models and language. The GSM (see Figure 3.1) highlights the important role of ongoing information and communication within the team, between the team and patient and family, and with other providers in overlapping systems of care. Professionals can contribute to successful interprofessional collaboration by organizing spaces and procedures for this interaction and communication to occur. For more natural integration of collaborative practice, we must: consider a change to the current, uni-professional models of education; intentionally find opportunities for collaborative visits, team rounds, and purposeful team meetings; facilitate education that automatically includes interprofessional collaboration as a vital skill and practice; include all members of the interprofessional team in pre- and post-licensure/certification palliative care educational programs and fellowships; allow all professions the opportunity to gain cross-domain competencies specific to hospice and palliative care; and provide education and training in team collaboration as a basic skill of palliative care practice.

A comprehensively staffed palliative care team is clinically beneficial and morally incumbent for successful and holistic palliative care. Successful cooperation between chaplains, nurses, physicians, social workers, and others who contribute to the plan of care is essential to the present and future success of palliative care. Collaboration between professions and testing and refining methods and models for synergistic cooperation are hallmarks of hospice and palliative care.

Discussion Questions

1. How do practice, education, research, and policy at your institution support or limit the integration of essential roles and team members?
2. In your practice, what do you need to learn about the roles, clinical practice, and values of the other professions with whom you work?
3. What role do you play in advocating for both your profession in palliative care and a fully staffed palliative care service?
4. What are the best strategies to address the domains of care as a single clinician on a team?
5. How are interprofessional education and collaboration possible on a single-clinician or small-team service?

References

1. Kamal AH, Bull JH, Swetz KM, Wolf SP, Shanafelt TD, Myers ER. Future of the palliative care workforce: preview to an impending crisis. *Am J Med*. 2017;130(2):113–114.
2. Harrison JE, Weber S, Jakob R, Chute CG. ICD-11: An international classification of diseases for the twenty-first century. *BMC Med Inform Decision Making*. 2021;21(6):1–10.
3. Berwick DM, Nolan TW, Whittington J. The triple aim: care, health, and cost. *Health Affairs*. 2008;27(3):759–769.
4. Bodenheimer T, Sinsky C. From triple to quadruple aim: care of the patient requires care of the provider. *Ann Fam Med*. 2014;12(6):573–576.
5. Bachynsky N. Implications for policy: The triple aim, quadruple aim, and interprofessional collaboration. Paper presented at: Nursing Forum, 2020.
6. Earnest M, Brandt B. Aligning practice redesign and interprofessional education to advance triple aim outcomes. *J Interprof Care*. 2014;28(6):497–500.
7. Wei H, Corbett RW, Ray J, Wei TL. A culture of caring: the essence of healthcare interprofessional collaboration. *J Interprof Care*. 2020;34(3):324–331.
8. Graham J, Ramirez A, Cull A, Finlay I, Hoy A, Richards M. Job stress and satisfaction among palliative physicians. *Palliat Med*. 1996;10(3):185–194.
9. Batorowicz B, Shepherd TA. Measuring the quality of transdisciplinary teams. *J Interprof Care*. 2008;22(6):612–620.
10. LaRocca-Pitts M. The board-certified chaplain as member of the transdisciplinary team: an epistemological approach to spiritual care. *J Study Spiritual*. 2019;9(2):99–109.
11. Jünger S, Pestinger M, Elsner F, Krumm N, Radbruch L. Criteria for successful multiprofessional cooperation in palliative care teams. *Palliat Med*. 2007;21(4):347–354.
12. Vyt A. Interprofessional and transdisciplinary teamwork in health care. *Diabetes Metab Res Rev*. 2008;24(S1):S106–S109.
13. Puchalski C, Ferrell B, Virani R, et al. Improving the quality of spiritual care as a dimension of palliative care: the report of the Consensus Conference. *J Palliat Med*. 2009;12(10):885–904.
14. National Consensus Project for Quality Palliative Care. *Clinical Practice Guidelines for Quality Palliative Care*. 4th ed. National Coalition for Hospice and Palliative Care; 2018.
15. Bahraini S, Gifford W, Graham ID, et al. The accuracy of measures in screening adults for spiritual suffering in health care settings: a systematic review. *Palliat Support Care*. 2020;18(1):89–102.
16. King SD, Fitchett G, Murphy PE, Pargament KI, Harrison DA, Loggers ET. Determining best methods to screen for religious/spiritual distress. *Support Care Cancer*. 2017;25(2):471–479.
17. Pullon S. Competence, respect and trust: Key features of successful interprofessional nurse-doctor relationships. *J Interprof Care*. 2008;22(2):133–147.
18. MacDonald MB, Bally JM, Ferguson LM, Murray BL, Fowler-Kerry SE, Anonson JM. Knowledge of the professional role of others: a key interprofessional competency. *Nurse Educ Pract*. 2010;10(4):238–242.
19. Blacker S, Deveau C. Social work and interprofessional collaboration in palliative care. *Progress Palliat Care*. 2010;18(4):237–243.
20. Federation of State Medical Boards. Physician licensure. Accessed August 12, 2022. https://www.fsmb.org/u.s.-medical-regulatory-trends-and-actions/u.s.-medical-licensing-and-disciplinary-data/physician-licensure/.Published 2022.
21. American Medical Association. Certification & licensure: Council on Medical Education reports. Accessed August 12, 2022, Published 2020. Accessed. https://www.ama-assn.org/councils/council-medical-education/certification-licensure-council-medical-education-reports.
22. The Association of the Theological School and the Commission of Accrediting. Standards of accreditation for the commission on accrediting of the association of theological schools. Published 2020. Accessed August 12, 2022. https://www.ats.edu/files/galleries/standards-of-accreditation.pdf.

23. UC San Diego Health. Clinical Pastoral Education. Accessed August 12, 2022. https://health.ucsd.edu/for-health-care-professionals/education-training/clinical-pastoral-education/Pages/default.aspx.

24. BCCI: Board of Chaplaincy Certification Inc. Palliative Care & Hospice Advanced Certification. Published 2022. Accessed August 12, 2022. https://bcci.professionalchaplains.org/content.asp?pl=25&contentid=25.

25. National Association of Catholic Chaplains. Palliative Care and Hospice Advanced Certification (PCHAC). Published 2022. Accessed August 12, 2022. https://www.nacc.org/certification/palliative-care-and-hospice-advanced-certification/.

26. Spiritual Care Association. Hospice and Palliative Care Specialty Certification (APBCC-HPC). Published 2022. Accessed August 12, 2022. https://www.spiritualcareassociation.org/apbcc-hpc.

27. Handzo G, Puchalski C. The role of the chaplain in palliative care. In Cherny NI, Fallon MT, Kaasa S, Portenoy RK, Currow DC, eds. *Oxford Textbook of Palliative Medicine*. 6th ed. Oxford University Press; 2021:198–205.

28. Jeuland J, Fitchett G, Schulman-Green D, Kapo J. Chaplains working in palliative care: who they are and what they do. *J Palliat Med*. 2017;20(5):502–508.

29. Abu-Raiya H, Pargament KI, Krause N. Religion as problem, religion as solution: religious buffers of the links between religious/spiritual struggles and well-being/mental health. *Qual Life Res*. 2016;25(5):1265–1274.

30. Balboni TA, Paulk ME, Balboni MJ, et al. Provision of spiritual care to patients with advanced cancer: associations with medical care and quality of life near death. *J Clin Oncol*. 2010;28(3):445.

31. Gillilan R, Qawi S, Weymiller AJ, Puchalski C. Spiritual distress and spiritual care in advanced heart failure. *Heart Failure Rev*. 2017;22(5):581–591.

32. Tarbi EC, Gramling R, Bradway C, Meghani SH. "If it's the time, it's the time": existential communication in naturally-occurring palliative care conversations with individuals with advanced cancer, their families, and clinicians. *Patient Educ Counsel*. 2021;104(12):2963–2968.

33. Davenport AA. Libera me, Domine: Christian roots of palliative care. *Perspect Biol Med*. 2016;59(4):507–516.

34. Masel EK, Schur S, Watzke HH. Life is uncertain. Death is certain: Buddhism and palliative care. *J Pain Symptom Manage*. 2012;44(2):307–312.

35. Schultz M, Baddarni K, Bar-Sela G. Reflections on palliative care from the Jewish and Islamic tradition. *Evid Based Complementary Altern Med*. 2012;2012:1–8.

36. Balboni TA, Fitchett G, Handzo GF, et al. State of the science of spirituality and palliative care research Part II: screening, assessment, and interventions. *J Pain Symptom Manage*. 2017;54(3):441–453.

37. Lucchetti G, Bassi RM, Lucchetti ALG. Taking spiritual history in clinical practice: a systematic review of instruments. *Explore*. 2013;9(3):159–170.

38. Fitchett G, Hisey Pierson AL, Hoffmeyer C, et al. Development of the PC-7, a quantifiable assessment of spiritual concerns of patients receiving palliative care near the end of life. *J Palliat Med*. 2020;23(2):248–253.

39. Kestenbaum A, McEniry KA, Friedman S, Kent J, Ma JD, Roeland EJ. Spiritual AIM: assessment and documentation of spiritual needs in patients with cancer. *J Health Care Chaplaincy*. 2021;28(4):566–577.

40. Handzo GF, Cobb M, Holmes C, Kelly E, Sinclair S. Outcomes for professional health care chaplaincy: an international call to action. *J Health Care Chaplaincy*. 2014;20(2):43–53.

41. Chow R, Tenenbaum L, Balboni TA, Prsic EH. Medical outcomes of oncology inpatients with and without chaplain spiritual care visit: the Yale New Haven Hospital experience. *JCO Oncol Pract*. 2022;18(3):e334–e338.

42. Balboni TA, VanderWeele TJ, Doan-Soares SD, et al. Spirituality in serious illness and health. *JAMA*. 2022;328(2):184–197.

43. Kwak J, Cho S, Handzo G, Hughes BP, Hasan SS, Luu A. The role and activities of board-certified chaplains in advance care planning. *Am J Hosp Palliat Med*. 2021;38(12):1495–1502.

44. Lee AC, McGinness CE, Levine S, O'Mahony S, Fitchett G. Using chaplains to facilitate advance care planning in medical practice. *JAMA Internal Med.* 2018;178(5):708–710.

45. Russell J, Quaack KR, Nunez J. Chaplain reported plans for end-of-life care conversations: role clarity for the spiritual care specialists. *J Health Care Chaplaincy.* 2022;29(4):337–352.

46. Colenda CC, Blazer DG. Review of religious variables in advance care planning for end-of-life care: consideration of faith as a new construct. *Am J Geriatr Psychiatry.* 2022;30(7):747–758.

47. Dempsey-Henofer H. Death without God: nonreligious perspectives on end-of-life care. *Divers Equal Health Care.* 2019;16(4):74–79.

48. Drillaud F, Saussac C, Keusch F, et al. The existential dimension of palliative care: the mirror effect of death on life. *Omega.* 2022;85(4):915–935.

49. Ernecoff NC, Curlin FA, Buddadhumaruk P, White DB. Health care professionals' responses to religious or spiritual statements by surrogate decision makers during goals-of-care discussions. *JAMA Internal Med.* 2015;175(10):1662–1669.

50. Heikkinen PJ, Roberts B. I see you: a chaplain case study on existential distress and transdisciplinary support. *J Health Care Chaplaincy.* 2022;16(3):1–18.

51. Lynch M, Dahlin C, Hultman T, Coakley EE. Palliative care nursing: defining the discipline? *J Hosp Palliat Nurs.* 2011;13(2):106–111.

52. Antonytheva S OA, Garnett A. Professional intimacy in nursing practice: a concept analysis. *Nurs Forum.* 2021;56(1):151–159.

53. Hagan TL, Xu J, Lopez RP, Bressler T. Nursing's role in leading palliative care: a call to action. *Nurse Educ Today.* 2018;61:216–219.

54. Hospice & Palliative Nurses Association. HPNA Value Statement—Hospice and Palliative Nursing. Published 2023. Accessed October 19, 2023. https://www.advancingexpertcare.org/wp-content/uploads/2023/08/HPNA-Statement-Value-Of-H.P.Nurse_.pdf

55. The United States Medical Licensing Examination. Federation of State Medical Boards and National Board of Medical Examiners. Published 2022. Accessed August 14, 2022. https://www.usmle.org/.

56. American Academy of Hospice and Palliative Medicine. A career in hospice and palliative medicine: Is it for you? Accessed August 14, 2022. http://aahpm.org/uploads/AAHPM16_Medical_Student_BroWEB.pdf.

57. Council on Social Work Education. Educational Policy and Accreditation Standards. Published 2022. Accessed August 28, 2022. https://www.cswe.org/accreditation/standards/2022-epas/.

58. National Association of Social Workers. Code of Ethics of the National Association of Social Workers. Published 2021. Accessed August 28, 2022. https://www.socialworkers.org/About/Ethics/Code-of-Ethics/Code-of-Ethics-English.

59. International Federation of Social Workers. Global Definition of Social Work. Published August 2014. Accessed September 11, 2023. https://www.ifsw.org/what-is-social-work/global-definition-of-social-work/

60. Head B, Peters B, Middleton A, Friedman C, Guman N. Results of a nationwide hospice and palliative care social work job analysis. *J Soc Work End Life Palliat Care.* 2019;15(1):16–33.

61. Social Security Act, Section 1861. 42 U.S.C. § 1395d; 42 U.S.C. § 1395f; 42 U.S.C. § 1395x. Published 1982. Accessed August 28, 2022. https://www.ssa.gov/OP_Home/ssact/title18/1861.htm.

62. Terry Altilio MS, Otis-Green S, Cagle JG, eds. *The Oxford Textbook of Palliative Social Work.* Oxford University Press; 2022.

63. Bosma H, Johnston M, Cadell S, et al. Creating social work competencies for practice in hospice palliative care. *Palliat Med.* 2010;24(1):79–87.

64. Glajchen M, Berkman C, Otis-Green S, et al. Defining core competencies for generalist-level palliative social work. *J Pain Symptom Manage.* 2018;56(6):886–892.

65. Sumser B, Leimena M, Altilio T. *Palliative Care: A Guide for Health Social Workers.* Oxford University Press; 2019.

66. National Association of Social Workers. NASW Standards for Palliative & End of Life Care. Published 2004. Accessed August 28, 2022. https://www.socialworkers.org/LinkClick.aspx?fileticket=xBMd58VwEhk%3D&portalid=0.

67. Sumser B, Remke S, Leimena M, Altilio T, Otis-Green S. The serendipitous survey: a look at primary and specialist palliative social work practice, preparation, and competence. *J Palliat Med.* 2015;18(10):881–883.

68. Jones B, Phillips F, Head BA, et al. Enhancing Collaborative Leadership in Palliative Social Work in Oncology. *J Soc Work End Life Palliat Care.* 2014;10(4):309–321.

69. Otis-Green S, Sidhu RK, Del Ferraro C, Ferrell B. Integrating social work into palliative care for lung cancer patients and families: a multidimensional approach. *J Psychosoc Oncol.* 2014;32(4):431–446.

70. Tuggey EM, Lewin WH. A multidisciplinary approach in providing transitional care for patients with advanced cancer. *Ann Palliat Med.* 2014;3(3):139–143.

71. O'Donnell A, Gonyea JG, Leff V. Social work involvement in palliative care heart failure research: a review of recent literature. *Curr Opin Support Palliat Care.* 2020;14(1):3.

72. Jones BL. Pediatric palliative and end-of-life care. *J Soc Work End Life Palliat Care.* 2006;1(4):35–62.

73. Remke SS, Schermer MM. Team collaboration in pediatric palliative care. *J Soc Work End Life Palliat Care.* 2012;8(4):286–296.

74. Lawson R. Palliative social work in the emergency department. *J Soc Work End Life Palliat Care.* 2012;8(4):120–134.

75. McCormick AJ, Engelberg R, Curtis JR. Social workers in palliative care assessing activities and barriers in the intensive care unit. *J Soc Work End Life Palliat Care.* 2007;8(4):929–937.

76. McCormick AJ, Stowell-Weiss P, Toms C, Engelberg R. Improving social work in intensive care unit palliative care: results of a quality improvement intervention. *J Soc Work End Life Palliat Care.* 2010;8(4):297–304.

77. Christophel Lichti JL, Cagle JG. Documenting the contributions of palliative care social work: testing the feasibility and utility of tracking clinical activities using medical records. *Soc Work Health Care.* 2020;59(4):257–272.

78. Yosick L, Gatto M, Crook RE, et al. Effects of a population health community-based palliative care program on cost and utilization. *J Palliat Med.* 2019;22(9):1075–1081.

79. Edmonds KP, Onderdonk C, Durazo C, Molavi-Kerner C, Soriano K, De Meules A. An exploratory study of demographics and outcomes for patients seen by specialist palliative care social work in the inpatient setting at an academic medical center. *J Pain Symptom Manage.* 2021;62(4):813–819.

80. Rosa WE, Anderson E, Applebaum AJ, Ferrell BR, Kestenbaum A, Nelson JE. Coronavirus disease 2019 as an opportunity to move toward transdisciplinary palliative care. *J Palliat Med.* 2020;23(10):1290–1291.

81. Youngwerth J, Twaddle M. Cultures of interdisciplinary teams: how to foster good dynamics. *J Palliat Med.* 2011;14(5):650–654.

82. Supper I, Catala O, Lustman M, Chemla C, Bourgueil Y, Letrilliart L. Interprofessional collaboration in primary health care: a review of facilitators and barriers perceived by involved actors. *J Public Health.* 2015;37(4):716–727.

83. Centers for Medicare & Medicaid Services. Fiscal Year (FY) 2022 Hospice Payment Rate Update Final Rule (CMS-1754-F). Updated July 29, 2021. Accessed August 14, 2022. https://www.cms.gov/newsroom/fact-sheets/fiscal-year-fy-2022-hospice-payment-rate-update-final-rule-cms-1754-f.

84. The Joint Commission. Palliative Care Certification. Updated 2022. Accessed August 14, 2022. https://www.jointcommission.org/accreditation-and-certification/certification/certifications-by-setting/hospital-certifications/palliative-care-certification/.

85. Rogers M, Heitner R. Latest Trends and Insights from the National Palliative Care Registry. Center to Advance Palliative Care National Seminar; 2019; Atlanta, GA.

86. Lyndes KA, Fitchett G, Berlinger N, Cadge W, Misasi J, Flanagan E. A survey of chaplains' roles in pediatric palliative care: integral members of the team. *J Health Care Chaplain.* 2012;18(1–2):74–93.

87. Balboni MJ, Sullivan A, Amobi A, et al. Why is spiritual care infrequent at the end of life? Spiritual care perceptions among patients, nurses, and physicians and the role of training. *J Clin Oncol.* 2013;31(4):461–467.

88. Russell-Babin K, Wurmser T. Transforming care through top-of-license practice. *Nurs Manage.* 2016;47(5):24–28.
89. Kestenbaum A, Fitchett G, Galchutt P, et al. Top ten tips palliative care clinicians should know about spirituality in serious illness. *J Palliat Med.* 2022;25(2):312–318.
90. Ambrose-Miller W, Ashcroft R. Challenges faced by social workers as members of interprofessional collaborative health care teams. *Health Soc Work.* 2016;41(2):101–109.
91. O'Connor M, Fisher C, Guilfoyle A. Interdisciplinary teams in palliative care: a critical reflection. *Int J Palliat Nurs.* 2006;12(3):132–137.
92. Al-Agba N, Bernard R. *Patients at Risk: The Rise of the Nurse Practitioner and Physician Assistant in Healthcare.* Universal-Publishers; 2020.
93. Khalili H, Price SL. From uniprofessionality to interprofessionality: dual vs dueling identities in healthcare. *J Interprof Care.* 2022;36(3):473–478.
94. Hafferty FW, Franks R. The hidden curriculum, ethics teaching, and the structure of medical education. *Acad Med.* 1994;69(11):861–871-871.
95. Trockel MT, Hamidi MS, Menon NK, et al. Self-valuation: attending to the most important instrument in the practice of medicine. *Mayo Clin Proceed.* 2019;94(10):2022–2031.
96. Schot E, Tummers L, Noordegraaf M. Working on working together: a systematic review on how healthcare professionals contribute to interprofessional collaboration. *J Interprof Care.* 2020;34(3):332–342.

4

Professional Identity and Interprofessional Tension

Ian B. Kwok and Bridget Sumser

Key Points

- Tension is a necessary result of teamwork. Tension can be a source of both creative stretching as well as discordant straining on interprofessional teams. Team tensions may threaten to undermine team dynamics if not properly addressed.
- An intentional process of learning about each profession's training, code of ethics, roles and responsibilities, scope of service, and foundational values provides the essential foundation on which team members build a sense of connection and belonging.
- While job roles and responsibilities can be blurred in transdisciplinary practice, a clear understanding of professional roles and expectations builds a team structure that promotes trust and interdependence.
- Professional relationships are enhanced through a mutual understanding of why individual team members choose to work in palliative and hospice care.
- The presence of trust and psychological safety is essential for successful team collaboration. Misunderstandings can be reduced when administrators and practitioners get to know the daily experience of each individual and profession on the team.
- Fully integrated interprofessional and transdisciplinary practice is still a novel concept for most teams. Group exploration of the evolving team best practices and code of ethics may highlight new opportunities and methods for collaboration.

Introduction

The palliative care team at a tertiary teaching hospital (social worker, chaplain, physician, and nurse) have been working together consistently for 3 years. The team *agrees on the principle of transdisciplinary* practice (see Chapter 3 for more on transdisciplinary practice) and collaborates on all aspects of care and care planning for all patients and families. They regularly see patients together in joint visits, as well as completing individual follow-ups as indicated. Rounds are led by a different profession every morning in an effort to share leadership and to model a flattened power hierarchy. As their census builds, this model becomes harder for the team to maintain. After morning rounds, the team physicians are inundated with new consult referrals. In an effort to respond as promptly as possible, the physicians quickly call the referring providers back and start to address the consults. Team communication and updates are then cut short. Some team members feel their input is not valued and feel excluded from the palliative care planning process. Negative assumptions and reactions among the team related to exclusion, perceptions of hierarchical decision-making, and questions about team member commitments and intentions replace collaboration.*

Why do interprofessional tensions, as illustrated in the above scenario, arise? How does tension, when unaddressed, lead to conflict? How do differences in professional roles, expectations, and values affect team cohesion? More broadly, how do institutional, societal, and cultural norms influence teams, and what can we do about it? This chapter examines these questions and describes common challenges to interprofessional teamwork. While every team is different and possesses its own unique, interpersonal dynamics, this chapter focuses on sources of team tension and conflict related to the interprofessional nature of the team itself, illustrated by common case examples within the context of health care institutions. The authors identify common sources of interprofessional team conflict, explored through the context of a sociological framework with an emphasis on the concepts of professional identity, organizational structures, power dynamics, and intersectionality. The chapter concludes with an exploration of best practices and strategies for naming and negotiating tensions and team distress within the context of a palliative care team.

Tension and Conflict

Tension, defined as a state in which individuals apply different personal values and experiences to a collaborative task,[1] resulting in divergent ideas and behaviors, is a necessary result of teamwork.[2] All interprofessional teams are made up of unique individuals with a diverse set of personal values, behaviors, and prior experiences.[3] These differences can be helpful, as they allow teams to approach their work from a variety of perspectives. However, unresolved team tensions can also result in conflict, antagonistic interactions caused by differing goals, values, perceptions, or

---

* The process this theory is pointing to is more accurately described as transprofessional, since it illustrates the collaboration and synergy between professions rather than disciplines. However, in this chapter and throughout the book, the term *transdisciplinary* is used since it is currently the word most commonly used in the literature to signify this form of team collaboration.

systemic barriers that may threaten to undermine team dynamics if not properly addressed.[4] In this way, tension can be a source of both creative stretching as well as discordant straining on interprofessional teams. The recognition and differentiation between common manifestations of tension and conflict are critical to effective team management.

While a common topic in business and organizational development literature,[5,6] the concept of group tension has not been well explored within the study of palliative care team functioning. Interprofessional palliative care teams are unique due to their context as specialized consult services within complex health care systems, combined with the inherent intimacy in working with those facing serious illness and death. The emotional and existential nature of the work is personal, fosters closeness between people, and at times can be incredibly private, as team members hold the hopes and fears, grief and joy, needs and wants of patients, families, and communities. The work of supporting people through physical, psychological, social, and spiritual realms requires vulnerability. This lends to moments of expressive sharing, heightened sensitivity, raw emotion, and unconscious behaviors. Recurrent and heightened emotional experiences of caring for those who are terminally ill or dying can greatly magnify the effects of interpersonal and group tensions, highlighting the need to learn how to recognize and address these tensions before they evolve into dysfunctional conflicts. Table 4.1 lists examples of tension and resulting conflict to highlight how tension may manifest within teams. The following section describes some of the main sources of tension affecting teams in palliative care settings.

Sources of Tension and Conflict

In an attempt to improve interprofessional communication, palliative care service leadership at a university hospital considers scheduling a weekly orientation to welcome rotating residents and medical students and to set expectations for team workflows. The intent behind the new meeting is well received by all team members. However, the social worker, nurse, and chaplain, who do not rotate off the service, express some concern with being assigned a disproportionate administrative burden of attending and facilitating the weekly orientation due to their continuous schedules. In addition, the scheduling of the meeting interferes with the social worker's ability to participate in the weekly social work department lecture series. These meetings eventually are combined with teaching rounds in order to best accommodate physician schedules, leading to meetings dominated by biomedical discussions, while other domains of palliative care and the roles of the social worker, nurse, and chaplain are often not explored and are even marginalized.

This example and the following sections explore significant individual and social forces that impact interprofessional tension and conflict. While the makeup of palliative care teams varies by location, the specialty has usually been defined

Table 4.1 Common Forms of Tension and Conflict on Palliative Care Teams

Tension	Conflict
Actual and perceived unequal authority among team members	Personal and profession-specific feeling of resentment due to not being respected, heard, or valued
Disparity in participation in and access to continuing education.	Indignation felt by team members with less access and resources, whose continuing education activities are limited to online modules, while colleagues with more resources enjoy in-person courses in travel settings that can be combined with leisure
Individual and professional priorities related to patients' domain-specific vs. holistic health needs	Disputes related to prioritizing clinical interventions after profession-specific assessment, i.e., providing immediate emotional support for a patient versus sharing medical information in the context of an imminent prognosis
Inequality in scheduling, protected non-clinical time, salary, and paid leave	Conflict related to professional status, career growth, and ability to emotionally sustain in the work. Resentment over unequal pay for equal work
Differing styles of workflow management and clinical assessment	Disagreement related to interpretation of clinical priorities, standards, and ethics
Differing styles of stress management and professional sustainability	Disputes related to ultimate power and authority in clinical and administrative decisions
Profession-specific cultural norms related to friendships with colleagues, time management, and expectations for participation in professional organizations	Criticism related to perceived nonprofessional behavior
Imbalance of health care responsibilities and privileges	Resentments related to required co-signatures; micro-managing within others' scope of practice; perceptions of unfairness
Traditional power structure and hierarchy	During challenging patient encounters, those in power look to each other rather than other qualified team members for input and leadership. Use of ill-informed, disrespectful or marginalizing language.

by 4 core[†] professions, both in this book and in the palliative care literature.[7] The ideal palliative care team is characterized by a flattened hierarchy, open communication and decision-making, shared responsibility, and close collaboration so that diverse needs can be met simultaneously.[8] In the example above, in a more transdisciplinary environment, the team members, including the administrator, would discuss their perspectives and priorities. They could set expectations for teaching rounds to integrate the most pertinent elements of clinical assessments to create a multilayered care plan; one that includes both focused counseling (emphasizing historical coping and current strengths) and as-needed medications

---

[†] In this book, we use the term "core" to refer to chaplains, nurses, physicians, and social workers who are all named as part of the interprofessional team for both the Medicare hospice guidelines and the NCP guidelines. This designation does not minimize the importance of other team members who contribute to the palliative care of patients and families.

to manage peak experiences of illness-related stress. Together, the administrator and clinical team could review productivity statistics and learner feedback, meet with the billing team to optimize documentation, and strategically plan workflows that fulfill the patient's, family's, and learner's holistic needs while meeting the financial targets of the service.

Professional Identity

The chaplain, on an outpatient clinic team, has been serving as the main palliative care clinician caring for a spouse who is facing the unfortunate decline of her partner due to a rapid progression of amyotrophic lateral sclerosis (ALS). After multiple individual discussions with the chaplain, the family asks the chaplain to convene a meeting with the neurology team to update the wife on the patient's condition in light of their wishes to "ensure that he lives as long as possible, at peace, and has time to feel positive energy and love from his spiritual teacher at the end." In the team pre-meeting, the neurology attending physician repeatedly turns to the palliative care nurse practitioner for input related to the patient's values. The chaplain attempts to interject with her experience of the family's understanding, but her thoughts are met with polite silence followed by a new topic. The chaplain is experienced in serious illness communication and facilitation of family meetings, but the nurse practitioner does not perceive her as skilled due to her limited perception of the role of a chaplain. The nurse practitioner agrees to facilitate the family meeting on the request of the attending physician, and afterward, encourages the chaplain to remain with the family for spiritual and emotional support. Although the chaplain welcomes the opportunity to support the family after the meeting, she feels out of integrity with her conscience since she missed the opportunity to facilitate the meeting while advocating for the family's stated values. Consequently, the patient's and family's expressed values were not considered in the goals of care discussion or care planning.

As the above scenario exemplifies, within a high-intensity health care environment, interprofessional tensions can quickly escalate. In these situations, the role of converging professional identities is a common source of tension, although considerable variation may exist. Each team member may feel pulled to a different aspect of the clinical demands, both as a function of what they see as most important (e.g., a new consult with uncontrolled symptoms or a patient's values and beliefs) and what they need personally to move forward (e.g., time with family to process a challenging death or a chance to leverage rapport with a family to successfully facilitate a treatment discussion). In addition, one's over-identification with a professional identity can supersede the sense of a personal self, accentuating the cognitive and emotional salience of these tensions. Higher levels of individual role identification can be an indicator of a lower level of overall team identification, but role identification can also compensate for a lower level of team identification in how successfully a team collects and retrieves knowledge.[9]

Furthermore, professional identities are affected by societal expectations. Patients and their care partners come with a unique understanding of health care interactions, which may be informed by prior experiences and media exposure within the content of individual and family culture.[10-12] These may include preconceived notions, bias, or stereotypes of professional roles (e.g., the physician as a distant medication prescriber, the nurse as a constantly available/deferential support, social worker as a gatekeeper of resources needed for logistical planning, or the chaplain as primarily there for religious prayer right before death).[13,14] Teams are likely to encounter difficult emotions expressed by patients and caregivers, and potentially a deep distrust of the health care industry, which can further strain one's sense of positive professional identity. For these reasons, the societal contexts of professional roles can contribute significantly to interprofessional tensions.

While the convergence of diverse professional identities can represent a challenge to teamwork in palliative care, tensions can be anticipated by identifying and acknowledging the roots of different clinical perspectives. For example, medical education tends to use deductive reasoning, while nursing education uses inductive reasoning. Professions focused on psycho-social-spiritual domains tend to learn using a process of reflection and action, focused on relationship building. Without recognizing the unique ways in which each profession is socialized, others may appear "wrong," as opposed to simply using a different approach. In the same way as palliative care clinicians are taught to approach each patient with cultural humility,[15,16] team members can benefit from approaching each other with respectful curiosity and appreciation for their unique foundations and values.

Organizational Structures

The home-based palliative care team notices that structural pressures to maximize billable visits and productivity have inadvertently diminished the time that the team has available to support a grieving family. To them, this feels like an unnecessary infringement on their autonomy and personal time management. The nurse on the team considers these structural pressures to reflect a lack of caring on the part of administration that interferes with the team's emotional presence.

This example and section explore how interprofessional roles interact within the structures of modern health care systems, representing major challenges to effective transdisciplinary teamwork in palliative care. As the previous scenario illustrates, team identities do not exist in a vacuum—they are defined by both complex personal narratives and their organizational environments. In addition to training differences, each interprofessional team member is contextualized by a unique blend of individual and institutional cultures.

Operational structures significantly affect palliative care teams. Each interprofessional role carries its own unique set of institutional expectations, which are based on historical practices that often misalign with transdisciplinarity. Operational structures encompass many aspects of daily workflows and professional demands, including work schedules, expectations for documentation, and incentive schemes for promotion. Notably, these vary significantly between professions. For example, in the nurse-led hospice service model, the nurse case manager's documentation, in most institutions, not only signals the clinical response to a consult referral for the hospice team but also serves as the main record for Medicare reimbursement. Cultivating a basic understanding of each team member's operational context is essential to defining realistic, culture-informed roles and responsibilities in interprofessional team settings.

Institutional habits of billing and hiring also affect the interaction, with physicians outnumbering other professions in many palliative care teams. Conversely, in rural community settings, a fully qualified palliative care physician may not be available, and palliative care services may be provided primarily by whoever is available and interested in palliative care. Palliative care teams in under-resourced areas may not be able to afford team members who are unable to bill for services. While quality patient care may be provided during a solo interaction, the absence of the interprofessional perspective negatively affects patient care if unaddressed. Societal and organizational values influence the environment in which all teams operate, and contribute to interprofessional tensions that may be misinterpreted as interpersonal deficits.

Power Dynamics

During a consult referral, the primary care physician directs all of his questions toward the palliative care physician, a male palliative care fellow. The fellow attempts to create a conversational opening for the palliative care social worker, a female team member with decades of experience, and other team members. Despite repeated attempts, the fellow still ends up dominating the discussion, and important issues remain unaddressed by the end of the meeting.

In this example, the palliative care team is limited by both institutional and societal perceptions of traditional hierarchies, based on a physician-centric model of care. Despite the physician's own aspiration toward interprofessional balance, the interaction is heavily influenced by the referring physician's expectations and bias. Furthermore, power dynamics related to the performative culture of medical education also play a role, as the fellow may be incentivized to make a positive impression on his attending physician by demonstrating his competence, inadvertently preventing other team members from participating in the conversation.

While hierarchies exist in all organized communities, health care teams are characterized by persistent, distinguishable patterns of power imbalance. The power imbalance is ubiquitous in all healthcare specialties, including in hospice and palliative care. These cultural systems of power have been ingrained in medical and health professions education and public perceptions, resulting in negative patient outcomes,[17] and representing conscious and subconscious barriers to achieving the balance of shared responsibility that is crucial for transdisciplinarity. Some of the power dynamics are inherent to the structure of the healthcare system.[18] For example, physicians are legally responsible for all care of the patient, and they are the first ones to receive legal action when something goes wrong. Some are evolutionary cultural patterns, such as team members respectfully referring to physicians with their professional title of "doctor" but not using professional titles with other members of the team.

Each profession is situated within systems of power, and this systemic trajectory exists along a spectrum from center to margin, analogous to the line characterizing race, class, gender identity, and so on.[19] Within the healthcare system, team members inevitably experience tensions resulting from these institutional and societal structures, which often play a significant role in team conflicts.[20-22] Despite some teams' best efforts to flatten the hierarchy and value each profession equally, the structures and policies of the healthcare system are deeply rooted, largely for financial reasons.[23] While the shared mission of palliative care teams can be overshadowed by the gradual accumulation of unaddressed hierarchical tensions, identifying their societal roots provides a larger context, which depersonalizes tension that can often feel personal and induce defenses.

Intersectionality

The hospice nurse describes the role of each member of the hospice team during the initial admission visit to a family. The patient is a Vietnam veteran in his late 70s who has been diagnosed with an aggressive form of pancreatic cancer. When the nurse describes the role of the social worker and the chaplain, the patient's wife states that they "do not need therapy" and "chaplains are for the end." The nurse determines that the team members' services won't be needed. The social worker reviews the intake forms and assesses that the patient has a history of acute post-traumatic stress disorder (PTSD) and substance use. The intake notes document that he is "terrified of dying with so many strangers in the house." The social worker identifies a number of differential diagnoses, including a trauma history. The chaplain learns from the admission paperwork that the patient "feels abandoned by God." At the next weekly interdisciplinary meeting, the nurse states that "the family declined psycho-social and spiritual care services so it will just be me that will see them." The patient's psycho-social and spiritual needs are unaddressed in the 2 weeks before he dies.

The complex interplay between professional identities and organizational power structures suggests that the appropriate analysis of team tensions should not be simplified to focus on isolated individual behaviors, but should consider a broader, multidimensional approach. The concept of intersectionality provides a conceptual model in which the interaction of interdependent factors affecting team tensions in healthcare can be considered.[24]

An individual's experiences are shaped not by a single axis of social division, be it race or gender or class, but by many axes that work together and influence each other.[25] The term *intersectionality*, based on the metaphor of an intersection, was coined by legal scholar Kimberlé Crenshaw in 1989 to encapsulate this multidimensional understanding of identity. Crenshaw wrote that traditional feminist ideas and anti-racist policies exclude Black women because they face overlapping discrimination unique to them.[26] An elemental tenet of intersectionality is the theory that social categories such as race, gender, and sexual orientation are not independent and unidimensional but rather overlapping, interdependent, and mutually constitutive systems of discrimination or disadvantage[27] (see Figure 4.1). An intersectional mindset considers how people navigate their agency in the context of multiple structures of power, such as patriarchy, colonialism, ageism, and ableism, which in turn shape their everyday activities and behavior. Intersectionality invites reflection related to the many identities, social locations, and experiences possible for each person. For example, intersectionality indicates that an individual's choice of profession is informed by their experience of other aspects of their identity. Professional choice is potentially a reflection of different values or interpretations of

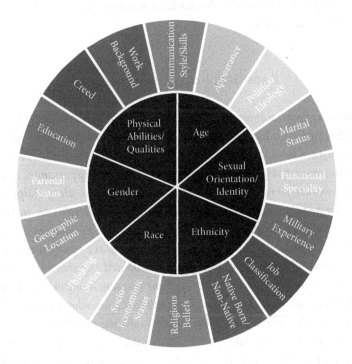

Figure 4.1. Intersectionality.

Adapted from Kathleen Clark, *Digging into Intersectionality*; https://www.identiversity.org/topics/lgbtq-identities/digging-into-intersectionality.

the same values. The choice to become a social worker versus a chaplain may highlight differing relationships to truth, spirituality, concepts of service, education, and social systems at large. Choice of profession therefore is layered and rich in personal story and lineage. These factors also affect the way the individual practices their chosen profession.

Professional identities in hospice and palliative care are compounded by the intersectional realities of each team member.[28] The complex intersection of how we experience the world through race, gender, class, religion, and spirituality may be challenging to integrate into a standardized team process, but must be acknowledged as the basis for how we operate professionally. These differences in social experience complicate and blur our understanding of how to interpret team interactions. Interpersonal versus professional and systemic conflicts are intrinsically linked, and it may be impossible to differentiate them.

Best Practices and Strategies for Managing Tension and Conflict

The science of teamwork in palliative care is still in its infancy, with little evidence supporting specific strategies for managing interprofessional team tensions and conflict. In this section, we have drawn from teamwork models that have been studied in other professional fields and have adapted them as examples for reflection and future directions.

Transdisciplinary Teamwork Model

The community hospital emergency department (ED) functions at a high level because of the collaborative leadership of the medical director and the nurse administrator. They have worked hard to develop respect and synergy among the ED team members, including the nursing staff, providers, phlebotomists, imaging personnel, case management social worker, consulting physicians, and the first responders. Hospital administration has asked the ED leadership team to integrate palliative care in their service, as they have received complaints from families when care provided in the ED was not aligned with the family's values. On several occasions, the family was not contacted before terminally ill and elderly patients were intubated and sent to the intensive care unit (ICU), and on another occasion, a patient was sent home on hospice with a significant other as caregiver, without a phone call to the son who was legally designated as the surrogate decision-maker on the patient's advance directive. The ED leadership team meets with the medical director and the chaplain administrator of the palliative care team, and asks the palliative care team to provide an "as-needed member of your team" to meet with patients and families in the ED for goals of care discussions to re-duce admissions.

Many frames have been applied to palliative care teamwork. Seaman et al.[29] note that teams are referred to as "multidisciplinary," "interdisciplinary," "interprofessional," and "transprofessional" interchangeably and indiscriminately. This confusion is seen as a major barrier to integrating collaborative practice into education and clinical settings. Using unclear terminology heightens the risk of reinforcing traditional hierarchies and power structures that can limit team ef-fectiveness to address the needs of the whole patient.[30] The concept of team has undergone a gradual shift from the siloed structure of multi- and interdisciplinary teams to a more interconnected structure proposed by a transdisciplinary team-work model.[31]

Transdisciplinary collaborative practice is particularly well-suited for interprofessional healthcare settings where diverse roles and responsibilities often overlap, as it supports complex, holistic problem-solving in the setting of serious illness.[32,33] This style of teamwork requires that each team member integrate a va-riety of interprofessional perspectives. For example, a nurse must frequently screen for and communicate a patient's psychosocial, spiritual, and existential needs to the appropriate team domain experts in addition to completing a medical screen and in-depth nursing assessment (see the Generalist-Specialist Assessment Model in Chapter 3).

The shared decision-making component of transdisciplinary teamwork requires the establishment of intentional processes to counteract interprofessional power imbalances. Transdisciplinary models often use a democratic process of decision-making in the spirit of holding all perspectives as equal. However, making space for all perspectives in decision-making is not sufficient, as it does not relieve the need for clearly defined clinical purpose, role descriptions and responsibilities, and a clearly defined and transparent leadership structure. Ideal team leadership for transdisciplinary collaboration requires interprofessional participation, dedicated training, time and compensation, and promotion of a culture of connection and belonging. Specific skills in mediation, cross-cultural communication, personal re-flection, feedback, and integration are essential in the management of dynamic and effective teams.[34]

Cross-Cultural Communication Styles

Communication is a central clinical skill and intervention in palliative care. While it is most commonly taught and practiced with clinical scenarios, applying ad-vanced communication techniques to team dynamics and conversations is essen-tial to mitigating tension. As a foundation, utilizing exploratory and open-ended questions, active listening, validation, and personal reflection can lead to better understanding and a greater sense of connection through challenging encounters.

A new attending physician becomes frustrated with the nurse manager and medical director of a growing outpatient palliative care clinic because he feels that the scheduled back-to-back virtual appointments do not provide enough time to replenish between sessions and adequately assess and treat all the domains of care for each patient. He is able to openly share his concern with his team members, and during the conversation, he is able to appreciate the overall service strategy behind this workflow and collaborate more closely with team members to meet the holistic needs of the patients.

The team has focused on co-creating a culture of open, honest feedback and active listening. When tensions arise related to workflow, the team members can access the team values of openness and honesty that have been habituated over time. Creating a mutual understanding through shared language assures that teams are clear when using common phrases in palliative care and team collaboration.

Professional dynamics and interactions can be assessed with a cross-cultural lens. As explored in prior sections, each team member's professional identity is shaped by different values, reinforced through differing models in training and orientation to professional role and responsibility. While palliative care teams are joined in mission, cultural variation can act as a barrier to understanding the different perspectives and interpretations of the same situation. Profession-specific culture can be explored when space is created to share stories of what it feels like to be a palliative care chaplain, social worker, nurse, and physician, or when opportunities are offered to shadow colleagues. A cross-cultural perspective suggests that team dynamics can benefit from applying a lens of cultural humility[35] to interprofessional interactions, while taking the time to diagnose and address discrepancies as a source of tensions.

James Hallenbeck explores the concept of high and low context cultures.[36] High context communication embeds a great amount of meaning in what is being said and is dependent on the precise situation at hand, while low context communication is more generalizable, explicit, and direct. In the setting of serious illness, patients and families are often positioned in a high context perspective, while clinical information may be presented in a low context format. For example, in sharing prognosis, care teams provide windows of time (hours to days, days to weeks, weeks to months) predicting life expectancy generally for a person in similar conditions. This is an example of *low context* communication. Patients and families receive this information with *high context*, considering personal aspects such as the roles they hold in their life, how they perceive time, relationships to control, spiritual and existential concepts, and stressors related to logistics.

While high context and low context systems are not diametrically opposed, it can be helpful to apply the differences of these contexts to each profession's common communication style. The high–low spectrum is not used to imply better or worse strategies, but rather is an opportunity to reflect on the cultural variation that may inform how we take in information in the service of patient care. Team members who do not share the same perspective on the high–low context continuum may naturally experience interprofessional tensions. Compared to other medical specialties, palliative care clinicians often deliberately attempt to weave together high and low context styles, providing information tailored to the context of the audience. However, when communicating outside of clinical encounters, team members may fall back on the default modes of their training and education, leading to tension and conflict over time. For example, rushed in rounds, a physician may refer to a patient via age, assumed gender, and diagnosis, skipping over high context details of personhood. Communication challenges can also arise from disconnects related to health literacy, pace of communication, role expectations, appropriate self-disclosure, and hidden agendas.[37]

Psychological Safety and Trust

The community-based palliative care (CBPC) team is affiliated with a hospice owned by the same organization that runs the hospital. The CBPC nurse practitioner frequently reaches out to the inpatient palliative care team when their patients are hospitalized, to provide a warm handoff and ensure continuity of care during the hospital stay. Conversely, when patients are discharged, the inpatient team members reach out to the CBPC team with updates regarding next steps in the care plan. Through regular joint staff meetings, transparent feedback methods, and interpersonal communication training, the team members of the inpatient and CBPC services have created a trusting environment where clinicians feel that they can share challenging feedback and be respected and heard. Recently, there have been a number of cases where the inpatient palliative care team felt that the CBPC service did not follow through on the emergency symptom management that they had promised families. Three families had expected a nurse to come to their home in the middle of the night when the patient was experiencing severe pain. The CBPC service had 24-hour phone coverage but was not staffed for 24-hour in-person support. Because of their investment in collective vulnerability and trust, members of the CBPC and inpatient palliative care team were prepared to discuss inter-service challenges and identify satisfying resolutions.

Transdisciplinary teamwork and high-quality communication are both contingent on the presence of psychological safety and team trust. Psychological safety in successful teams, studied in the business and education literature, is the presence of a shared belief among team members that the team is safe for interpersonal risk-taking. This type of safety is a central mechanism which determines collective learning and positive team-level performance.[38] In addition to psychological safety, team trust, defined as "the shared willingness of the team members to be vulnerable to the actions of the other team members based on the shared expectation that the other team members will perform particular actions that are important to the team, irrespective of the ability to monitor or control the other team members"[39(p1152)] is associated with successful group learning and outcomes.

According to Brauer et al,[40] 5 main categories of perceived trustworthiness in teams are antecedents of team trust. Perceived trustworthiness includes the concepts of ability, benevolence, integrity, predictability, and transparency. When team trust was present, team members were willing to engage in risk-taking behaviors, defined as team members' actions reflecting the shared willingness of the team members to be vulnerable to the actions of the other team members. In addition, a recent meta-analysis of organizational outcomes has shown that team trust is positively related with team-related attitudes, information processing in teams, and team performance.[41,42] Tensions are inevitable in interprofessional teamwork, and an intentional process of reflecting on these tensions requires the facilitation of a safe holding space with the specific intention of acknowledging the challenges of interprofessional teamwork. These tensions must be normalized in order for team members to express themselves honestly within the complex interplay of organizational hierarchies and operational incentive schemes.

Time, planning, and thoughtful leadership are needed to ensure a psychologically safe and trust-building space on a consistent basis. Tools such as regular debriefing and effective feedback systems can allow for the consideration of the wider context of intersectional power dynamics, and contribute to healthier, more productive teams. Daniel Coyle, in his book *The Culture Code*,[43] which focuses on the characteristics of highly successful groups, identifies the principles of personal safety, shared vulnerability, and clear purpose as common characteristics of all high-functioning teams.

Conclusion

Interprofessional team dynamics are infused with complex professional identities, cultural variation, and intersectional differences. Team dynamics are magnified by the hierarchical power structure of the healthcare system. Unlike interpersonal aspects of teamwork on an individual level, these structural influences must be addressed on a systemic level. Despite these challenges, effective team leadership can foster an environment of inclusiveness, belonging, and curiosity. Psychological safety is foundational in creating the container that facilitates this sensitive and relational work.

Discussion Questions

1. How well do you understand the training and background of your team members?
2. What comprises a professional identity? What aspects of your identity outside of your profession inform your perspective?
3. What tensions and conflicts do you encounter at work? How does your team approach conflict?
4. How do societal and institutional cultures and norms influence our efforts at collaboration?

References

1. Bochatay N, Bajwa N, Cullati S, et al. A multilevel analysis of professional conflicts in health care teams: insight for future training. *Acad Med.* 2017;92: S84–S92 (11S Association of American Medical Colleges Learn Serve Lead: Proceedings of the 56th Annual Research in Medical Education Sessions).
2. Sam R, Barley WC, Ruge-Jones L, Poole MS. Tacking amid tensions: using oscillation to enable creativity in diverse team Wilson. *J Appl Behav Sci.* 2022;58(1):5–28
3. Kling J. Tension in teams. *Harvard Business Review.* January 14, 2009. Accessed August 15, 2022. https://hbr.org/2009/01/tension-in-teams.html.
4. Meier C, Beresford L. The palliative care team. *J Palliat Med.* 2008;11(5):677–681.
5. Greer L, Van Bunderen L, Yu S. The dysfunctions of power in teams: a review and emergent conflict perspective. *Res Organ Behav.* 2017;37:103–124.
6. Behfar K, Peterson RS, Mannix EA, Trochim WMK. The critical role of conflict resolution in teams: a close look at the links between conflict type, conflict management strategies, and team outcomes. *J Appl Psychol.* 2008;93(1):170–188.
7. Spetz J, Dudley N, Trupin L, Rogers M, Meier DE, Dumanovsky T. Few hospital palliative care programs meet national staffing recommendations. *Health Affairs.* 2016 Sep;35(9):1690–1697.
8. Daly D, Matzel SC. Building a transdisciplinary approach to palliative care in an acute care setting. *OMEGA.* 2013;67(1-2):43–51.
9. Liao J, O'Brien AT, Jimmieson NL, Restubog SL. Predicting transactive memory system in multidisciplinary teams: the interplay between team and professional identities. *J Bus Res.* 2015;68(5):965–977.
10. Ayotte BJ, Allaire JC, Bosworth H. The associations of patient demographic characteristics and health information recall: the mediating role of health literacy. *Neuropsychol Dev Cogn B Aging Neuropsychol Cogn.* 2009 Jul;16(4):419–432.
11. Maricic M, Stojanovic G, Pazun V, et al. Relationship between socio-demographic characteristics, reproductive health behaviors, and health literacy of women in Serbia. *Front Public Health.* 2021 Apr 29;9:629051.
12. Rivera-Romero O, Gabarron E, Miron-Shatz T, Petersen C, Denecke K. Social media, digital health literacy, and digital ethics in the light of health equity. *Yearb Med Inform.* 2022 Aug;31(1):82–87.
13. Girvin J, Jackson D, Hutchinson M. Contemporary public perceptions of nursing: a systematic review and narrative synthesis of the international research evidence. *J Nurs Manage.* 2016;24(8):994–1006.
14. Dopelt K, Bachner YG, Urkin J, Yahav Z, Davidovitch N, Barach P. Perceptions of Practicing Physicians and Members of the Public on the Attributes of a "Good Doctor". *Healthcare.* 2022;10(1):73.

15. Tervalon M, Murray-García J. Cultural humility versus cultural competence: a critical distinction in defining physician training outcomes in multicultural education. *J Health Care Poor Underserv*. 1998;9(2):117–125.

16. Yeager KA, Bauer-Wu S. Cultural humility: essential foundation for clinical researchers. *Appl Nurs Res*. 2013;26(4):251–256.

17. Bould MD, Sutherland S, Sydor DT, Naik V, Friedman Z. Residents' reluctance to challenge negative hierarchy in the operating room: a qualitative study. *Can J Anaesth*. 2015 Jun;62(6):576–586.

18. Samra R, Hankivsky O. Adopting an intersectionality framework to address power and equity in medicine. *Lancet (British)*. 2021;397(10277):857–859.

19. Altilio T, Otis-Green A, Cagle JG. Guess who's coming to dinner? The evolving identity of palliative social workers. In Higgins PC, ed. *The Oxford Textbook of Palliative Social Work*. 2nd ed. Oxford University Press; 2022:65–76; https://doi.org/10.1093/med/9780197537 855.003.0006.

20. Cahn PS. How interprofessional collaborative practice can help dismantle systemic racism. *J Interprof Care*. 2020;34(4):431–434.

21. Moadel AB, Papalezova K, Milner G, Gipson-Fine A, Kalnicki S. A systemic look at professional burnout and well-being within an urban cancer center as a roadmap to recovery. *J Clin Oncol*. 2022;40(Suppl 16):11017–11017.

22. Gabay G, Netzer D, Elhanany A. Shared trust of resident physicians in top-management and professional burnout: a cross-sectional study towards capacity for patient-focussed care, peer support and job expectations. *Int J Health Plan Manage*. 2022;37(4):2395–2409.

23. Berwick DM, Nolan TW, Whittington J. The triple aim: care, health, and cost. *Health Aff (Millwood)*. 2008 May–Jun;27(3):759–769.

24. Samra R, Hankivsky O. Adopting an intersectionality framework to address power and equity in medicine. *Lancet (British)*. 2021;397(10277):857–859.

25. Collins PH, Bilge S. *Intersectionality*. Polity Press; 2016:2.

26. Crenshaw K. Demarginalizing the intersection of race and sex: a Black feminist critique of antidiscrimination doctrine, feminist theory and antiracist politics. *Univ Chicago Legal Forum*. 1989;1:139–167.

27. Crenshaw KW. Mapping the margins: Intersectionality, identity politics, and violence against women of color. *Stanford Law Rev*. 1991;43(6):1241–1299.

28. Lavaysse LM, Probst TM, Arena DF. Is more always merrier? Intersectionality as an antecedent of job insecurity. *Int J Environ Res Public Health*. 2018;15(11):2559.

29. Seaman JB, Lakin JR, Anderson E, Bernacki R, Candrian C, Cotter VT, DeSanto-Madeya S, Epstein AS, Kestenbaum A, Izumi S, Sumser B, Tjia J, Hurd CJ. Interdisciplinary or Interprofessional: Why Terminology in Teamwork Matters to Hospice and Palliative Care. *J Palliat Med*. 2020 Sep;23(9):1157–1158.

30. World Health Organization. Palliative care. Updated 2022. Accessed August 15, 2022. https://www.who.int/news-room/fact-sheets/detail/palliative-care.

31. Otis-Green S, Ferrell B, Spolum M, et al. An overview of the ACE Project—Advocating for Clinical Excellence: transdisciplinary palliative care education. *J Cancer Educ*. 2009;24(2):120–126.

32. Altilio T, Leimena M, Sumser B. In: Sumser B, Leimena ML, Altilio T, eds. *Palliative Care: A Guide for Health Social Workers*. Oxford University Press; 2019:13.

33. Rosa WE, Anderson E, Applebaum AJ, Ferrell BR, Kestenbaum A, Nelson JE. Coronavirus disease 2019 as an opportunity to move toward transdisciplinary palliative care. *J Palliat Med*. 2020;23(10):1290–1291.

34. Dahlin C, Coyne P, Goldberg J, Vaughan L. Palliative care leadership. *J Palliat Care*. 2018;34(1):21–28.

35. Tervalon M, Murray-García J. Cultural humility versus cultural competence: a critical distinction in defining physician training outcomes in multicultural education. *J Health Care Poor Underserv*. 1998;9(2):117–125.

36. Hallenbeck J. High context illness and dying in a low context medical world. *Am J Hosp Palliat Med*. 2006;23(2):113–118.

37. Wittenberg-Lyles E, Goldsmith J, Ferrell B, Ragan SL. *Communication in Palliative Nursing*. Oxford University Press; 2013.

38. Kim S, Lee H, Connerton TP. How psychological safety affects team performance: mediating role of efficacy and learning behavior. *Front Psychol*. 2020;11:1581–1581.

39. Breuer C, Hüffmeier J, Hertel G. Does trust matter more in virtual teams? A meta-analysis of trust and team effectiveness considering virtuality and documentation as moderators. *J Appl Psychol*. 2016;101(8):1151–1177; 1152.

40. Breuer, C Hüffmeier J, Hibben F, Hertel G. Trust in teams: a taxonomy of perceived trust-worthiness factors and risk-taking behaviors in face-to-face and virtual teams. *Human Relat (New York)*. 2020;73(1):3–34.

41. Colquitt, JA, Scott, BA, LePine, JA. Trust, trustworthiness, and trust propensity: a meta-analytic test of their unique relationship with risk-taking and job performance. *J Appl Psychol*. 2007;92(4):909–927.

42. De Jong BA, Dirks KT. Beyond shared perceptions of trust and monitoring in teams: implications of asymmetry and dissensus. *J Appl Psychol*. 2012;97(2):391–406.

43. Coyle D. *The Culture Code: The Secrets of Highly Successful Groups*. Bantam; 2018.

5

Theories and Frameworks Relevant
to Interprofessional Collaboration

Deborah Witt Sherman and Andrea L. Pfeifle

Key Points

- Theory organizes, connects, and structures knowledge to support scholarly inquiry and the formulation of frameworks that support knowledge dissemination.
- Improving healthcare quality demands theoretically grounded thinking and interprofessional cross-disciplinary collaboration of health professionals in administration, education, practice, research, and scholarship.
- The World Health Organization's (WHO) Framework for Action on Interprofessional Education and Collaborative Practice offers a clarion call to generate evidence of the education and clinical outcomes of interprofessional education and collaborative practice in healthcare.
- Institutions of higher learning are being called to lead transformational change in healthcare education, beginning with the definition of core competencies for interprofessional collaborative practice to guide curricular design, core content, and evaluation of educational and practice outcomes.
- A number of theoretical frameworks are relevant to understanding interprofessional collaboration in healthcare. These include *Framework for Action on Interprofessional Education and Collaborative Practice*[1]; *Triple Aim*[2]; *Interprofessional Education Collaborative's Core Competencies for Interprofessional Collaborative Practice*[3-5]; *Canadian Interprofessional Health Collaborative National Interprofessional Competency Framework*[6]; and *Interprofessional Learning Continuum.*[7]
- Palliative care requires a comprehensive interprofessional approach and the integration of varying theoretical perspectives to develop a comprehensive, effective, and compassionate plan of care.

A theory, as a set of interrelated concepts, definitions, and propositions, explains, describes, predicts, or controls a phenomenon of interest, event, or situation. Many clinicians are not conscious of the extent to which they use theory in practice, or translate the findings from tested theories into clinical practice. Health professionals theorize during patient care when they make assessments, synthesize findings, hypothesize about antecedents to conditions (i.e., risk factors), consider the relationship among variables, select interventions, and evaluate outcomes or consequences related to health. Health professions, as practice disciplines, develop and test theories to describe and predict phenomena, test interventions to determine their value in achieving defined outcomes, and create practice change.[8]

Interprofessional members of a team may have unique theoretical/conceptual frameworks that guide their professional assessments and development of an intervention plan. In providing collaborative care, the knowledge and theories from diverse professionals must be synthesized to guide practice. Theories which have been created and tested in one profession may also inform the care provided by another profession, as the concepts and theories are borrowed or adapted.[8] This is particularly relevant to the use of theory in providing interprofessional care and conducting interprofessional research. This chapter provides an introduction to the value of theoretical thinking for the interprofessional team, explores relevant theories and frameworks, and addresses their potential application to palliative care.

Theoretical Thinking of the Interprofessional Team

Theory organizes, connects, and structures knowledge. Goodson defines "theorizing or theoretical thinking as a dynamic process of asking and answering specific types of questions."[9(p76)] Theoretical questions ask why, how, when, where, or what, and these questions lead to answers that structure logical explanations sought by a discipline.* Theorizing leads health professionals to ask questions, to question the status quo, to seek answers, and to build narratives and logical structures for the answers and questions.[9]

Theories have meaning and validity or truth within a specific context, such as the social, cultural, or historical context.[10] Theoretical thinking is closely tied to clinical practice, as the ongoing iterative process of action and reflection during and after clinical encounters leads to refinement of the clinician's thought processes about the phenomenon.[9] Theorizing is an interplay between questions and answers, and the constant dialogue of action and reflection is inherent in theory and practice. The theories or theoretical frameworks relevant and embraced by a profession or discipline have value in defining the scope of practice, while influencing the education and socialization of its professionals.[11]

---

* Although often used interchangeably, "discipline" refers to a branch of knowledge, while "profession" refers to an occupation that requires special education and/or prolonged training and a formal qualification. In this book, we have attempted to standardize the use of the term "profession" when referring to occupations such as chaplaincy, medicine, nursing, and social work, but occasionally the term "discipline" is used, especially when focused on the theory and knowledge development of the professions.

One of the most significant trends in academia, clinical practice, and research over the course of the past half century, greatly stimulated by government and foundation funding policies, has been the movement to larger projects carried out by teams of healthcare educators, clinicians, or researchers from multiple disciplines. As the emphasis on these cross-disciplinary projects has grown, new terminology has emerged to describe these types of collaborations. In the social sciences, these projects are often referred to as "transdisciplinary collaborations"; in research, they are referred to as "team science"; and in the health fields, they are referred to as "interprofessional collaborations."[12-14]

Over the past 40 years, the importance of theory has been emphasized for its use in knowledge translation. Clinicians are expected to appraise research and to understand how theory development and testing not only guide individual professional knowledge, but also guide and evaluate the care offered through interprofessional collaboration. Rycroft-Malone encourages interprofessional collaboration in the endeavors of education, research, and clinical practice.[15] The use and testing of theories relevant to palliative care, conducted by interprofessional scholarly teams, are important to move forward the evidence base of palliative care. For example, humanistic theory guides the team in addressing the physical, social, and spiritual needs of patients in an attempt to alleviate suffering. Theories related to symptom assessment and management also guide clinicians in the relief of suffering.

Complexity science is an emerging paradigm that offers a new approach to viewing healthcare and healthcare organizations.[16] Complexity science is an emerging approach to research using a collection of theories and conceptual tools, rather than being grounded in a single theory. Theoretical concepts of complexity move science beyond linear, positivist reductionism, to ideas related to nested systems from person, family, community, healthcare units, and organizations to healthcare delivery systems, engaging scholars, researchers, and clinicians in a new paradigm of interdisciplinary study and collaboration.[16] In an Institute of Medicine report published 20 years ago, the complexity of healthcare was recognized as a factor leading to unpredictability and variability of healthcare outcomes, relevant across micro, meso, and macro system levels.[17] Such complexity demands the best thinking and interprofessional cross-disciplinary collaboration of health professionals in administration, education, practice, and research/scholarship.

Professions with both unique and shared competencies can name a central phenomenon of interest, perhaps the care of a particular patient with a clinical problem, and use a theoretical perspective to guide their interprofessional work together. As an example, discipline-specific and synthesized perspectives may provide a theoretical lens that guides clinical assessments and generates related clinical questions. Furthermore, interprofessional team members may hypothesize regarding factors that influence the phenomenon, propose relationships to be considered and evaluated, and recommend or consider potential interventions to achieve desirable health outcomes. The theorizing and thinking inherent in interprofessional collaboration may not only guide clinical practice, but also be foundational to professional and interprofessional education in academia, and in the arena of clinical practice across healthcare settings. Additionally, theorizing by interprofessional colleagues is extremely important in guiding research, the questions asked, the theory to be tested, and the actual design and methodology of any given research study that can inform evidence-based practice.[18]

Frameworks Relevant to Interprofessional Collaboration in Healthcare

The World Health Organization's (WHO) Framework for Action on Interprofessional Education and Collaborative Practice provided a structure inextricably connecting education and practice and made several recommendations for educators, policymakers, and healthcare providers.[1] Given major significant issues of preventable mortality and morbidity, increasing medical errors, inadequacies in costly and fragmented systems of care, as well as lack of patient-centered care,[19,20] interprofessional collaboration is deemed critical to clinicians, researchers, professional groups, and governments.[21,22]

Institutions of higher learning are being called to lead transformational change in healthcare education, beginning with a review of the curriculum and educational outcomes of the various health professions and areas where interprofessional collaboration naturally align. In accordance with the Interprofessional Education Collaborative, health professions educational programs are encouraged to integrate core competencies for collaborative practice, embedding essential content of interprofessional communication, patient-family centered care, role clarification, collaborative leadership, and conflict resolution into curricula, including program and course outcomes, teaching-learning approaches, and assessment strategies.[4] Each of these important concepts may be identified in an extant conceptual and theoretical framework which guides the education of health professional students and courses related to interprofessional care.

The Institute of Medicine (IOM) report challenges existing educational systems to prepare future clinicians with the skills of interprofessional collaboration, given the growing body of evidence that well-planned interprofessional learning is the antecedent of patient-centered, cost-effective, efficient, safer, timelier, and more equitable healthcare.[23,24] Through interprofessional education and training, health professionals recognize shared values and codes of conduct, and a move from a sense of independence to interdependence in providing healthcare.[24] This paradigm shift in the education of health professionals emphasizes the critical fit between interprofessional education and real-world interprofessional collaborative practice across healthcare settings.[24,25]

A number of conceptual frameworks are relevant to interprofessional collaboration in healthcare. These include *Triple Aim*[2]; *Framework for Action on Interprofessional Education and Collaborative Practice*[1]; *Interprofessional Education Collaborative's Core Competencies for Interprofessional Collaborative Practice*[3-5]; *Canadian Interprofessional Health Collaborative National Interprofessional Competency Framework*[6]; and *Interprofessional Learning Continuum*.[26] Table

Table 5.1 Summary of Interprofessional Collaboration Frameworks

Framework	Sponsoring Organization	Authors	Key Concepts
IHI Triple Aim	Institute for Healthcare Improvement	Berwick et al.[2]	Describes optimized health system performance as simultaneously achieving improved patient experience, improved population health, and increased cost effectiveness
Framework for Action on Interprofessional Education and Collaborative Practice	World Health Organization	WHO[1]	Shapes successful integration of interprofessional education, collaborative teamwork, and integrated health and education policies
Interprofessional Collaborative Practice Competencies	Interprofessional Education Collaborative	IPEC[4]; IPEC[3]; IPEC[5]	Guides curriculum development across health professions education programs to address four core competencies for interprofessional collaborative practice: values/ethics, roles and responsibilities, interprofessional communication, and teams and teamwork
National Interprofessional Competency Framework	Canadian Interprofessional Health Collaborative	CIHC[6]	Describes 6 essential collaborative practice competencies: patient-centered care, communication, role clarification, conflict resolution, team functioning, and collaborative leadership
Interprofessional Learning Continuum	Institute of Medicine	IOM[7]	Guides the study of interprofessional education across the education-to-practice continuum by describing interrelationships across individual learning-, health-, and system-related outcomes and major enabling and interfering factors, such as professional culture, institutional culture, workforce policy, and financing policy

5.1 includes a summary of each of these frameworks, subsequently described in more detail in the paragraphs that follow, alongside their potential relevance to interprofessional collaboration. Readers desiring additional detail are directed to the source documents for each.

Triple Aim Framework

The Triple Aim framework was developed by the Institute for Healthcare Improvement in Cambridge, Massachusetts (www.ihi.org), as an approach to optimizing health system performance. The framework includes 3 dimensions, all of which must be developed simultaneously to achieve quality healthcare outcomes:

- Improving the patient experience of care;
- Improving the health of populations; and
- Reducing the per capita cost of healthcare.

The Triple Aim framework purports that organizations and communities that attain the Triple Aim will have improved coordination of care and reduced burden of illness (see Figure 5.1). Additional research regarding whether the triple aims are achieved when care is offered by an interprofessional palliative care team would be of value, as often they are studied as separate outcomes. Regardless, the Triple Aim is often described as the penultimate intended outcome of interprofessional education and practice.[26,27]

Importantly, Bodenheimer and Sinsky recommended that the Triple Aim be expanded to a Quadruple Aim, adding the goal of improving the work life of healthcare providers, including clinicians and staff.[28]

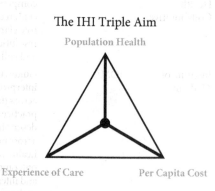

The IHI Triple Aim

Population Health

Experience of Care   Per Capita Cost

Figure 5.1 Triple Aim framework.

The IHI Triple Aim framework was developed by the Institute for Healthcare Improvement in Boston, Massachusetts (www.ihi.org).

WHO Report: Framework for Action on Interprofessional Education and Collaborative Practice

The World Health Organization's *Framework for Action on Interprofessional Education and Collaborative Practice* defines interprofessional education as "when students from two or more professions learn about, from and with each other to enable effective collaboration and improve health outcomes," and identifies it as a necessary step in preparing a "collaborative practice-ready" health workforce prepared to respond to local health needs and improve health outcomes.[1(p 13)]

The report describes key mechanisms that shape successful integration of interprofessional education, collaborative teamwork, and integrated health and education policies. Further, it outlines a series of action items for educators, policymakers, and decision-makers to apply within the local context to support their implementation. The report also suggests a number of mechanisms that shape how interprofessional education is developed and delivered that are relevant to interprofessional education within palliative care settings (see Figure 5.2). These include educator mechanisms (faculty development, administrative leadership, institutional support, practice champions, and specific learning outcomes) and curricular mechanisms (logistics and scheduling, program content, mandatory participation, integration of adult learning principles, and contextual learning).

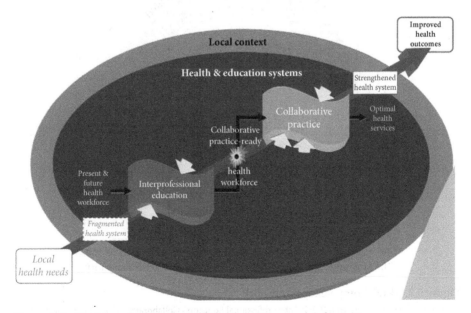

Figure 5.2. Health and education systems from Framework for Action.

Reproduced with permission from World Health Organization, *Framework for Action on Interprofessional Education & Collaborative Practice*, produced by the Health Professionals Network Nursing and Midwifery Office within the Department of Human Resources for Health, p. 9, copyright 2010.

Interprofessional Education Collaborative (IPEC) Core Competencies for Interprofessional Collaborative Practice

In 2009, 6 national associations of schools of health professions formed the Interprofessional Education Collaborative (IPEC) to promote and encourage efforts to advance interprofessional learning experiences that help prepare future health professionals for enhanced team-based care of patients and improved population health outcomes. The collaborative, representing dentistry, nursing, medicine, osteopathic medicine, pharmacy, and public health, convened an expert panel of representatives from each of the 6 IPEC sponsor professions to create core competencies for interprofessional collaborative practice, to guide curriculum development across health professions schools. The competencies and implementation recommendations subsequently were published in the 2011 Core Competencies for Interprofessional Collaborative Practice[4] and revised in 2016.[5] The 2016 version organizes the competencies within a singular domain of interprofessional collaboration that encompasses 4 topical areas, as follows (see Figure 5.3).

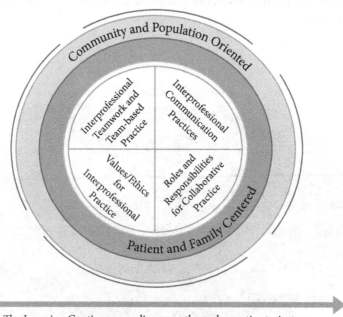

Figure 5.3. IPEC Competency framework.

Reprinted with permission from IPEC®: Interprofessional Education Collaborative, *Core Competencies for Interprofessional Collaborative Practice: 2016 Update.*

- Values/Ethics for Interprofessional Practice
  - o Work with individuals of other professions to maintain a climate of mutual respect and shared values.
- Roles and Responsibilities
  - o Use the knowledge of one's own role and those of other professions to appropriately assess and address the healthcare needs of patients and to promote and advance the health of populations.
- Interprofessional Communication
  - o Communicate with patients, families, communities, and professionals in health and other fields in a responsive and responsible manner that supports a team approach to the promotion and maintenance of health and the prevention and treatment of disease.
- Teams and Teamwork
  - o Work effectively in different team roles to plan, deliver, and evaluate patient/population-centered care and population health programs and policies that are safe, timely, efficient, effective, and equitable.

The competencies have been broadly disseminated, and provide a basis for planning and evaluation of interprofessional practice and education initiatives. Having such a shared taxonomy among the health professions serves to guide, streamline, and synergize educational planning and implementation, as well as to support related assessment and evaluation efforts. Because interprofessional practice and education are inextricably connected and the ideal state has been described by the National Center for Interprofessional Practice and Education as "a deeply connected, integrated learning system to transform education and care together" (https://nexusipe.org/informing/about-nexus), the four topics have formed the basis of education, practice, and assessment designed to improve a number of care models, and have application in palliative care.

Canadian Interprofessional Health Collaborative (CIHC) National Interprofessional Competency Framework

The Canadian Interprofessional Health Collaborative's (CIHC) *National Interprofessional Competency Framework*[6] describes a framework for interprofessional learning, much like a layered elliptical, so as to illustrate its flexible and dynamic nature. It includes clear definitions of the components of interprofessional practice and their interrelationships.[6]

The framework itself comprises 6 competency domains for collaborative practice (see Figure 5.4). Two all-encompassing domains, of interprofessional communication and patient/client/family/community-centered care, support four additional

CIHC National Competency Framework

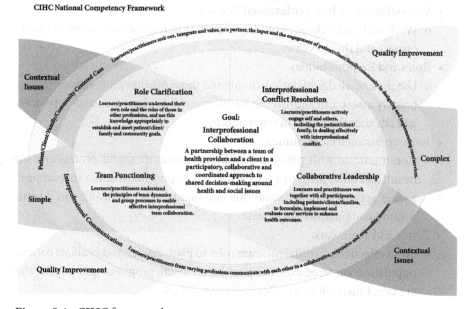

Figure 5.4. CIHC framework.

Reprinted with permission from Canadian Interprofessional Health Collaborative, *A National Interprofessional Competency Framework*, 2010.

domains of role clarification, team functioning, interprofessional communication, and collaborative leadership. In total, the CIHC framework comprises a set of competencies that require the development and integration of attitudes, behaviors, values, and judgments necessary for collaborative practice.[6]

The primary purpose of the framework is to inform educators of the relevant principles and content that should be included in an interprofessional education program. It can also be applied to research, policy, and practice.

The CIHC framework is one of the first to describe the acquisition of collaborative competencies as a developmental process, and interprofessional learning as a continuum. This approach has been integrated into practice redesign, curriculum design, and accrediting requirements for health professions education and has application for educators, accreditors, learners, clinicians, researchers, and policymakers engaged in palliative care. The complexity of the situation and the context for care should heavily influence the way in which it is used.

Interprofessional Learning Continuum (IPLC)

The interprofessional learning continuum (IPLC) model[7] was developed by a panel of experts convened by the Institute of Medicine (IOM), as the Committee on Measuring the Impact of Interprofessional Education on Collaborative

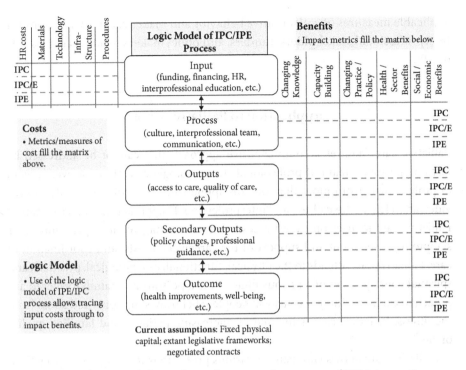

Figure 5.5. A framework for analysis of return on investment of IPE interventions or collaborative care approaches.

HR = human resources; IPC = interprofessional collaboration; IPE = interprofessional education.

Source: Nason E. The "ROI" in "team": Return on investment analysis framework, indicators and data for IPC and IPE. Ontario, Canada: Institute on Governance; 2011. Used with kind permission of the Institute on Governance and the Health Education Task Force.

Practice and Patient Outcomes. The model is intended to guide the study of interprofessional education across the full education-to-practice continuum. It includes and addresses the interrelationships across a broad array of individual learning-, health-, and system-related outcomes and major enabling and interfering factors, such as professional culture, institutional culture, workforce policy, and financing policy.

Measuring the Impact of Interprofessional Education on Collaborative Practice and Patient Outcomes[7] describes an interprofessional learning continuum and the vision that team members share a team identity and work closely together to solve problems and improve delivery of care. In addition to an illustration of the IPLC model in figure 3-2 of that publication[7], the report authors observe that thoughtful, well-designed studies are needed to demonstrate the association between interprofessional education and care outcomes. But these studies cannot be conducted without an understanding of the methods and measurements needed to conduct such an analysis. The report describes a conceptual model for evaluating IPE that can be adapted to particular settings in which it is applied, such as in palliative care See Figure 5.5. It also addresses the lack of broadly applicable measures of collaborative behavior and makes recommendations for interprofessional stakeholders, funders, and policymakers to advance the study of IPE.

Application to Palliative Care

Palliative care requires a comprehensive approach that cannot be addressed by just one person, a team of professionals from a single discipline, or even a team of professionals from more than one discipline who are working serially to provide care. Hence, the call for an "interprofessional" approach in palliative care.[20] Palliative care focuses on expert assessment and management of pain and other symptoms, assessment and support of the caregivers' needs, and coordination of care. Palliative care attends to the physical, functional, psychological, practical, and spiritual consequences of a serious illness. It is a person- and family-centered approach to care, providing seriously ill people relief from symptoms and stress from the illness. Palliative care is focused on increasing patients' and families' quality of life.[29]

Palliative care allows clinicians of various professions to bring their specialized competencies and expertise to focus on serious and complex health problems. Palliative care clinicians combine their clinical expertise and judgment with the best evidence available through research and an understanding of the preferences of patients and families, a process known as evidence-based care.[20] Although discipline-specific theories indicate a professional's commitment to the advancement of their discipline, allowing their ability to practice to the full extent of their scope of practice, there is a need for optimal team cooperation, collaboration, and the application of a shared theoretical lens which synthesizes knowledge from various health disciplines.[18]

Since the first publication of the National Consensus Project (NCP) Guidelines for Quality Palliative Care in 2004, and with each revision of the NCP Guidelines in 2008, 2013, and 2018, there has been increasing recognition of the importance of interprofessional collaboration and teamwork in palliative care's national framework. This conceptual framework consists of 8 domains that guide clinical practice, education, and research.[28] Based on the NCP Guidelines, the National Quality Forum (NQF) released *A National Framework and Preferred Practices for Palliative and Hospice Care Quality* in recognition of the palliative care services increasingly being rendered within the healthcare system. This report endorsed the framework of preferred practices to improve hospice and palliative care and has been utilized as the first step in developing quality measures.[30] The NCP and NQF have formalized the concept of palliative care, have differentiated palliative care from other types of care, and have summarized the theoretical structure of palliative care in 8 domains of care: (1) structure and processes of care; (2) physical aspects; (3) psychological and psychiatric; (4) social; (5) spiritual, religious, and existential; (6) cultural; (7) care of the imminently dying patient; and (8) ethical and legal.[28–29] See Chapter 1 for a thorough discussion of these domains.

In interprofessional palliative care, middle-range theories may guide assessments, interventions, and research. Middle-range theories are theories that are more specific in focus to describe, explore, or predict phenomena of interest, rather than grand theories which are abstract in nature.[30] When palliative care team members collaborate in developing a comprehensive, effective, and compassionate plan of care, as identified in the first domain of "structure and processes of care,"[29] middle-range theories are of value as they have testable propositions (the relationship of one concept to another) which are relevant to specific phenomena or clinical problems in palliative care. In Table 5.2, various middle-range theories developed by nurses and other health professionals have been examined in relation to the domains of the NCP/NQF framework for quality palliative care. The identified middle-range theories may informally or formally be applied to the development and evaluation of a patients' and families' plan of care, curriculum development in education, or in guiding a research project.

Case Vignette to Illustrate Interprofessional Palliative Care and the Application of Concepts from Relevant Conceptual Frameworks or Theories

The following vignette helps readers to understand the complexity of care for persons with serious, chronic, progressive, and life-threatening illness. Care offered by an interprofessional team of healthcare providers ensures that the patient's physical, emotional, social, and spiritual needs are met, along with the needs of the family.

Setting: Veterans Administration Medical Center; Rehabilitation Unit
Patient: 29-year-old Hispanic male discharged from acute care unit to rehab unit with referral to the Palliative Care Service given the need for comprehensive, holistic care for chronic life-limiting illness.
Military History: Army, deployment to Afghanistan
Palliative Care Interprofessional Team: Patient and family, medicine, nursing and advanced practice nursing, communication speech disorders, occupational therapy, physical therapy, 3rd year physical therapy student, recreation therapy, pharmacy, 4th year pharmacy student, social work, social work intern, dietetics, and chaplaincy
Diagnoses: Traumatic brain injury and left lower leg amputation by ID explosion, anterograde amnesia, executive function deficits (cognitive flexibility, planning, self-regulation, organization, impulsivity, and distractibility), chronic neuropathic pain, PTSD, depression

Interprofessional Team Collaboration includes:

1. Completion of a comprehensive health history, identifying chief complaints, review of systems (symptom identification), physical examination, and review of laboratory data and diagnostic tests;
2. Determination and prioritization of diagnoses/clinical problems;
3. Development of an interprofessional treatment plan, to include pharmacologic, nonpharmacologic, and complementary interventions, further diagnostic and laboratory testing needed, relevant education and training, and necessary referrals;
4. Review and revise a plan of care to obtain all team members' acceptance of the problems identified and their roles in attaining defined goals;
5. Pharmacy student provision of recommendations to the team for medication reconciliation under the supervision of the pharmacist;
6. Physical therapy student with supervision provides recommendations to the team: education and training for family and caregivers in transfers; range of motion; positioning; general mobility; and strengthening exercises;
7. Social worker and student intern recommendation of psychosocial and mental health interventions including counseling, resource appropriation, medical treatment for depression, and caregiver support and respite;
8. Chaplain recommendation of spiritual interventions in collaboration with patient's personal pastor;
9. Evaluation of healthcare outcomes for both patients and families, as well as outcomes related to the interprofessional team, such as burnout, or the institution itself, such as length of stay and associated cost; and
10. All team members work together toward shared goal setting and discharge planning for transfer to home with ongoing palliative care support.

Interprofessional Collaborative Care Process:

1. The patient and his family share their goals and concerns with the team;
2. Each discipline reviews the available clinical data from their professional perspectives and determines additional assessment data needed; for example, Medicine, Nursing, Communication Science Disorders, and Occupational Therapy were interested in the head and neck examination to determine hearing acuity, speech perception, and discrimination; Medicine, Nursing, Physical Therapy, OT, and Recreation Therapy focus on functional assessment and mobility; Chaplaincy and Social Work focus on psychological, social, and spiritual well-being;
3. The interprofessional team convenes to determine additional needs, such as further detailed evaluation of his attention, memory, executive functioning, an oral-facial examination of motor speech abilities, and swallow testing;

4. Recommendations are made regarding instruments that would provide further specific clinical data. Team members alerted to the fact that the results of these further clinical tests would support the possible diagnoses which have relevance to interprofessional care;

5. Ongoing team meetings reflect not only an understanding of shared knowledge and competencies, but also the elimination of redundancies in care, collaborative treatment approaches, and an appreciation of the complexity of the case and the unique laser-focused assessment and examination required by other health professions in providing comprehensive, effective, and compassionate treatment options and interventions.

Relevant Theoretical Frameworks to Guide and Inform Interprofessional Care:

1. The World Health Organization Framework for Action on Interprofessional Education and Collaborative Practice (2010) provides a framework for contextualized interprofessional collaboration in palliative care and the successful integration of interprofessional education into the care model;

2. Interprofessional Education Collaborative (2016) core competencies guide effective interprofessional collaborative practice to include values and ethics for interprofessional collaboration, interprofessional communication, teams and teamwork, and role clarification and responsibilities;

3. The Canadian Interprofessional Collaborative Framework (2010) provides additional context for interprofessional care and education in the areas of patient-centered care and collaborative leadership;

4. The Institute of Medicine Report (2015) conceptual model for evaluating IPE guides the definition of health-related and individual learning outcomes and promotes principles for effective teamwork, such as the recognition of shared values, codes of conduct of interprofessional team members, and interdependence in providing quality healthcare;

5. The National Consensus Project/National Quality Forum Framework and Preferred Practices for Palliative and Hospice Care Quality (2004, 2008, 2013, 2018) is used to address all domains: structures and processes of care; physical aspects; psychological and psychiatric; social; spiritual, religious, existential; cultural; care of the dying; and ethical-legal aspects;

6. Application of mid-range theories: pain, symptom assessment and management; social support, resilience, suffering, spiritual care, and cultural competence;

7. The incorporation of students into the interprofessional team and the integration of education and practice in the clinical environment enables team practice addressing multiple layers of care needs and supports the patient and his family's goals; therapy supports the Triple Aim outcome of creating a better experience, improving health, and reducing costs.

Table 5.2 Middle-Range Theories Relevant to the Domains of Palliative Care Offered through Interprofessional Collaboration

Domain of Palliative Care	Theory	Authors	Key Concepts
1. Structures and processes	Modeling and role modeling	Schultz[31]	Modeling, role modeling, facilitation, nurturance, unconditional acceptance
	Relationship-based care	Stewart[32]	Leadership, outcomes measurement, resources, patient care delivery, professional nursing, teamwork
2. Physical	Pain: Balancing analgesia and side effects	Good[33]	Multimodal therapy, attentive care, patient participation
	Unpleasant symptoms	Lenz and Pugh[34]	symptoms, influencing factors, performance outcomes
	Symptom management	Bender et al.[35]	symptom experience, symptom management, symptom status outcomes
3. Psychological/ Psychiatric	Chronic sorrow	Eakes[36]	Loss experience, disparity, chronic sorrow, management methods
	Resilience	Haase and Phillips[37]	Distress, defensive coping, courageous coping, family environment, social integration, derived meaning
4. Social	Social support	Schaffer[38]	Social activity, support function, social appraisals, coping processes, health and mental health outcomes
	Caregiving dynamics	Williams[39]	commitment, expectation management, and role negotiation
	Social determinants of health	Baker[40]	Age, sex, constitutional factors, individual lifestyle factors, social and community networks, living and working conditions, socioeconomic, cultural and environmental conditions
5. Spiritual/ Existential	Spiritual care	Burkhart and Hogan[41]	Patient cure, decision to engage, spiritual intervention, emotional response, search for meaning, formation of spiritual memory and spiritual well-being
	Suffering	Morse[42]	enduring to die, transition, emotional suffering, releases, failure, acceptance, self-reformulation
	Self-transcendence	Reed[43]	self-transcendence, vulnerability, well-being, personal and conceptual factors

Table 5.2 Continued

Domain of Palliative Care	Theory	Authors	Key Concepts
6. Cultural	Cultural competence	Purnell[44]	Heritage, communication, family roles and organizations, workforce issues, biocultural ecology, high-risk health behaviors, nutrition, pregnancy practices, death rituals, spirituality, healthcare practices, clinicians
7. Care of the dying	Health-related quality of life Comfort	Sandou, Bredow, and Peterson[45] Kolcaba[46]	Health and function, socioeconomic, psychological/spiritual, family domains relief, ease, transcendence, physical, psychospiritual, social and environmental comfort
8. Ethical/Legal	Health equity and health disparities	Baker[40]	Quality of healthcare, difference, clinical appropriateness and need, patient preferences, operation of healthcare symptoms, legal and regulatory climate, discrimination, biases, stereotyping, uncertainty, disparity

Conclusion

This chapter describes how theories and frameworks inform the knowledge base of a profession and are foundational to education, research, and practice. Health professionals do not usually think of themselves as "theorists," but in reality they integrate knowledge from the physical, biological, and human sciences to assess clinical situations, and develop hypotheses, diagnoses, and differential diagnoses. Then, with empirical evidence from a physical examination, patient/family interviews, and laboratory and diagnostic data, health professionals determine a comprehensive, compassionate, and effective plan of care. However, the complexity of health problems requires the integration of knowledge and the expertise of many health professionals to provide quality care.

This chapter has briefly summarized theories and conceptual frameworks that are important for the integration of interprofessional education and collaboration in healthcare and specifically in palliative care. The use of these theories and frameworks can support practitioners and educators navigating the array of issues that they encounter in planning, implementing, and evaluating interprofessional collaborative care across various settings.

Discussion Questions

1. Compare and contrast the competency frameworks developed by the Interprofessional Education Collaborative and the Canadian Interprofessional Health Collaborative to describe their similarities and differences. Further consider whether or not they might be combined to create an integrated competency framework describing interprofessional collaborative practice.

2. Theoretical underpinnings are essential prerequisites to interprofessional practice and education. Describe how one or more of the theories or frameworks presented in this chapter are relevant to palliative care.

3. Discuss the shared competencies of health professionals on a palliative care team considering physical, emotional, social, cultural, and spiritual/existential/religious domains of palliative care as identified in the National Consensus Project for Quality Palliative Care Guidelines.[28]

4. Develop a case study of a patient experiencing traumatic brain injury and their family as the unit of care. Identify which members of the interprofessional palliative care team may lead in addressing the following clinical problems: neuropathic pain, depression, caregiving dynamics, and social support. Explain how various mid-range theories identified in this chapter may guide clinical assessment and interventions offered by the interprofessional palliative care team.

References

1. World Health Organization. *Framework for Action on Interprofessional Education and Collaborative Practice*. World Health Organization; 2010.
2. Berwick D, Nolan T, Whittington J. The Triple Aim: care, health and cost. *Health Affairs*. 2008;27(3):759–769.
3. Interprofessional Education Collaborative (IPEC). *Core Competencies for Interprofessional Collaborative Practice: Report of an Expert Panel*. Interprofessional Education Collaborative; 2015.
4. Interprofessional Education Collaborative Expert Panel. *Core Competencies for Interprofessional Collaborative Practice: Report of an Expert Panel*. Interprofessional Education Collaborative; 2011.
5. Interprofessional Education Collaborative. *Core Competencies for Interprofessional Education to Advance Triple Aim Outcomes*. Interprofessional Education Collaborative; 2016.
6. Orchard C, Bainbridge L, Bassendowski S, Stevenson K, Wagner SJ, Weinberg L, Curran V, Di Loreto L, Sawatsky-Girling B. *A National Interprofessional Competency Framework*. Canadian Interprofessional Health Collaborative. Published 2010. Accessed February 17, 2021. https://phabc.org/wp-content/uploads/2015/07/CIHC-National-Interprofessional-Competency-Framework.pdf.
7. Committee on Measuring the Impact of Interprofessional Education on Collaborative Practice and Patient Outcomes; Board on Global Health; Institute of Medicine. *Measuring the Impact of Interprofessional Education on Collaborative Practice and Patient Outcomes*. Washington (DC): National Academies Press (US); 2015.

8. Ellis R. The practitioner as theorist. In: Reed P, Shearer N, eds. *Perspectives on Nursing Theory*. Lippincott Williams & Wilkins; 2012:56–61.

9. Goodson P. Theory as practice. In: Butts J, Rich K, eds. *Philosophies and Theories for Advanced Nursing Practice*. 3rd ed. Jones & Bartlett; 2018:75–79.

10. Edberg M. *Social and Behavioral Theory in Public Health*. Jones and Bartlett; 2007.

11. Glanz K, Burke L, Rimer B. Health behavior theories. In: Butts J, Rich K, eds. *Philosophies and Theories for Advanced Nursing Practice*. 2nd ed. Jones & Bartlett; 2015:235–253.

12. Chamberlain-Saloun J, Mills J, Kim U. Terminology used to describe healthcare teams: an integrative review of literature. *J Multidiscip Healthc*. 2013;6:65–74.

13. Choi B, Pak A. Multidisciplinarity, interdisciplinarity and transdisciplinarity in health research, services, education and policy: 1. Definitions, objectives, and evidence of effectiveness. *Clin Invest Med*. 2006;29(6):351–364.

14. Little M, Hill C, Ware K, et al. Team science as interprofessional collaborative research practice: a systematic review of the science of team science literature. *J Investig Med*. 2017;65(1):15–22.

15. Rycroft-Malone J. Theory and knowledge translation: setting some coordinates. In: Reed P, Shearer N, eds. *Perspectives on Nursing Theory*. 6th ed. Lippincott Williams & Wilkins; 2012:111–120.

16. Engebretson J, Hickey J. Complexity science and complex adaptive systems In: Butts J, Rich K, eds. *Philosophies and Theories for Advanced Nursing Practice*. 2nd ed. Jones & Bartlett; 2015.

17. Institute of Medicine. *Crossing the Quality Chasm: A New Health System for the 21st Century*. National Academy Press;2001.

18. Sherman DW, Maitra K, Hough M, et al. Illustrating and analyzing the processes of interprofessional collaboration: lessons learned from palliative care in deconstructing the concept. *J Palliat Med*. 2017;20(3):227–234.

19. Olenick M, Allen L, Smego R. Interprofessional education: Concept analysis. *Adv Med Educ Pract*. 2010;1:1–10.

20. Sherman DW, Bookbinder M. Palliative care: a response to the need for health care reform in America. In: Matzo M, Sherman DW, eds. *Palliative Care Nursing: Quality Care through the End of Life*. 5th ed. Springer; 2019:19–33.

21. Sherman DW. Interprofessional collaboration. In: Matzo M, Sherman DW, eds. *Palliative Care Nursing: Quality Care through the End of Life*. 5th ed. Springer; 2019:37–47.

22. Gilbert JHV, Yan J, Hoffman SJ. A WHO report: Framework for action on interprofessional education and collaborative practice. *J Allied Health*. 2010;39(3):196–197.

23. Institute of Medicine. *Health Professions Education: A Bridge to Quality*. National Academies Press;2003.

24. Karstadt L. Does interprofessional education provide a global template? *Br J Nurs*. 2012;21(9):522.

25. Milton C. Ethical issues surrounding interprofessional collaboration. *Nurs Sci Q*. 2012;26(4):316–318.

26. Earnest M, Brandt B. Aligning practice redesign and interprofessional education to advance triple aim outcomes. *J Interprof Care*. 2014;28(6):497–500.

27. Bodenheimer T, Sinsky C. From triple to quadruple aim: care of the patient requires care of the provider. *Ann Fam Med*. 2014;12(6):573–575.

28. National Consensus Project for Quality Palliative Care. *Clinical Practice Guidelines for Quality Palliative Care*. NCP; 2018.

29. National Quality Forum. *A National Framework and Preferred Practices for Palliative and Hospice Care Quality*. NQF; 2016.

30. Smith MJ, Liehr PR. *Middle Range Theories in Nursing*. 4th ed. Springer; 2018.

31. Schultz E. Modeling and role-modeling. In: Peterson S, Bredow T, eds. *Middle Range Theories: Application to Nursing Research and Practice*. 4th ed. Wolters Kluwer; 2017:177–195.

32. Stewart M. Models and theories focused on competencies and skills. In: Butts J, Rich K, eds. *Philosophies and Theories for Advanced Nursing Practice*. 3rd ed. Jones & Bartlett; 2018:519–543.

33. Good M. Pain: a balance between analgesia and side effects. In: Peterson S, Bredow T, eds. *Middle Range Theories: Application to Nursing Research and Practice*. 4th ed. Wolters Kluwer; 2018:49–63.

34. Lenz E, Pugh L. Theory of unpleasant symptoms. In: Smith MJ, Liehr PR, eds. *Middle Range Theory for Nursing*. Springer; 2018:165–196.

35. Bender M, Jonson S, Franch L, Lee K. Theory of symptom management. In: Smith M, Liehr P, eds. *Middle Range Theories in Nursing*. Springer; 2018:41–164.

36. Eakes G. Chronic sorrow. In: Peterson S, Bredow T, eds. *Middle Range Theories: Applications to Nursing Research and Practice*. Wolters Kluwer; 2017:107–115.

37. Haase J, Phillips C. Resilience. In: Peterson S, Bredow T, eds. *Middle Range Theories: Applications to Nursing Research and Practice*. Wolters Kluwer; 2017:259–278.

38. Schaffer M. Social support. In: Peterson S, Bredow T, eds. *Middle Range Theories: Application to Nursing Research and Practice*. 4th ed. Wolters Kluwer; 2017:117–135.

39. Williams L. Theory of caregiving dynamics. In: Smith MJ, Liehr PR, eds. *Middle Range Theory for Nursing*. 3rd ed. Springer; 2014:309–327.

40. Baker T. Theories focused on health equity and health disparities. In: Butts J, Rich K, eds. *Philosophies and Theories for Advanced Nursing Practice*. 3rd ed. Jones & Bartlett; 2018:393–421.

41. Burkhart L, Hogan N. Spiritual care in nursing practice. In: Peterson S, Bredow T, eds. *Middle Range Theories: Application to Nursing Research and Practice*. 4th ed. Wolters Kluwer; 2017:106–115.

42. Morse J. The praxis theory of suffering. In: Butts J, Rich K, eds. *Philosophies and Theories for Advanced Nursing Practice*. Jones & Bartlett; 2018:603–632.

43. Reed P. Theory of self-transcendence. In: Smith MJ, Liehr PR, eds. *Middle Range Theory for Nursing*. Springer; 2018:109–139.

44. Purnell L. Models and theories focused on culture. In: Butts J, Rich K, eds. *Philosophies and Theories for Advanced Nursing Practice*. 3rd ed. Jones & Bartlett; 2018:565–601.

45. Sandou K, Bredow T, Peterson S. Health-related quality of life. In: Peterson S, Bredow T, eds. *Middle Range Theories: Application to Nursing Research and Practice*. 4th ed. Wolters Kluwer; 2017:212–238.

46. Kolcaba L. Comfort. In: Peterson S, Bredow T, eds. *Middle Range Theories: Application to Nursing Research and Practice*. 4th ed. Wolters Kluwer; 2017:196–211.

6

Principles of Interprofessional Education Applied to Palliative Care

Barbara L. Jones, Jennifer Currin-McCulloch, and Regina M. Fink

Key Points

- Palliative care can and should be taught using principles of interprofessional education.
- Real-world simulations of palliative care clinical scenarios enhance learners' understanding of interprofessional palliative care skills.
- Palliative care education must incorporate the core competencies of interprofessional education.
- Palliative care can be a leader in models of interprofessional education.
- Interprofessional faculty, representing the core palliative care professions, must collaborate to develop and teach palliative care curricula based on palliative care core competencies while providing mentorship to interprofessional learners.

Introduction

Palliative care is essentially an interprofessional practice that is designed to improve patient and family quality of life through coordinated, compassionate, collaborative care.[1,2] Palliative care is a limited resource in many healthcare settings due to a shortage of qualified and certified palliative care professionals. While primary care providers often advocate for and implement *primary* palliative care interventions in their work, they lack evidence-based palliative care knowledge and skills to deliver quality *specialty* palliative care, resulting in significant practice variation. Often, this is due to limited access to well-defined palliative care content in the 4 core* professions of nursing, medical, social work, and chaplaincy/spiritual care curricula. To increase availability of a skilled palliative care workforce with expertise in working on an interprofessional team, a comprehensive interprofessional palliative care educational

---

* In this book, we use the term "core" to refer to chaplains, nurses, physicians, and social workers, who are all named as part of the interprofessional team for both the Medicare hospice guidelines and the NCP guidelines. This designation does not minimize the importance of other team members who contribute to the palliative care of patients and families.

program encourages learners from various professions or fields of study (disciplines) to learn together and have a deeper appreciation of their various roles while fostering professional and personal growth within each other.[3] Learning together as interprofessional student cohorts reflects the goal of palliative care teamwork and is a new paradigm that strengthens the students' resolution to interweave their various perspectives and deliver exceptional interprofessional care in real-world settings. This chapter focuses on the basic principles of interprofessional palliative care curriculum design by a team of professionals from core palliative care disciplines,[†] competency development, innovative teaching and educational strategies, and evaluation. After introducing 2 exemplar educational programs, we discuss Kern's 6-step approach to curriculum development, which provides a framework for exploring principles of interprofessional palliative care curriculum development, with additional emphasis on assessment and evaluation. Interprofessional palliative care education is important to realizing the quadruple aim (enhancing the seriously ill patient's experience, improving population health, reducing costs, improving quality of life for healthcare providers and staff) and guiding collaborative practice.[1]

Interprofessional Education Program Exemplars

Exemplar 1: Colorado

The Interprofessional Master of Science in Palliative Care (MSPC) 33-credit program and the Interprofessional Palliative Care Certificate (IPCC) 12-credit program at the University of Colorado Anschutz Medical Campus, supported by a broad coalition including the Graduate School, College of Nursing, School of Pharmacy, and School of Medicine, provides interprofessional education to nurses, physicians and physician assistants, social workers, chaplains/spiritual care providers, pharmacists, and psychologists.[3] Campus-wide interprofessional workgroups convened to develop the mission, vision, and goals of the program; these were ultimately approved by University of Colorado Board of Regents. The curriculum, designed by an interprofessional faculty comprising nurses, physicians, physician assistants, pharmacists, psychologists, social workers, chaplains/spiritual care providers, and experts in biomedical ethics, humanities, and communications, was guided by 9 core competencies (Box 6.1), based on the National Consensus Project for Quality Palliative Care, National Quality Forum, and Hospice and Palliative Nurses' Association (HPNA) core competencies.[4-6] The online curriculum focuses on interprofessional teamwork, communication skills, and practical application of biomedical, psychological, social, spiritual, and ethical

---

[†] Although often used interchangeably, "discipline" refers to a branch of knowledge, while "profession" refers to an occupation that requires special education and/or prolonged training and a formal qualification. In this book, we have attempted to standardize the use of the term "profession" when referring to occupations such as chaplaincy, medicine, nursing, and social work, but occasionally the term "discipline" is used, especially when focused on the theory and knowledge development of the professions.

Box 6.1. University of Colorado Master of Science
in Palliative Care, Core Competencies of the Palliative Care
Community Specialist and Crosswalk to NQF Consensus and
HPNA Competencies

1. Communications Skills
   The Palliative Care Community Specialist demonstrates expertise in
   relationship-centered communication theory and skills to gather and
   share information, negotiate shared decision-making and plans of
   care, and sustain relationships with palliative care patients/families,
   interdisciplinary teams, and other healthcare professionals.
   NQF 1, 2, 3, 4, 5, 6, 7, 8   HPNA 8

2. Expert Symptom Management Skills (Pain and Non-pain)
   The Palliative Care Community Specialist demonstrates expert clinical/
   psycho-social-spiritual judgment in performing a comprehensive patient
   assessment, leading to diagnosis development, implementation, and
   ongoing reassessment with modification of effective, evidence-based care
   plans utilizing the skills and expertise of the IDT, for all distressing pain
   and non-pain symptoms experienced by patients with any serious illness.
   NQF 2, 7   HPNA 1, 4, 9

3. Ethics, Advocacy, and Legal Aspects of Care
   The PCCS incorporates knowledge of ethical and legal aspects of palliative
   care by engaging ethical issues in end-of-life care, exhibiting the highest
   professional standards, and by understanding legal aspects of care so that
   they can advocate for patients'/families' access to optimal palliative care.
   NQF 1, 6, 8   HPNA 2, 3

4. Spiritual, Religious, and Existential Aspects of Care
   As part of the IDT, the Palliative Care Community Specialist demonstrates
   and promotes spiritually sensitive care, respecting diversity in all forms,
   for patients/families and other healthcare professionals.
   NQF 5, 6   HPNA 4, 6

5. Social and Cultural Aspects of Care
   As part of the IDT, the Palliative Care Community Specialist demonstrates
   respect for diverse communities through cultural humility, recognizing
   how social and economic barriers and challenges impact the delivery of
   health care services.
   NQF 4, 6   HPNA 3, 4, 5, 6

6. Psychological Aspects of Care
   As part of the IDT, the Palliative Care Community Specialist effectively
   addresses psychological concerns, promotes access to expanded resources
   for all patients/families living with any serious illness, and ensures self-care.
   NQF 3, 6   HPNA 2, 4, 5, 8

Box 14.4 Continued

---

7. Palliative Care Integration for Patients throughout the Course of any Serious Illness in all Venues
   The Palliative Care Community Specialist effectively advocates to provide evidence-based palliative care for patients/families and supports and develops expanded resources for all patients/families living with any serious illness.
   NQF 1, 4, 6, 8   HPNA 2, 3, 4, 7, 9
8. Effective Palliative Care Educator
   The Palliative Care Community Specialist demonstrates knowledge, skills, and applies adult learning principles when providing palliative care education to patients/families, healthcare professionals, and the community.
   NQF 1, 4, 6, 8   HPNA 2, 3, 4, 5, 7, 9
9. Systems Thinking
   The Palliative Care Community Specialist demonstrates understanding of the healthcare system to effectively manage and utilize resources to support patients/families living with any serious illness and advocates for the reform of healthcare systems to provide optimal palliative care.
   NQF 1, 8   HPNA 2, 4, 5, 9

---

content. The pedagogical approach is narrative-based and emulates the in-person clinical experience, with patient cases progressing throughout the curriculum that set the stage for the presentation of weekly materials. Faculty and students are highly engaged in the materials and the integrated and interprofessional nature of the curriculum. In MSPC Capstone coursework (6 credits), students are mentored by faculty to apply what they have learned to their work settings by designing and implementing a Capstone project (e.g., evidence-based practice, quality improvement, program development/evaluation, needs assessment, education) and sharing results through a professional abstract and poster presentation to faculty and colleagues. They may also present their work at a professional palliative care meeting. The MSPC and IPCC programs provide the opportunity for palliative care providers who have *clinically worked* together for many years to now *teach, mentor, and develop* students together.

Exemplar 2: Texas

The Foundations for Interprofessional Collaborative Practice (FICP) course emerged from a history of interprofessional collaboration at The University of Texas at Austin. Originally training students in cohorts of 25, the interprofessional education program expanded to include annual student cohorts of over 260 students as a collaborative pedagogical initiative between the university's Dell Medical School, School of Nursing, College of Pharmacy, and Steve Hicks School of Social Work. This longitudinal interprofessional course, delivered over 2 semesters, incorporates the Interprofessional Education Collaborative (IPEC) core competencies and includes modules that focus on roles and responsibilities, implicit bias, team communication in addiction care, error prevention and disclosure, and team communication in palliative care. The final 2 class modules center on building interprofessional skills for leading palliative care family meetings, discussing goals of care, practicing patient and family role-plays, as well as learning from panelists with extensive experience in pediatric and adult palliative care interprofessional collaborative practice. The culmination of the course centers on a palliative care simulated family meeting that engages actors to play patients' caregivers. This simulation, often acknowledged by students as the hallmark of their interprofessional identity development, provides interprofessional teams the opportunity to apply their course learning in a simulated hospital room setting with an actor who brings a realistic challenge to the development of an end-of-life care plan.[7]

Curriculum Development

When designing interprofessional palliative care education, Kern et al's 6-step model for medical education offers a systematic approach for developing curriculum.[8] The initial step involves performing a problem identification in which one assesses the current health professions' education system, provider competencies, and systemic gaps in healthcare, while also envisioning the structure of an ideal strategy for growth. After completing this step, a targeted needs assessment delves deeper into the unique needs of the targeted institution and its learners. Developing goals and objectives for the educational program helps to clarify measurable outcomes to guide the implementation and evaluation of program implementation. Through the design of educational strategies, the planning team decides the specific content and educational methods of delivering the course content. The implementation phase includes educational intervention delivery and the attainment of institutional investment and resource acquisition. Lastly, the systematic approach includes the development of strategies for evaluation and feedback of the curriculum, key personnel, and instructors. While Kern's approach was developed for medical education, it offers a step-wise approach to curriculum development that could include the specific expertise of all healthcare professionals involved in interprofessional palliative care education. Because each profession brings its own strengths, it is crucial to include educational pedagogy, theory, and skills from nursing, social work, spiritual care, psychology, pharmacy, and other healthcare professional education.

Step 1: Problem Identification

If one were to apply Kern's model to interprofessional education, the first step would entail institutions performing a comprehensive exploration of national and/

or community-level health professions' education programs to determine gaps in training, and systemic and societal barriers that may impede the provision of equitable, high-quality healthcare. Within interprofessional education, a problem assessment may include the acknowledgment of an integrated training system that fails to equitably incorporate voices from each profession or that centers on physical health without integrating social determinants of health. After this general assessment, institutions brainstorm an ideal interprofessional educational model that intentionally cultivates a more socially responsive clinician training and engaged community response to enhance individual and community-level well-being.

Step 2: Needs Assessment

To gauge potential student educational needs and demands, a needs assessment survey may be used to assess knowledge, awareness, and available educational resources related to palliative care in various professions' practice settings. The ultimate goal of conducting a needs assessment is to inform the development of an interprofessional palliative care program for healthcare learners and professionals. Previously developed needs assessment instruments have assessed palliative care knowledge, services provided, barriers to palliative care delivery, staff education offered, and resources that would be helpful to improve palliative care knowledge, attitudes, and skills. [9-11] Several questions ask what respondents would like to learn about palliative care and how they prefer to receive that information. Other questions could focus on what would make it possible for providers and professionals to enroll as students or participate in a palliative care educational offering. Additionally, assessing and understanding learners' interests and the barriers they face can provide insights to possible solutions for overcoming challenges.

Prior to the development of the interprofessional MSPC and IPCC programs at the University of Colorado Anschutz Medical Campus, an electronic survey methodology was used to survey professionals representing multiple disciplines, using blog postings, websites, and listservs.[3] Most respondents were mid-career professionals who had a desire to move into hospice and palliative care as part of their practice. Survey results informed initial interprofessional program development.

Interprofessional Competencies

Standards and competencies are essential to define professional practice. Competencies characterize the knowledge, skills, and attitudes that must be demonstrated to provide safe, consistent, quality, evidence-based, and compassionate care.[4] Achievement of defined competencies can be enhanced through training, education, and professional development and correlates with positive job performance and improved patient outcomes.[12] Many organizations and programs representing various professions document profession-specific palliative care competencies (Table 6.1); [4-6,13-20] yet, interprofessional collaborative practice is the ideal approach to team-based palliative care.[2,21,22]

Table 6.1 Palliative Care Core Competencies by Organization and Specialty

NQF/NCP	EAPC	HPNA	G-CARES	AAHPM	US Medical Licensing Examination (USMLE)	Canadian SW	NASW	Spiritual Care EAPC
Domain 1: Structure and Processes of Care	1. Apply the core constituents of palliative care in the setting where patients and families are based.	1. Clinical judgment	1. Articulate the value of palliative care as a basic human right at a local, national, and global level.	1. Patient and family care	1. Pain and symptom management	1. Advocacy	1. Ethics and Values	1. Demonstrate the reflective capacity to consider the importance of spirituality in one's own life
Domain 2: Physical Aspects of Care	2. Enhance physical comfort throughout patients' disease trajectories.	2. Advocacy and ethics	2. Advocate for access to palliative care and hospice services as standard practice in all clinical, community, and technology-mediated (telehealth) settings.	3. Medical knowledge	2. Communication	2. Assessment	2. Knowledge	2. Recognize the importance of spirituality in the life of the patients, and understand the patients' and families' spiritual, existential and religious needs, respecting their choice not to focus on this aspect of care.

(continued)

Table 6.1 Continued

NQF/NCP	EAPC	HPNA	G-CARES	AAHPM	US Medical Licensing Examination (USMLE)	Canadian SW	NASW	Spiritual Care EAPC
Domain 3: Psychological and Psychiatric Aspects	3. Meet patients' psychological needs	3. Professionalism	3. Contribute to creating, critiquing, translating, and evaluating the evidence base for primary palliative care	3. Practice-based learning and improvement	3. Psychosocial, spiritual, and cultural aspects of care	3. Care delivery	3. Assessment	3. Integrate the patients' and families' and caregivers' spiritual needs in the care plan and document SC provision.
Domain 4: Social Aspects of Care	4. Meet patients' social needs	4. Collaboration	4. Identify the dynamic changes in population demographics, healthcare economics, service delivery, caregiving demands, and financial impact of serious illness	4. Interpersonal and communication skills	4. Terminal care and bereavement	4. Care planning	4. Intervention and treatment planning	4. Be conscious of the boundaries that may need to be respected in terms of culture, ritual, and traditions.
Domain 5: Spiritual, Religious, and Existential Aspects of Care	5. Meet patients' spiritual needs	5. Systems thinking	5. Promote social justice, equity, and equality for the seriously ill within clinical and educational settings, professional organizations, and state and national legislatures.	5. Professionalism	5. Palliative care principles and practice	5. Community capacity building	5. Attitude and self-awareness	

Domain 6: Cultural Aspects of Care	6. Respond to the needs of family carers in relation to short-, medium- and long-term patient care goals.	6. Cultural and spiritual competence	6. Communicate and collaborate with organizational and policy leaders to eliminate health disparities and financial and regulatory barriers related to palliative care.	6. Systems-based practice	6. Confirmation	6. Empowerment and advocacy
Domain 7: Care of the Patient Nearing the End of Life	7. Respond to the challenges of clinical and ethical decision-making in palliative care	7. Facilitation of learning	7. Educate consumers, stakeholders, community leaders, policymakers, and healthcare providers regarding patient and family, professional, and system outcomes related to the provision of primary palliative care.		7. Decision-making	7. Documentation

(continued)

Table 6.1 Continued

NQF/NCP	EAPC	HPNA	G-CARES	AAHPM	US Medical Licensing Examination (USMLE)	Canadian SW	NASW	Spiritual Care EAPC
Domain 8: Ethical and Legal Aspects of Care	8. Practice comprehensive care coordination and interdisciplinary teamwork across all settings where palliative care is offered.	8. Communication	8. Role-model resiliency and sustainability to patient/family and interprofessional healthcare providers, demonstrating strategies for coping with suffering, loss, and moral distress associated with serious illness.			8. Education and research	8. Interdisciplinary teamwork	
	9. Develop interpersonal and communication skills appropriate to palliative care.	9. Evidence-based practice and research				9. Information sharing	9. Cultural competence	
	10. Practice self-awareness and undergo continuing professional development.					10. Interdisciplinary team	10. Continuing education	
						11. Self-reflective practice	11. Supervision, leadership, and training	

Sources: AACN; Arnold et al.; Best et al.; Bosma et al.; Carey et al.; Ferrell et al.; Jacono et al.; NASW; NQF.[8-17]

In an effort to provide a consistent framework for palliative care practice and education, 8 domains and structures of high-quality palliative care have been comprehensively described by the National Quality Forum (NQF) in 2006[6] and have been endorsed by the National Consensus Project (NCP) for Quality Palliative Care (see Chapter 1 for a detailed description of the NCP Guidelines).[5] In addition, IPEC developed core competencies to serve as guidelines for training students in interprofessional collaborative practice.[23] The IPEC core competencies center on 4 domains: interprofessional teamwork and team-based practice, interprofessional communication, roles and responsibility for collaborative practice, and values and ethics for interprofessional practice (see Chapter 5).[23] These competencies map strongly to the goals of interprofessional palliative care practice, but there has been little discussion of how specifically to teach these IPEC competencies in palliative care education.

Most palliative care professional organizations offer their own guidelines for interprofessional palliative care practice specific to their profession. Some examples include the American Academy of Hospice and Palliative Medicine (AAHPM), the Hospice and Palliative Nurses Association (HPNA), the Social Work Hospice and Palliative Care Network (SWHPN), the Association of Professional Chaplains (APC), and the National Association of Catholic Chaplains (NACC). In 2013, the European Association for Palliative Care (EAPC) White Paper on core competencies addressed substantive competencies for clinical palliative care practice that are important and mutual for *all* health and psychosocial care professionals and practitioners to achieve, irrespective of specific professional background.[18] These competencies offer a framework for the development of robust palliative care education programs and inform curriculum development. A program that does not delineate interprofessional competencies is unlikely to provide the required knowledge, skills, and characteristics needed to inform quality palliative care practice. Standards of excellence for interprofessional educational programs designed to prepare clinicians to provide palliative care have been proposed.[24]

Step 3: Goals and Objectives

When determining course goals and objectives, course developers should consider the needs of their specific learners and learning environment, overall course goals and program competencies, as well as the objectives to meet the needs across professions and programs. Sample goals might focus on supporting students in their interprofessional identity development and profession-specific confidence, while also augmenting their understanding of the clinical responsibilities and strengths of other health professions on the palliative care team. These goals change depending upon whether the targeted learners are pre-clinical, clinical, or practicing professionals. The introduction of practice skills in the provision of interprofessional palliative care should highlight strategies for developing a person-centered framework for engaging patients and families in palliative care. Curricula should also engage students in exploring their implicit biases, as well as stereotypes they hold about their own profession and other health professions. Lastly, the course should center on perspectives toward healthcare from the individual and family perspective, as well as the larger systemic social, political, and environmental factors that influence palliative care access and treatment provision.

Through incorporating a Bloom's taxonomy lens, course developers can implement multiple layers of activities and instructional formats that appeal to the learning preferences and needs of all students and focus on cognitive, affective, and active domains.[25] Using Bloom's taxonomy to formulate learning objectives sets the stage for faculty to plan and deliver instruction and design ways to assess outcomes, and for students to understand the purpose of the pedagogical interchange.[26]

Step 4: Teaching Modalities and Educational Strategies

To most effectively engage students in interprofessional palliative care learning environments, curriculum developers must incorporate a variety of instructional modalities. The complex nature of palliative care delivery requires that students have exposure to learning activities that highlight real-life challenges students may encounter in everyday clinical and professional practice. Some common instructional strategies include case scenarios, simulations, standardized patients, role-plays, and panels of palliative care professionals or patient and family caregivers. Key facets of palliative care education include screening for and understanding the needs of patients and families, developing patient- and family-centered care plans, discussing advance care planning, and building communication techniques for difficult dialogues and conversations. Team-based role-plays and simulations provide students with opportunities to practice leading discussions about patients' and families' values, meaning, and preferences; quality of life; desires for medical treatment or changes in course of treatment; end-of-life care plans; and challenging family discussions. Professional actors as simulated patients or caregivers add an additional layer of realism and challenge for student-based interprofessional teams in navigating case scenarios. Role-plays can be accomplished online through video conferences, student-developed videotapes that respond to prompts and dialogues, or case studies that have been audio- or videotaped for asynchronous viewing. Interdisciplinary team conferences about patient and family case studies that emulate patient/family care conferences can be attended through video conferencing.

Step 5: Implementation

During the implementation phase, program leaders need to garner endorsement from key administrative and departmental leaders who can support the accrual of vital resources such as funding, classroom space, course instructors, and classroom resources. Programs should also consider the overall learning climate and processes for creating a safe, trusting, and equitable learning environment.

Learning Climate

To foster truly engaged interprofessional palliative care education, attention must be paid to the structural and systemic power differences among healthcare professions. In order to be truly interprofessional, the climate must privilege all of the voices equally and allow for leadership to come from all participating professions. Often seen as an exemplar in interprofessional teamwork, palliative care teams intentionally focus on the additive and synergistic value of each individual's personal and professional expertise.[1] Nursing and social work, specifically, have provided guidance on how to lead interprofessional palliative care education and practice.[27,28] Specific interprofessional training in implicit bias, structural inequality, and health disparities for healthcare professionals enhances the ability of teams to provide the most equitable care to all, especially during the serious illness experience when patients and families are so vulnerable.

To facilitate the growth of all professionals in difficult topic areas, the learning climate must include an element of trust and safety. Building personal rapport and camaraderie is essential before tackling more difficult skills and topics such as communication, role conflict, inequity, or bias. This type of climate can be created by leading with patient-focused education, beginning the pedagogy by listening to patient voices to establish the shared goals of care. Small, interprofessional student teams with attentive, well-trained facilitators can enhance the building of trust and communication. Activities where all members of the team are safe to share their understanding and to grow together are essential to a positive learning climate. The level of interprofessional teamwork and trust required to carry out activities should broaden over the course, potentially mirroring students' level of confidence in their skills and value as an interprofessional team member. Building in an element of fun and shared challenge can help a team unify as they begin to better understand each other's roles and responsibilities. Simulations utilizing standardized patients can be an effective pedagogical tool to engage interprofessional learners in enacting the lessons from their shared learning.

Step 6: Evaluation and Feedback

Student Assessment

Evaluation, assessment, and feedback enable both faculty and learners to monitor progress toward realizing learning objectives, and can be approached in various ways. Formative assessment refers to tools or instruments that identify misunderstandings, difficulties, and learning gaps and assess how to close those gaps. Formative assessments evaluate the learner's abilities *throughout* the coursework and includes evaluation of the instructor or the module, whereas summative assessments are used to evaluate student learning or proficiency at the conclusion of a program.[29] Ideally, each student should be evaluated before, during, and after the program to assess for learning and growth areas during student progression. A comprehensive evaluation process may be accomplished through a program analysis that can include standard course evaluations, semistructured interviews and/or focus groups facilitated by advisors, and learner self-assessments on interprofessional palliative care skills/tasks throughout the program's formal training, communication skills exercises, discussion boards, assignment submissions, and problem-solving case studies. Adapted from Weissman et al,[30] Table 6.2 is an example of the University of Colorado Anschutz Medical Campus MSPC self-assessment that learners have completed over the program's course (pre-, mid-, and post-program).[3] These learner self-assessments ensure that students achieve the outlined competences and also measure if students have become employed in a palliative care work setting. Course evaluations and student feedback about faculty teaching methods also contribute to course and content improvement. The Interprofessional Collaborative Competencies Attainment Survey (ICCAS), a 20-item, learner self-assessment tool commonly utilized in interprofessional courses, measures student collaboration, communication, roles and responsibilities, collaborative patient- and family-centered approach, conflict management/resolution, and team functioning.[31]

Formative and summative assessment of students' interprofessional palliative care growth may also include the incorporation of role-play activities. In-class team-based role-plays of palliative care clinical scenarios provide a safe setting to address end-of-life ethics and communication, roles in family meetings, as well as team comfort in discussing potentially emotionally distressing case scenarios. Through the inclusion of actors in simulated patient role-plays or the use of video clips and critique, student teams can test their clinical skills in unpredictable patient/family interactions. These activities enable students to explore leadership roles and the shared responsibility of developing patient care plans.[7] The addition of team debriefs through watching and evaluating videos of their interprofessional patient/family interactions facilitate students' reflection on their strengths and areas for growth. Course instructors and/or team facilitators also serve vital roles in providing in-the-moment feedback on student and group performance in implementing interprofessional practice skills. This real-time feedback enables students to dialogue about their strengths, and consider their potential for personal and interprofessional growth.

Another method to evaluate student interprofessional growth is the use of qualitative assessments tools such as journal entries, focus groups, open-ended survey items on assessments, critical reflections, or narrative self-assessments. These qualitative approaches pair well with quantitative measures in providing students opportunities to reflect on their personal and interprofessional growth. Post-course focus groups can provide course leaders with insight into student impressions of

Table 6.2 University of Colorado Anschutz Medical Campus MSPC Student Survey Self-Assessment of Competence in Palliative Care Skills

For each item there are 2 responses.

Response 1: Now. Select the response that best reflects your competence to perform each patient/family interaction or patient management skill at the time of the assessment—pre,- mid-, or post-program.

Response 2: Look Back. Select the response that best reflects your self-assessed competence to perform each patient/family interaction or patient management skill **before** you started the MSPC course of study.

Item #	Item	I need basic instruction.	I feel competent to perform with close supervision or coaching.	I feel competent to perform with minimal supervision.	I feel competent to perform independently.	I feel competent to perform independently and teach others.
1	Perform a whole-person patient assessment	1	2	3	4	5
2	Collaborate effectively with the interdisciplinary team to create a care plan to address physical, psychological, social, practical, and spiritual needs	1	2	3	4	5
3	Talk with patient/family about prognosis	1	2	3	4	5
4	Give bad news to a patient/family	1	2	3	4	5
5	Collaborate effectively with an interdisciplinary team to optimize patient/family comfort	1	2	3	4	5
6	Coordinate care across settings using written and verbal communications	1	2	3	4	5
7	Perform a pain assessment	1	2	3	4	5
8	Manage use of oral opioid analgesics	1	2	3	4	5
9	Manage use of parenteral opioid analgesics	1	2	3	4	5
10	Titrate opioid doses for optimal pain relief	1	2	3	4	5
11	Manage use of adjuvant analgesics (e.g., tricyclics, steroids, anticonvulsants)	1	2	3	4	5

Table 6.2 Continued

Item #	Item	I need basic instruction.	I feel competent to perform with close supervision or coaching.	I feel competent to perform with minimal supervision.	I feel competent to perform independently.	I feel competent to perform independently and teach others.
12	Assess and manage delirium	1	2	3	4	5
13	Assess and manage dyspnea	1	2	3	4	5
14	Assess and manage nausea and vomiting	1	2	3	4	5
15	Assess and manage constipation	1	2	3	4	5
16	Assess and manage sleep disturbances	1	2	3	4	5
17	Assess and manage depression	1	2	3	4	5
18	Identify a patient who is imminently dying	1	2	3	4	5
19	Assess patient decision-making capacity	1	2	3	4	5
20	Discuss a shift in treatment approach (goals of care) from curative to comfort care	1	2	3	4	5
21	Discuss advance directives with patients/families	1	2	3	4	5
22	Discuss do-not-resuscitate (DNR) orders with patients/families	1	2	3	4	5
23	Discuss requests for physician assisted death	1	2	3	4	5
24	Ensure comfort during withdrawal of mechanical ventilation	1	2	3	4	5
25	Discuss use and withdrawal of non-beneficial treatments (e.g., antibiotics, hydration, non-oral feedings, routine medications)	1	2	3	4	5
26	Conduct a family conference to discuss end-of-life decisions	1	2	3	4	5

Table 6.2 Continued

Item #	Item	I need basic instruction.	I feel competent to perform with close supervision or coaching.	I feel competent to perform with minimal supervision.	I feel competent to perform independently.	I feel competent to perform independently and teach others.
27	Discuss home hospice referral	1	2	3	4	5
28	Recognize and address suicide risk	1	2	3	4	5
29	Assess and address psychosocial concerns (anxiety, grief, financial worries)	1	2	3	4	5
30	Communicate effectively in highly emotive clinical situations	1	2	3	4	5
31	Initiate communications with other physicians and staff regarding end-of-life care	1	2	3	4	5
32	Initiate a conversation with patient/family about spirituality	1	2	3	4	5
33	Recognize and address spiritual distress/existential suffering	1	2	3	4	5
34	Recognize and access spiritual resources	1	2	3	4	5
35	Create a care plan that reflects cultural values and practices (e.g., dietary needs, rituals)	1	2	3	4	5
36	Address communication barriers (e.g., language, literacy, sensory impairments) that limit patient/family comprehension of current situation and care plan	1	2	3	4	5
37	Discuss integrative modalities with patients/families	1	2	3	4	5

(*continued*)

Table 6.2 Continued

Item #	Item	I need basic instruction.	I feel competent to perform with close supervision or coaching.	I feel competent to perform with minimal supervision.	I feel competent to perform independently.	I feel competent to perform independently and teach others.
38	Identify ethical issues affecting patient/family	1	2	3	4	5
39	Know when you need to call for an ethics consultation	1	2	3	4	5

Adapted from Weissman DE, Ambuel B, Norton AJ, et al. A survey of competencies and concerns in end-of-life care for physician trainees. *J Pain Symptom Manage.* 1998;15:82–90.

instructional methods, curriculum, and their own growth resulting from their team-based learning. Semi-structured mid- and/or post-course reflection assignments offer students the ability to assimilate their own personal and interprofessional development, areas of growth, insight, and potential to engage their skills in future interprofessional palliative care practice. The University of Texas at Austin's FICP incorporated summative assessment across all professions in the form of a post-course semi-structured reflection assignment. This qualitative evaluation of students' learning aimed to capture the nuances of growth and insight that a quantitative survey might not capture. Although not all healthcare professional schools from the course have completed their analysis, the social work profession published findings from a thematic analysis of 133 BSW and MSW level students' post-course reflections.[7] Findings from the study revealed 4 key themes: the whole is greater than the sum of its parts; taking leadership roles; finding one's voice; and future practice. These themes reflect social work students' enhanced understanding of the additive strength of the team's combined interprofessional skills; their ability to practice leadership roles with the team and during simulated case scenarios; their acknowledgment of their value on the team; and their keen interest in carrying their acquired interprofessional skills into future practice.

Finally, the Kirkpatrick Model (Figure 6.1),[32] a commonly used method to evaluate the effectiveness of training programs and learning solutions, has been used to evaluate the MSPC and the IPCC educational programs at the University of Colorado Anschutz Medical Campus. The Kirkpatrick Model has 4 levels: (1) reaction, (2) learning, (3) behavior, and (4) results.[32] In Level 1, evaluating reaction describes student perceptions or satisfaction with the program. Level 2, learning, occurs when knowledge has increased, attitudes have changed, and/or there is improvement in skill acquisition. Level 3, behavior or application of the learning, is an indication as to how on-the-job behavior has changed due to the program. Level 4,

THE KIRKPATRICK MODEL

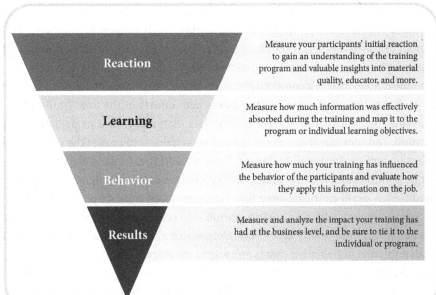

Figure 6.1. The Kirkpatrick Model.

results, determines a program's impact on organizational benefits and the final results that occur. In the palliative care area, level 4 evaluates whether the learning transfers to the clinical setting and improves patient outcomes. Consideration of Level 4 in the Kirkpatrick Model from the beginning can guide program development and identify the results that students and faculty wish to achieve.[32]

Curriculum Evaluation

Curriculum evaluation must be continually performed to ensure student learning, curricular effectiveness, evidence-based changes to courses and pedagogy, and achievement of program competencies and educational outcomes. As faculty continually improve the curriculum using a multitude of teaching and assessment strategies, effectiveness of student learning is ensured. Three assessment milestones regarding curriculum assessment have been identified. First, student course evaluations and surveys must be reviewed by program directors in order to make appropriate modifications to courses or curriculum. Second, an annual review of the program's core competencies ensures that courses are mapped to the competencies using various assessment methodologies. For example, some assignments and evaluation methods may include individual written and videotaped dialogues and reflections; verbal and written educational presentations; case study integration, including patient- and family-centered care plans; communications skills demonstration in simulated practice settings; family meetings; and capstone (end of course) projects. In the University of Colorado MSPC program, students apply what they have learned to the real world through the design and implementation of a systems change project (e.g., quality improvement, education, needs assessment, program development or evaluation) in their work setting. Each student is assigned a faculty mentor based on their topic choice. After project implementation, the student presents a professional abstract and poster to their colleagues and program faculty.

The third milestone is a comprehensive review of programmatic objectives. This final review is the culmination of the assessment efforts of the first 2 milestones. The evaluation process utilizes assessment data, national trends in palliative care education, and input from faculty and other stakeholders to ensure the curriculum is effective and professionally relevant. Results of all these assessment milestones must be communicated to all faculty so that changes can be made, as appropriate. In addition, a significant challenge that faces educators is the impact of an educational program on palliative care integration into real-world settings and its effect on patients and their family caregivers. Determining whether students have taken on a new job role in palliative care is one way to measure the program's impact.

An additional method for utilizing real-time assessments to enhance course development is the use of "Just in Time (JIT) Faculty Training and Debriefs" directly before and after each educational session. These JIT prepare faculty immediately before a class to facilitate the interprofessional activities and dialogues, and engage faculty in an immediate post-session debriefing to capture the effectiveness of teaching methods, curriculum, and student responses to activities. This immediate debriefing also allows faculty to take the pulse of students' emotional well-being, seek consultation from other faculty about challenges in student team dynamics, and explore ways to prepare for upcoming sessions or future renditions of the course. Course leadership can then adjust or iterate the pedagogical approach "just in time" to support constant quality improvement.

Conclusion

Palliative care is and has always been a team-based approach to meeting patients' and families' needs to optimize quality of life and reduce suffering. While palliative care, as a field, has been a leader in developing interprofessional models of care that include medical, psychosocial, and spiritual aspects of care, there are few specific guidelines for interprofessional palliative care team training. As palliative care education continues to evolve, it is essential to incorporate the pedagogical evidence from interprofessional collaborative care and team-based learning to train professionals together before they are in practice. Palliative care is inherently interprofessional in nature. Future interprofessional education efforts should include palliative care cases, skills, and simulations to enhance the awareness of palliative care skills across health professional learners. Similarly, palliative care education efforts benefit from incorporating the interprofessional collaborative core competencies. The future of interprofessional palliative care education should include more explicit and evidence-based teaching of interprofessional collaborative practice that includes all of the voices on the team, including those of patients and families.

Discussion Questions

1. What is essential for healthcare professional and pre-professional students to learn interprofessional palliative care?
2. What methods can be used to assess learners in interprofessional palliative care training programs?
3. How do simulations and standardized patients enhance the interprofessional learning experiences for students?
4. How can patients and family caregivers provide feedback and be included as team members in the interprofessional learning experience?

Resources

- American Academy of Hospice and Palliative Medicine (AAHPM): http://aahpm.org/
- Center to Advance Palliative Care (CAPC): https://www.capc.org/
- Hospice and Palliative Nurses Association (HPNA): https://advancingexpertcare.org/
- Interprofessional Education Collaborative (IPEC): https://www.ipecollaborative.org/
- National Center for Interprofessional Practice and Education: https://nexusipe.org
- Social Work Hospice and Palliative Care Network (SWHPN): https://www.swhpn.org/
- Spiritual Care Association: https://www.spiritualcareassociation.org/resources.html
- The CSU Shiley Haynes Institute for Palliative Care: https://csupalliativecare.org/career-development/

References

1. Seaman JB, Lakin JR, Anderson E, et al. Interdisciplinary or interprofessional: why terminology in teamwork matters to hospice and palliative care. *J Palliat Med.* 2020;23(9):1157–1158.
2. World Health Organization. *Framework for Action on Interprofessional Education and Collaborative Practice.* 2010. Accessed November 14, 2020. https://www.who.int/publications/i/item/framework-for-action-on-interprofessional-education-collaborative-practice.

3. Fink RM, Arora K, Gleason SE, et al. Interprofessional master of science in palliative care: on becoming a palliative care community specialist. *J Palliat Med.* 2020;23(10):1370–1376.

4. Hospice and Palliative Nurses Association. *Competencies for the Hospice and Palliative APN.* 2nd ed. HPNA; 2014.

5. Ferrell BR, Twaddle ML, Melnick A, Meier DE. National consensus project clinical practice guidelines for quality palliative care guidelines. *J Palliat Med.* 2018;21(12):1684–1689.

6. National Quality Forum. *National Voluntary Consensus Standards for Palliative Care and End-of-Life Care.* 2006. Accessed November 14, 2020. https://www.qualityforum.org/Proje cts/Palliative_Care_and_End-of-Life_Care.aspx

7. Jones B, Currin-McCulloch J, Petruzzi L, Phillips F, Kaushik S, Smith B. Transformative teams in health care: enhancing social work student identity, voice, and leadership in a longitudinal Interprofessional Education (IPE) course. *Adv Soc Work.* 2020;20(2):424–439.

8. Thomas PA, Kern DE, Hughes MT, Chen BY, editors. *Curriculum Development for Medical Education: A Six-Step Approach.* JHU Press; 2016.

9. Fink RM, Oman KS, Youngwerth J, Bryant LL. A palliative care needs assessment of rural hospitals. *J Palliat Med.* 2013;16(6):638–644.

10. Silbermann M, Fink RM, Min SJ, et al. Evaluating palliative care needs in Middle Eastern countries. *J Palliat Med.* 2015;18(1):18–25.

11. Coats H, Paganelli T, Starks H, et al. A community needs assessment for the development of an interprofessional palliative care training curriculum. *J Palliat Med.* 2017;20(3):235–240. doi:10.1089/jpm.2016.0321

12. McConigley R, Aoun S, Kristjanson L, et al. Implementation and evaluation of an education program to guide palliative care for people with motor neurone disease. *Palliat Med.* 2012;26(8):994–1000.

13. American Association of Colleges of Nursing. *Graduate Competencies and Recommendations for Educating Nursing Students (G-CARES).* AACN; 2019. https://www.aacnnursing.org/Port als/42/ELNEC/PDF/Graduate-CARES.pdf.

14. Arnold R, Billings JA, Block SD, et al. *Hospice and Palliative Medicine Core Competencies.* Version 2.3. American Academy of Hospice and Palliative Medicine; 2009.

15. Best M, Leget C, Goodhead A, Paal P. An EAPC white paper on multi-disciplinary education for spiritual care in palliative care. *BMC Palliat Care.* 2020;19(1):9.

16. Bosma H, Johnston M, Cadell S, et al. Canadian social work competencies for hospice palliative care: a framework to guide education and practice at the generalist and specialist levels 2008. *Preuzeto s.* Accessed November 14, 2020. http://cms.virtualhospice.ca/Web/CVH/Ass ets/Social_Work_Competencies_July_2009_20150708134353.pdf (16.4.2019).

17. Carey EC, Paniagua M, Morrison LJ, et al. Palliative care competencies and readiness for independent practice: a report on the American Academy of Hospice and Palliative Medicine review of the US Medical Licensing Step Examinations. *J Pain Symptom Manage.* 2018;56(3):371–378.

18. Gamondi C, Larkin PJ, Payne S. Core competencies in palliative care Part 1 & 2. *Eur J Palliat Care.* 2013;20(2):86–91.

19. Jacono B, Young L, Baker C, et al. Developing palliative care competencies for the education of entry level baccalaureate prepared Canadian nurses. *Int J Nurs Ed Scholar.* 2011;15;8(1).

20. National Association of Social Workers. *NASW Standards for Social Work Practice in Palliative and End of Life Care.* NASW; 2004.

21. Kwak J, Jamal A, Jones B, Timmerman G, Hughes B, Fry L. An interprofessional approach to advance care planning. *J Pain Symptom Manage.* 2022;39(3):321–331. https://doi.org/ 10.1177/10499091211019316

22. Nedjat-Haiem FR, Carrion IV, Gonzalez K, Ell K, Thompson B, Mishra SI. Exploring health care providers' views about initiating end-of-life care communication. *Am J Hosp Palliat Med.* 2017;34(4):308–317.

23. Interprofessional Education Collaborative. Core Competencies for Interprofessional Collaborative Practice: 2016 Update. IPEC; 2016. Accessed October 29, 2020. https://nebula. wsimg.com/2f68a39520b03336b41038c370497473?AccessKeyId=DC06780E69ED19E2B 3A5&disposition=0&alloworigin=1.

24. Donesky D, Dooernbos A, Fink RM, Kitko L, Bailey FA, Hurd C. Excellence in post-licensure interprofessional palliative care education: consensus through a Delphi survey *J Palliat Nurs.* 2020;22(1):17–25.

25. Sosniak LA. *Bloom's Taxonomy.* Anderson LW, ed. University of Chicago Press; 1994.

26. Anderson LW, Bloom BS. *A Taxonomy for Learning, Teaching, and Assessing: A Revision of Bloom's Taxonomy of Educational Objectives.* Longman; 2001.

27. Blacker S, Head BA, Jones BL, Remke SS, Supiano K. Advancing hospice and palliative care social work leadership in interprofessional education and practice. *J Soc Work End Life Palliat Care.* 2016;12(4):316–330.

28. Jones B, Phillips F. Social work and interprofessional education in health care: a call for continued leadership. *J Soc Work Ed.* 2016;52(1):18–29.

29. Theall M, Franklin JL. Assessing teaching practices and effectiveness for formative purposes. In: Gillespie KJ, Robertson D, and Associates, eds. *A guide to faculty development. 2nd ed.* Jossey-Bass; 2010:Chapter 10, 151–168.

30. Weissman DE, Ambuel B, Norton AJ, et al. A survey of competencies and concerns in end-of-life care for physician trainees. *J Pain Symptom Manage* 1998;15:82–90.

31. Schmitz CC, Radosevich DM, Jardine P, MacDonald CJ, Trumpower D, Archibald D. The Interprofessional Collaborative Competency Attainment Survey (ICCAS): a replication validation study. *J Interprof Care.* 2017;31(1):28–34.

32. Kirkpatrick DL. Evaluation of training. In: Craig RL, Bittel LR, eds. *Training and Development Handbook.* McGraw Hill; 1967:87–112. Kirkpatrick website: https://www.kirkpatrickpartn ers.com/Our-Philosophy.

7

State of the Evidence for Interprofessional Education in Palliative Care

Tara J. Schapmire and Mark P. Pfeifer

Key Points

- To date, studies have shown feasibility and wide acceptance, with some success at improving collaboration and communication.
- While evidence for the value of interprofessional education (IPE) in palliative care is growing rapidly, the body of work presented generally reveals small sample sizes, self-selected trainees, self-reported outcomes, frequent low evaluation-response rates, and minimal longitudinal outcome measures.
- The most commonly measured outcomes are course evaluation/satisfaction, knowledge, attitudes/perception, and competence/skills, all in the areas of palliative and end-of-life care, collaboration, and communication. Patient outcomes have not been measured.
- Future studies should improve size and scale, the dependable use of validated evaluation instruments and objective outcome measures.

Introduction

Since its creation in 2001, the National Consensus Project for Quality Palliative Care (NCP)[1] has inspired excellence in palliative and hospice care from the clinical practice level to the programmatic level, and all the way "upstream" to the educational level. Clinical research on the impact of palliative care has increasingly offered promise toward the attainment of the triple aim of healthcare[2]: enhancing patient experience,[3-6] improving population health,[7] and reducing costs.[6,8-13] According to the World Health Organization (WHO), interprofessional education (IPE) is an experience that "occurs when students from 2 or more professions learn about, from, and with each other."[14] Unfortunately, most health professional education still occurs in discipline*-specific silos, with minimal interaction among professions. Competencies, strategies, and accreditation requirements for IPE are clearly outlined[15,16]; however, developing and implementing IPE activities at the grassroots level challenges institutions. Crowded curricula, differing academic calendars, disparate cultures between disciplines, and logistical issues are some barriers which may seem insurmountable.[17] After almost 20 years of "upstream" efforts to create quality interprofessional palliative care educational opportunities in both academic and clinical settings, questions remain: Are they effective? Do they improve practice and patient care? This chapter attempts to answer these questions by exploring the state of the science of interprofessional palliative care education.

Methods

Our purpose was to review the impact of palliative care IPE interventional studies on learner and/or patient outcomes for pre- and post-licensure healthcare learners. The literature search for this chapter utilized 3 databases: PubMed, ClinicalKey, and Cochrane. Search terms and controlled vocabulary included "palliative care," "palliative medicine," "education," "training," "interprofessional education," and "interdisciplinary education." Articles in languages other than English or not translated into English were excluded. The initial search resulted in 294 articles. The authors reviewed abstracts and selected articles published between 2001 and 2020 that presented an interactive interprofessional palliative care educational intervention targeted to learners in at least 2 professions, and measured learner or patient outcomes. Eligible study designs included quantitative, qualitative, and mixed methods. This resulted in 80 full articles reviewed. Full article reviews revealed studies reporting education on interprofessional practice but that did not have actual IPE curriculum as defined above. These studies reported educational interventions where trainees learned *about* each other through online modules or lectures that were not reported as explicitly interactive; we excluded these as non-IPE, as learners did not learn *from and with* each other. The 41 articles meeting inclusion criteria are reviewed here.

In our experience in mentoring faculty teams who wish to create palliative IPE learning experiences at their own institutions, we find that many teams start the process thinking, "We have X learners in X disciplines in X level training programs (undergraduate/graduate/clinical, etc.), so what can we do?" Because of that entry

---

* Although often used interchangeably, "discipline" refers to a branch of knowledge, while "profession" refers to an occupation that requires special education and/or prolonged training and a formal qualification. In this book, we have attempted to standardize the use of the term "profession" when referring to occupations such as chaplaincy, medicine, nursing, and social work, but occasionally the term "discipline" is used, especially when focused on the theory and knowledge development of the professions.

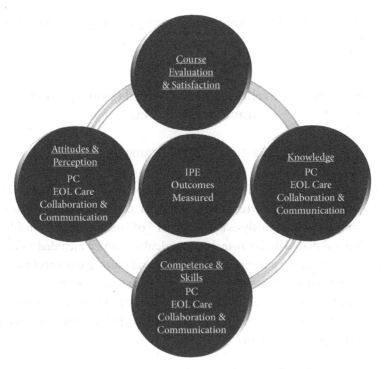

Figure 7.1. Most common IPE outcomes measured across all studies.

point, we divided our studies by the target learner population so that readers could go directly to the studies most relevant to their own learners. The first section of this review is focused on palliative care IPE offered in academic settings; we highlight the literature by educational level and according to the predominant outcomes measured. The second section is focused on palliative care IPE offered in the clinical setting. Due to the diversity of the targeted learner groups in clinical settings, we present the literature by professional specialty/clinical settings. Outcomes measured in all studies tend to fall in the areas of course evaluation/satisfaction, knowledge, attitudes/perception, and competence/skills, all in the areas of palliative and end-of-life care (PC/EOL), and collaboration and/or communication. Figure 7.1 highlights these outcomes.

Evidence for Interprofessional Academic Education in Palliative Care

Academic institutions have offered a variety of examples of interprofessional palliative care curricula, both with undergraduate and graduate learners. Most outcomes measured were program feasibility and/or learner knowledge or attitudes, with none focusing on patient outcomes. There were 14 studies aimed at undergraduate or mixed undergraduate/graduate learners and 8 studies aimed at graduate-level learners. They are presented here in those groups and by the outcomes they measured.

Undergraduate Prelicensure and Mixed (Undergraduate/Graduate) Programs

Satisfaction/Course Evaluation

While some studies included measures of satisfaction or course evaluation among their outcomes, only one reported solely on learner satisfaction and course evaluation. This mixed methods analysis by Grey et al[18] of satisfaction with an advance-care planning and shared decision-making curriculum, which included video and a role-playing workshop for advanced year medical and nursing students ($n = 85$), revealed good to excellent ratings regarding the meeting of course objectives, clinical relevance, teaching effectiveness, and overall workshop experience. Other studies may have reported these outcomes, but they were included with other outcomes and are presented in later sections.

Attitudes/Perception

Three studies focused on attitudes and perception related to palliative care (PC), end-of-life (EOL) care topics, or PC/EOL-related collaboration and/or communication. They used a variety of methods and highlight various examples of ways to improve these targeted outcomes.

A small study by Fairchild et al[19] examined the effectiveness of a 6-week, multidisciplinary, team-based, clinical placement in supportive oncology for learners in medicine, nutrition, occupational- and physio-therapy, and speech-language pathology ($n = 8$). Descriptive statistics revealed growth from pre- to post-test and sustained growth at 6 months on attitudes toward IPE and health professions.

Fineberg et al[20] conducted a quasi-experimental, longitudinal study analyzing the impact of a 4-session palliative care training program for medical and social work students that included didactics, experiential, interactive exercises covering stereotypes and roles, and role-played family conferences in the intervention group ($n = 45$) compared to a control group ($n = 26$). Self-administered surveys completed at baseline and at 3 months post-intervention revealed that perceived role understanding significantly improved for the intervention group compared to the control group, and gains were maintained at 3 months.

A small repeated-measures study by Sinha et al[21] examined a student-run series of 3 interactive workshops designed to foster a reflective and collaborative approach to EOL care through art, science, and standardized patients. Students in medicine and nursing ($n = 38$) completed a survey created by researchers exploring attitudes about collaboration, EOL issues, and the value of good EOL care at baseline, immediately after the last workshop, and at 6 months post-workshop. While there were no differences between medicine and nursing student average scores, the composite average scores for both groups improved significantly from pre- to post-test, and differences were sustained or higher at 6 months.

Multiple Outcomes

Ten studies highlighted examples of methods using multiple targeted outcomes. They vary in size, disciplines included, and educational modalities used, while offering insight into successful implementation efforts with many variables. A U.S. NIH-funded initiative by Head et al[22] sought to create and widely disseminate a comprehensive, mandatory oncology palliative care curriculum for learners in graduate chaplain residency, undergraduate medicine and nursing, and graduate social work programs. The multimodal curriculum included online case-based modules, a clinical rotation with a palliative care team, a reflective writing session, and an interdisciplinary case management experience using simulated role plays and video prompts. A mixed methods analysis with 373 learners revealed significant improvement in palliative care knowledge, skills, and readiness for IPE. Learners appreciated the experiential aspects, including observation of clinical palliative care teams and team-based skills practice with other learners.

A pilot mixed-methods study by Bradway et al[23] presented an analysis of a group of 73 learners in chaplaincy, medicine, nursing, pharmacy, physical and occupational therapies, and social work on self-reported level of confidence in interprofessional palliative care communication, behavior change, and professional identity after a workshop that included pre-readings and videos, and mock team meetings with standardized patients. Significant post-workshop growth occurred in self-reported level of confidence in interprofessional palliative care communication. Learners identified areas of behavior change and professional identity in written comments, in addition to providing faculty with feedback for future workshops.

Ellman et al[24] reported an analysis of the impact of a bimodal curriculum teaching spiritual and cultural aspects of palliative care, combining readings and online learning with a 90-minute live, interactive, small-group, problem-based simulation for students in divinity, medicine, nursing, and social work. They evaluated student self-reports of curriculum effectiveness at meeting objectives and increasing knowledge. Free text responses to online reflections ($n = 217$) indicated that learners recognized important issues beyond their discipline, the roles of other professionals on the team, and the importance of collaboration. Post-workshop questionnaires ($n = 309$) indicated learner perception that learning objectives were met. Trainees found the workshop useful and of high quality.

In a study by Erickson et al[25] aimed at improving communication and collaboration skills among medical and nursing students ($n = 136$), analysis of a 90-minute workshop on difficult discussions revealed learner growth on attitudes toward teamwork, but mixed results on confidence in communication/collaboration. Medical students did not significantly improve in attitudes toward physician-nurse collaboration or self-efficacy in communication, while nursing students improved significantly in both.

In a small, mixed methods study, Kaasalainen et al[26] conducted an analysis of a 5-day palliative care workshop that included small group problem-based sessions, as well as a Team Observed Structured Clinical Exam (TOSCE) among 25 learners in chaplaincy, medicine, nursing, occupational therapy and physiotherapy, and social work. Quantitative results indicated significant growth in readiness for IPE and perceptions of professional identity and team understanding from pre- to post-workshop. Qualitative results highlighted the value of learning about each other, learning to learn together, learning the benefits of IPE, and learning the possibilities of more collaborative practice.

An evaluation by Price et al[27] of a full-day, interactive workshop for nursing and midwifery students ($n = 73$), aimed at improving awareness of EOL care for infants in conjunction with the support of their families, used a mixed-methods design. Learners had significant growth in self-reported confidence after the intervention. Qualitative data revealed an appreciation for perinatal/neonatal palliative care, learning together, and impact on future practice.

The impact of a 2-session interprofessional, interactive, team-based, problem-based learning module on palliative EOL care on over 1000 learners in medicine, nursing, pharmacy, nutrition, physical therapy, clinical psychology, and social work was explored over 3 years by McKee et al.[28] Post-intervention satisfaction, including usefulness of curriculum, enjoyment, and facilitator effectiveness, were moderately high to very high. A retrospective self-assessment of knowledge of palliative care and other professions revealed statistically significant gains.

A small pilot pre- and post-analysis by Hall et al[29] of a synchronous online module on total pain assessed attitudes and satisfaction among 20 learners in medicine, nursing, physiotherapy and spiritual care. While attitude scores improved, they were not statistically significant, possibly due to a small sample size. Learners were satisfied with the experience and, in a 3-month follow-up survey, reported sustained value and indicated that they were applying what they learned in practice.

Prelock et al[30] compared the impact by discipline of an in-person film discussion focused on EOL care for 162 learners in undergraduate and graduate medicine, nursing, physical therapy, social work, and speech-language pathology. Using post-intervention evaluation of self-reported competency for interprofessional practice, few significant differences were found between the disciplines. Open-ended questions revealed that learners found the experience to be valuable.

A pilot study by Saylor et al[31] measured self-efficacy, attitudes toward physician-nurse collaboration, and interprofessional competencies as outcomes of a palliative care simulation among 104 learners in medicine and nursing. Overall mean and within-group (experience and discipline) self-efficacy scores improved significantly. Attitudes improved significantly overall, but not within groups by experience or discipline. Significant differences in nurse and physician evaluator TOSCE scores existed, though there were inconsistencies between evaluation methods.

Graduate Programs

While most studies reported on mixed levels of education among learners—which can be challenging in the creation of learning experiences that are relevant and useful to all learners—these 8 focused on graduate programs and provide insight into the use of higher-level curricula with their learners. One study offers an example of how to study career progression following a learning experience, while 3 highlight models aimed at improving competence and skills. The largest subgroup of 4 studies examined multiple outcomes.

Career Progression

One study by Koffman and Higginson[32] examined the impact of an interprofessional course in palliative care on career progression for 44 learners in mostly medicine and nursing who ranged from 1 to 6 years post course completion. A large majority of learners were practicing in palliative care, and most showed progression in terms of clinical responsibilities and positions as well. Qualitative data revealed learner appreciation for broadened thinking, challenging misconceptions, enhancing teamwork, professional networks, and confidence.

Competence/Skills

A study by Fink et al[33] of the impact of a mostly online interprofessional Master of Science program in palliative care on 66 learners showed improved self-reported palliative care competence. Learners included mostly nurses, with very small numbers in medicine, pharmacy, physician assistant programs, psychology, social work, and spiritual care.

Bays et al[34] reported on an experiential communications workshop, led by newly trained facilitators, on learners in medicine residency and nurse practitioner programs. They used a pre-post design measuring communication behavior in recorded standardized patient encounters. Recordings were coded for effective communication behaviors, and 145 trainees' scores improved in 8 of 11 coded behaviors.

An interprofessional simulation on withdrawal of life-sustaining measures aimed at improving team communication skills of 11 interprofessional teams of students representing medicine, nursing, and social work was evaluated by Lippe et al.[35] The 3-phase simulation required teams to communicate with the patient, family, and one another in the care of a seriously ill patient at the end of life. Team communication in the filmed simulations was analyzed by researchers using a communication behavior checklist. Results revealed fair to good communication across the 9 communication domains.

Multiple Outcomes

A U.S. Health Resources and Services Administration (HRSA)–funded study by Gellis et al[36] of a simulation-based geriatric palliative care training, targeting 111 learners in chaplaincy, medicine, nursing, occupational therapy, pharmacy, and social work, used a mix of pre- and post-measures as well as post- only, while also comparing those who participated in the simulation to those who only observed. Measures included attitudes toward healthcare teams (pre/post), communication self-efficacy (pre/post), interprofessional collaboration (post), and training satisfaction. Growth in attitudes and self-efficacy was statistically significant from pre- to post-test. Collaboration in 3 of 4 subscales was significantly better for the participant learners than it was for observer learners. Most participants were satisfied with the training.

A mixed methods study of TeamTalk by Donesky et al,[37] a series of interactive communication workshops including small group discussion, reflection, and high-fidelity simulation, reported on 61 learners in chaplaincy, medicine, and nursing. Attitudes toward interprofessional collaboration improved from pre- to post-test for all learners (only measured in year 2), while no individual professional group differences were found. Mixed, but encouraging, results were found for perceived self-efficacy in communication. Qualitative data documented learner appreciation for the opportunity to explore their professional roles together and with other professions.

Sixty-one learners in mostly medicine and nursing were evaluated by Lakin et al[38] for the impact of a multimodal curriculum for quality improvement as part of a palliative care fellowship program. Course assignments revealed improvement in targeted skills, knowledge, and attitudes, and course assessments demonstrated satisfaction. Significance levels were not reported.

A mixed methods study by Lee et al[39] evaluated the use of a virtual reality world educational environment (Second Life) for teaching palliative care among 35 interprofessional graduate learners in medicine, nursing, nutrition, physical therapy, and social work. Feasibility and acceptability were confirmed, with mixed significance with regard to self-reported attitudes toward teams, readiness for interprofessional learning, interprofessional collaboration, and team skills and fitness.

Table 7.1 Most Common Features of PC/EOL IPE Initiatives[18-39] for Academic Settings, 2001–2020

Program Goals	Pilot/Feasibility Studies
Primary content	Communication and collaboration
Methods	Multimodal curricula with online modules/videos and readings culminating in workshops using role-play and/or simulations
Duration	Less than a year
Trainees	Learners in all health professions, predominantly nursing and medicine
Outcome measures	Mix of satisfaction and self-reported attitude/perception, knowledge, and self-efficacy/confidence outcomes
Patient outcomes	Not measured

Summary of Academic Efforts

Overall, several themes came to light for IPE interventions in academic settings (Table 7.1). Most studies were pilot and feasibility programs with a mix of satisfaction and self-reported self-efficacy/confidence outcomes. Multimodal curricula with online modules/videos and readings culminating in workshops using role plays and/or simulations were a common method for training.[20,22-24,26,30,33,36-39] Longitudinal efforts were rare.[19-21,32] Communication and collaboration (in PC/EOL care) were popular content topics.[19-28,30,31,33-37,39] Nursing and medicine were the largest group of learners, and most studies enrolled small to modestly sized groups for analysis.

Outcomes were evaluated by a mix of validated and nonvalidated instruments that were predominantly self-reported. Patient outcomes were not reported. Attitudes/perception,[19-27,29-31,36,37,39] knowledge,[22,26,28,38] and competence/skills[22,30,31,33-35,37-39] were the most commonly reported trainee outcomes, and learners generally found the learning experiences favorable in these trials. The studies reported by Head et al,[22] Ellman et al,[24] McKee et al,[28] Lippe et al,[35] Gellis et al,[36] and Donesky et al[37] offer the most promising examples of research on academic palliative care IPE interventions due to their larger study sizes, mixed educational methods, and multimodal evaluation.

Evidence for Interprofessional Clinical Education in Palliative Care

The majority of IPE programs in palliative care target prelicensure students in academic programs, but clinician-focused programs are increasing based on the collective perceived value of interprofessional practice. Compared to academic initiatives, programs designed for practicing clinicians to date are almost exclusively voluntary, self-selected by interested trainees. This particularly impacts both the mix of trainee disciplines and the evaluation of the programs' value. Programs for clinicians are frequently designed to allow optimal integration into busy full-time clinician schedules.

Nineteen IPE studies published from 2001 to 2020 met the criteria outlined previously: an IPE intervention for clinicians with measured outcomes. These studies focused on diverse clinical settings and are presented in those settings.

Primary Palliative Care

The largest number of IPE interventions were aimed at primary palliative care education for all clinicians. In a large study of interdisciplinary teams ($n = 105$ teams, $n = 372$ learners), Friedman et al[40] showed that a 5-hour program that included simulated patients improved confidence and understanding in carrying out goals-of-care (GOC) conversations. The clinical team, typically 4 clinicians, including a nurse, physician, and social worker minimally, completed the course together. Outcomes were self-reported and included one qualitative and one quantitative general question 3 months following the program. A minority of trainees (24%) completed this outcome analysis, with the qualitative responses revealing the major themes of improved communication and increased awareness. Details are not provided on how learners measured improved patient outcomes, but two-thirds of learners said the program accomplished that goal. The authors considered this a pilot study to guide future efforts.

Similarly, Brighton et al[41] found that a half-day communication workshop for nurses, physicians, social workers, and other clinicians showed significant improvement in a cohort of 550 respondents in self-reported confidence, knowledge, and skill in caring for seriously ill patients. The pre-test/post-test method used learner evaluations immediately after the workshop. Role-play was highlighted by trainees as an effective learning tool.

Focusing on spiritual care for patients with advanced illness, Puchalski et al[42] carried out a 2.5-day course that trained pairs of clinicians (chaplains or spiritual care–trained social workers with either nurses or physicians) from the same institution for a train-the-trainer spiritual care initiative. The 48 teams, from 19 U.S. states and 10 other countries, included goal development and institutional leadership to support home institution program growth. Videos and simulated patients augmented the didactic material. Six scheduled phone calls supported the teams' implementations for 1 year after the workshop. While quantitative and qualitative outcomes were only measured by course evaluations, the workshop was rated favorably. The achievement of home institution program goals was not detailed.

Also focusing on palliative care communication, Papadakos et al[43] followed a needs assessment with a pilot study aimed at improving difficult conversations with cancer patients. The 1-month course enrolled and evaluated 40 chaplains, nurses, physicians, social workers, and other clinicians and was held 3 times. After online modules, a simulated patient IPE session addressed specific skills. Trainees self-reported improved competence and confidence in these communication skills.

In a small ($n = 18$) focus-group evaluation of a 3-day course to improve communication and interpersonal skills, Andrew et al[44] showed learners gaining confidence in communication skills but also hindered in transferring those skills to practice by time issues and work environments. Learners in this study were self-selected experienced clinicians, 83% of whom were nurses, who sought out the course voluntarily. Conclusions regarding IPE value itself are limited, as all but 3 of the learners were nurses.

Using IPE to promote collaborative practice, Grymonpre et al[45] evaluated clinicians on 4 inpatient units, including geriatrics and palliative care. The staff of 2 clinical units (orthopedics and internal medicine) received explicit training in IPE and collaborative team practice in preparation for placement of learners on their units. The clinical staff of 2 other units (geriatrics and palliative care) served as controls. The 4 units were dissimilar at baseline. Following training, validated instruments measuring collaborative practice outcomes were not significantly different between the intervention and control groups, despite clinicians reporting benefit from the training. Learner outcomes were not reported. The authors propose that study methodologies due to "real world challenges" and the complexities of drivers of interprofessional collaboration might explain the lack of impact of the intervention on clinical teams.

Specialty Palliative Care

Five studies focused IPE on clinicians in active palliative care practice. In a Chicago multi-institutional initiative, O'Mahony et al[46] reported a longitudinal multi-modal training program for employed clinicians practicing or wanting to practice in palliative care. An application process selected 26 clinicians, largely nurses, physicians, social workers, and chaplains, who completed the program with 4 major components: in-person interprofessional sessions, online learning, clinical mentors with shadowing, and a performance improvement project for their institution. The program was funded by a foundation, and a $5,000 stipend was provided to each trainee when completed. Nonvalidated measures showed improvement in confidence and more frequent use of new palliative care skills. Qualitative analysis supported the multimodal design and interprofessional training. This program has one of the strongest IPE designs to date.

Starks et al[47] reported a pilot study for an eventual palliative care graduate certification program that uses IPE. Twenty-four trainees with clinical experience in palliative care were selected from 99 applicants for a 9-month mixed methodology curriculum to improve palliative care communication, teamwork, and integration in health system environments. The trainees were active clinicians in nursing, medicine, social work, and chaplaincy. The curriculum consisted of 16 webinars, 8 online modules, 4 in-person workshops, and reflective exercises. Qualitative and quantitative analysis showed very significant self-reported improvement in all 3 focused domains.

Acknowledging crowded clinician work schedules, Podgurski et al[48] assessed the value of IPE integrated into standing conferences. The brief intervention focused on improving mindfulness levels in a palliative care academic practice. Five monthly 1-hour sessions for 29 nurses, physicians, physician assistants, and social workers were completed. Post-tests after the training and 7 months later showed increased mindfulness practices but no reduction in clinician burnout, using validated evaluation instruments. The training was feasible in this "workday" model and was valued by trainees.

Two workshop-based initiatives also reported success using IPE. Wittenberg et al[49] adapted the online COMFORT™ SM communication curriculum into a 2-day workshop for interprofessional clinical palliative care teams statewide in California. The 7 modules focused on specific communication skills with role-play, and via a train-the-trainer approach led to implementation of new programs at the trainees' home institutions. Fifty-eight trainees from 29 teams were competitively selected and represented chaplaincy, nursing, medicine, psychology, and social work. Course evaluation showed the training was well received. Nine-month follow-up reported the additional training of 962 clinicians at the trainees' institutions, largely integrated into existing palliative care meetings.

In a smaller-scale program with content focused on breathlessness in advanced illness, Shaw et al[50] held a 3-day workshop for nurses, nurse practitioners, healthcare assistants, and health trainers and advisors ($n = 30$). The content focused on practical clinical skills. Immediate post-tests showed increased confidence and self-reported knowledge.

Critical Care

Two studies addressed critical care clinicians. In a multimodal educational intervention focusing on EOL communication, family meetings, and clinician distress for 200 intensive care unit (ICU) staff, Gordon et al[51] showed that an 8-hour session with simulated patients and small group training improved self-reported abilities in patient care. Nurses predominantly made up the 200-person cohort, with some pharmacy, chaplaincy, and physicians mixed in. Twelve sessions were offered over a year and underwent qualitative and quantitative analysis. This is one of the few clinical IPE programs that was mandatory for some learners.

A small educational intervention by Graham et al[52] for ICU staff ($n = 27$) consisting primarily of nurses and respiratory therapists, with 2 physicians and 1 physical therapist, used focus groups, online learning, and in-person sessions in a 7-hour program targeting general EOL and palliative care knowledge and skills.

Fewer than half of the trainees completed evaluations, and the majority who did were nurses, diminishing the strength of the conclusions that such a program was accepted and feasible for an IPE learner group.

Rural Health

Rural health was the focus of 2 studies. Campion-Smith et al[53] completed a qualitative analysis 5 months following a semi-structured 2-hour evening workshop that sought to evaluate whether workshop skills translated into changes in clinical practice. The learners, largely physicians ($n = 12$) with 5 nurses and 2 social workers, were self-selected and shared stories around their work in palliative care using a facilitated discussion. This small study was evaluated by transcripts of follow-up phone calls and showed the majority of trainees felt more confident in their patient and family interaction skills after the workshop, and that the single brief session did impact their practice.

Kortes-Miller et al[54] used on-site small-group learning led by trained local facilitators in an effort to improve palliative care delivery in rural long-term care facilities in Canada. The content was delivered in multiple 2.5-hour evening sessions, with 15 total hours of training. Specific palliative care content was based on surveying learners' needs in advance. Nurses made up most learners, with aides and therapists also engaged. Outcomes were measured only by trainee feedback and reported generalized increase in comfort and confidence in delivering palliative care.

Geriatrics and Long-Term Care

Two other studies addressed geriatrics and long-term-care clinicians more generally. Lally et al,[55] in an effort to impact the care of frail elderly in an accountable care organization network, implemented a 2-arm curriculum in geriatrics for primary care practices that included a module on palliative care. The content included an emphasis on GOC discussions. Training was via 1-hour in-person sessions held at the ambulatory practice sites. Physicians made up most of the trainees, but nurses and office managers were involved. The intervention was variable, driven by each practice's choice in content and attendees, but all included the GOC session. Overall, 19 sessions were carried out over 5 practices. In a second arm, large interdisciplinary sessions for clinical managers, primarily with nursing backgrounds, engaged 173 trainees in 10 sessions. Evaluation instruments were unvalidated pre- and immediate post-test. Post-test scores showed a significant increase in confidence and self-reported geriatric and palliative care knowledge. Patient outcomes were not measured. Separately, Solberg et al[56] held a half-day geriatric boot camp that included a brief palliative care module. This IPE-focused training included 44 self-selected clinicians, with 77% reporting that the interprofessional aspect of the training was beneficial. Trainees were largely nurses but included a few social workers and physicians and one physical therapist.

Pediatrics

Two studies addressed IPE in pediatric palliative care. Friedrichsdorf et al[57] reported results from the design and implementation of a U.S. National Institutes of Health–funded initiative to widely disseminate a primary palliative care program in pediatrics. Their focus was on pediatric hematology/oncology clinicians and was derived in part from the adult Education in Palliative and End-of-Life Care (EPEC) program. The EPEC-Pediatrics program had trained more than 900 interdisciplinary clinicians, primarily nurses and physicians, by 2019. It had reached 58 countries and was available in 3 languages. The program consisted of 24 modules, and mixed online learning with a 1–2-day in-person training conference to address knowledge, attitude, and skills. Trainees self-reported improvement in all 3 of these goals. Patient outcome improvements were anticipated by trainees but not measured.

Also focusing on pediatric palliative care, a small study (10 evaluations) by Nicholl et al[58] trained chaplains, nurses, social workers, and a physiotherapist using stand-alone modules. The modules were interprofessional, but the interaction level between learners was not fully described. Trainees reported quantitative opinions via standard college course evaluations and through open-ended qualitative feedback. Strengths and weaknesses of the course were elaborated to help design future initiatives.

Summary of Interprofessional Educational Efforts
for Practicing Clinicians

Taken as a whole, these IPE interventions[40 58] for clinicians have several overarching themes (see Table 7.2). Study goals were frequently focused on evaluating feasibility and acceptance and were often self-described as pilots. Workshops were a common method for training, often supported by online modules and small group sessions. Longitudinal efforts were the exception. Role-playing and simulated patients or families were perceived as very useful by trainees. Several initiatives blended geriatrics and palliative care IPE. Content for the IPE was dominantly aimed at improving communication and interprofessional team function. Learners were predominantly nurses, and all but a few studies enrolled small to modestly sized cohorts.

With a few exceptions, outcomes were self-reported and evaluated largely by nonvalidated instruments. Patient outcomes were not reported, and increased

Table 7.2 Most Common Features of PC/EOL IPE Initiatives[40-58] for Practicing Clinicians, 2001–2020

Program goals	Testing feasibility and acceptance
Primary content	Communication and team function
Methods	Workshops, small groups, online modules
Duration	Less than a year
Trainees	Self-selected clinicians of 3 or more disciplines, predominantly nurses
Outcome measures	Unvalidated instruments regarding satisfaction and self-assessment of confidence, knowledge, and skills
Patient outcomes	Not measured

knowledge and skills were often assumed to predict improved patient care. Confidence, knowledge, and skills were the most reported trainee outcomes and were universally favorable in these trials. Many studies were described as interprofessional but were dominated by one professional group, with little opportunity for collaboration among professions, and did not include measures of interprofessional collaboration in the evaluation plan. The studies reported by Friedman et al,[40] Brighton et al,[41] O'Mahony et al,[46] and Starks et al[47] provide especially strong models of IPE initiatives for clinicians.

Conclusion

Evidence for the value of IPE in palliative care is growing rapidly. To date, studies have shown feasibility and wide acceptance, with some success at improving collaboration and communication. In general, the body of work reveals small sample sizes, self-selected trainees, self-reported outcomes, frequent low evaluation-response rates, and minimal longitudinal outcome measures. Research with clinical teams is weaker than in academic settings due to even smaller sample sizes. Overall, sample pre- to post-group comparisons were often significant, while comparisons between groups of professions often failed to show significance; this seemed likely due to disparate or small sample sizes within professions or possibly because groups improved similarly. Patient outcomes have not been measured. Given the nature of these early studies, broad conclusions must be restrained, while the groundwork is in place for the design of more rigorous studies. Looking forward, the solid base of these studies and their straightforward outcomes build the foundation for the inevitable growth of more IPE efforts.

The characteristics of successful interprofessional palliative care educational interventions we reviewed included some common elements They were designed and facilitated by interprofessional faculty representatives of the disciplines of the targeted learners; they had interprofessional faculty well trained in IPE facilitation;

and there were regular opportunities for cross-training with colleagues. Curriculum objectives were aligned with accreditation requirements and included multimodal pedagogy focused on allowing learners to learn about, from, and with each other. Role-plays, team simulation, and actual clinical learning experiences were supportive methodologies.

Future studies should improve size and scale, the dependable use of validated evaluation instruments, and objective outcome measures. Key measures will include interprofessional collaboration and patient impact. The engagement of even more diverse and balanced professions/disciplines will be essential. Also going forward, robust faculty development programs that include both IPE and educational leadership training will need to continue and grow in scale.

Interprofessional education for palliative care has made major strides in the past 20 years and provides the direction and lessons for the development of more extensive and robust IPE initiatives. While the studies reviewed here reflect the challenges and barriers of this work, the results are essential to improve the care of patients with advanced illness.

Discussion Questions

1. Reflect on 3 lessons learned from the studies presented.
2. Discuss the challenges of measuring patient outcomes associated with IPE efforts and think of approaches to overcome them.
3. If you were to create a palliative IPE effort in your own institution, reflect on the following (considering strengths and weaknesses, opportunities, and threats within your own institution):
   a. Who would you target in terms of faculty and learners?
   b. What palliative care concepts might you teach?
   c. How might you teach those concepts (online, workshops, semester courses, etc.), and how would you measure the impact of your educational intervention?
   d. Where might you do this (consider location/space needed)?
   e. When should it take place for all of your learners (consider when in the curriculum and when in the academic year)?

Acknowledgments

The authors wish to thank Ansley Stuart, Clinical Librarian, Kornhauser Library, at the University of Louisville for her assistance with our literature search.

References

1. National Consensus Project for Quality Palliative Care. Clinical Practice Guidelines for Quality Palliative Care. National Coalition for Hospice and Palliative Care. Published 2018. Accessed August 3, 2020. https://www.nationalcoalitionhpc.org/ncp/.

2. Institute for Healthcare Improvement. The IHI Triple Aim for Healthcare. Published 2020. Accessed September 4, 2020. http://www.ihi.org/Engage/Initiatives/TripleAim/Pages/defa ult.aspx.

3. Casarett D, Shreve S, Luhrs C, et al. Measuring families' perceptions of care across a health care system: preliminary experience with the Family Assessment of Treatment at End of Life Short Form (FATE-S). *J Pain Symptom Manage*. 2010;40(6):801–809.

4. Temel JS, Greer JA, Muzikansky A, et al. Early palliative care for patients with metastatic non–small-cell lung cancer. *NEJM*. 2010;363(8):733–742.

5. Bakitas M, Lyons KD, Hegel MT, et al. Effects of a palliative care intervention on clinical outcomes in patients with advanced cancer: the Project ENABLE II randomized controlled trial. *JAMA*. 2009;302(7):741–749.

6. Greer JA, Jackson VA, Meier DE, Temmel JS. Early integration of palliative care services with standard oncology care for patients with advanced cancer. *CA Cancer J Clin*. 2013;63(5):350–362.

7. Spettell CM, Rawlins WS, Krakauer R, et al. A comprehensive case management program to improve palliative care. *J Palliat Med*. 2009;12(9):827–832.

8. Lustbader D, Mudra M, Romano C, et al. The impact of a home-based palliative care program in an accountable care organization. *J Palliat Med*. 2017;20(1):23–28.

9. Krakauer R, Spettell CM, Reisman L, Wade MJ. Opportunities to improve the quality of care for advanced illness. *Health Aff*. 2009;28(5):1357–1359.

10. May P, Normand C, Cassel JB, et al. Economics of palliative care for hospitalized adults with serious illness: a meta-analysis. *JAMA Intern Med*. 2018;178(6):820–829.

11. Scibetta C, Kerr K, McGuire J, Rabow MW. The costs of waiting: implications of the timing of palliative care consultation among a cohort of decedents at a comprehensive cancer center. *J Palliat Med*. 2016;19(1):69–75.

12. Khandelwal N, Kross EK, Engelberg RA, Coe NB, Long AC, Randall Curtis J. Estimating the effect of palliative care interventions and advance care planning on ICU utilization: a systematic review. *Crit Care Med*. 2015;43(5):1102–1111.

13. Cassel B, Garrido M, May P, Del Fabbro E, Noreika D. Impact of specialist palliative care on re-admissions: a competing risks analysis to take mortality into account (TH341A). *J Pain Symptom Manage*. 2018;55(2):581.

14. World Health Organization. Framework for Action on Interprofessional Education & Collaborative Practice. World Health Organization. Published 2010. Accessed February 21, 2013. https://www.who.int/publications/i/item/framework-for-action-on-interprofessional-education-collaborative-practice.

15. Interprofessional Education Collaborative Expert Panel. *Core Competencies for Interprofessional Collaborative Practice: Report of an Expert Panel*. Interprofessional Education Collaborative; 2011.

16. World Health Organization. *Framework for Action on Interprofessional Education and Collaborative Practice*. World Health Organization Department of Human Resources for Health; 2010.

17. Head BA, Schapmire T, Hermann C, et al. The Interdisciplinary Curriculum for Oncology Palliative Care Education (iCOPE): meeting the challenge of interprofessional education. *J Palliat Med*. 2014;17(10):1107–1114.

18. Grey C, Constantine L, Baugh GM, Lindenberger E. Advance care planning and shared decision-making: an interprofessional role-playing workshop for medical and nursing students. *MedEdPORTAL*. 2017;13:10644.

19. Fairchild A, Watanabe S, Chambers C, Yurick J, Lem L, Tachynski P. Initiation of a multi-disciplinary summer studentship in palliative and supportive care in oncology. *J Multidiscip Healthc*. 2012;5:231–239.

20. Fineberg IC, Wenger NS, Forrow L. Interdisciplinary education: evaluation of a palliative care training intervention for pre-professionals. *Acad Med*. 2004;79(8):769–776.

21. Sinha P, Murphy SP, Becker CM, et al. A novel interprofessional approach to end-of-life care education: a pilot study. *J Interprof Care*. 2015;29(6):643–645.

22. Head BA, Schapmire T, Earnshaw L, et al. Evaluation of an interdisciplinary curriculum teaching team-based palliative care integration in oncology. *J Cancer Educ*. 2016;31(2):358–365.

23. Bradway C, Cotter VT, Darrah NJ, et al. An interprofessional education simulation workshop: health professions learning palliative care communication. *J Nurs Educ*. 2018;57(8):493–497.

24. Ellman MS, Schulman-Green D, Blatt L, et al. Using online learning and interactive simulation to teach spiritual and cultural aspects of palliative care to interprofessional students. *J Palliat Med*. 2012;15(11):1240–1247.

25. Erickson JM, Blackhall L, Brashers V, Varhegyi N. An interprofessional workshop for students to improve communication and collaboration skills in end-of-life care. *Am J Hosp Palliat Care*. 2015;32(8):876–880.

26. Kaasalainen S, Willison K, Wickson-Griffiths A, Taniguchi A. The evaluation of a national interprofessional palliative care workshop. *J Interprof Care*. 2015;29(5):494–496.

27. Price JE, Mendizabal-Espinosa RM, Podsiadly E, Marshall-Lucette S, Marshall JE. Perinatal/neonatal palliative care: effecting improved knowledge and multi-professional practice of midwifery and children's nursing students through an inter-professional education initiative. *Nurse Educ Pract*. 2019;40:102611.

28. McKee N, D'Eon M, Trinder K. Problem-based learning for inter-professional education: evidence from an inter-professional PBL module on palliative care. *Can Med Educ J*. 2013;4(1):e35–e48.

29. Hall P, Weaver L, Willett TG. Addressing suffering through an inter-professional online module: learning with, from, and about each other. *J Palliat Care*. 2011;27(3):244–246.

30. Prelock PA, Melvin C, Lemieux N, Melekis K, Velleman S, Favro MA. One team-patient, family, and health care providers: an interprofessional education activity providing collaborative and palliative care. *Semin Speech Lang*. 2017;38(5):350–359.

31. Saylor J, Vernoony S, Selekman J, Cowperthwait A. Interprofessional education using a palliative care simulation. *Nurse Educ*. 2016;41(3):125–129.

32. Koffman J, Higginson IJ. Assessing the effectiveness and acceptability of interprofessional palliative care education. *J Palliat Care*. 2005;21(4):262–269.

33. Fink RM, Arora K, Gleason SE, et al. Interprofessional master of science in palliative care: on becoming a palliative care community specialist. *J Palliat Med*. 2019.

34. Bays AM, Engelberg RA, Back AL, et al. Interprofessional communication skills training for serious illness: evaluation of a small-group, simulated patient intervention. *J Palliat Med*. 2014;17(2):159–166.

35. Lippe M, Stanley A, Ricamato A, Halli-Tierney A, McKinney R. Exploring end-of-life care team communication: an interprofessional simulation study. *Am J Hosp Palliat Care*. 2020;37(1):65–71.

36. Gellis ZD, Kim E, Hadley D, et al. Evaluation of interprofessional health care team communication simulation in geriatric palliative care. *Gerontol Geriatr Educ*. 2019;40(1):30–42.

37. Donesky D, Anderson WG, Joseph RD, Sumser B, Reid TT. TeamTalk: interprofessional team development and communication skills training. *J Palliat Med*. 2020;23(1):40–47.

38. Lakin JR, Brannen EN, Bernacki RE, Jones E. A curriculum in quality improvement for interprofessional palliative care trainees. *Am J Hosp Palliat Care*. 2020;37(1):41–45.

39. Lee AL, DeBest M, Koeniger-Donohue R, Strowman SR, Mitchell SE. The feasibility and acceptability of using virtual world technology for interprofessional education in palliative care: a mixed methods study. *J Interprof Care*. 2020;34(4):461–471.

40. Friedman MI, Attivissimo LA, Kiszko KB, Rimar A, Yezzo PM, Torroella Carney M. The development and piloting of a goals of care conversation education program for an advanced illness population. *Gerontol Geriatr Educ*. 2020;41(1):52–62.

41. Brighton LJ, Selman LE, Gough N, et al. "Difficult conversations": evaluation of multiprofessional training. *BMJ Support Palliat Care*. 2018;8(1):45–48.

42. Puchalski C, Jafari N, Buller H, Haythorn T, Jacobs C, Ferrell B. Interprofessional spiritual care education curriculum: a milestone toward the provision of spiritual care. *J Palliat Med*. 2020;23(6):777–784.

43. Papadakos CT, Stringer T, Papadakos J, et al. Effectiveness of a multiprofessional, online and simulation-based difficult conversations training program on self-perceived competence of oncology healthcare provider trainees. *J Cancer Educ*. 2020;36(5):1030–1038.

44. Andrew J, Taylor C. Follow-up evaluation of a course to develop effective communication and relationship skills for palliative care. *Int J Palliat Nurs*. 2012;18(9):457–463.

45. Grymonpre R, Bowman S, Rippin-Sisler C, et al. Every team needs a coach: training for interprofessional clinical placements. *J Interprof Care*. 2016;30(5):559–566.

46. O'Mahony S, Baron A, Ansari A, et al. Expanding the interdisciplinary palliative medicine workforce: a longitudinal education and mentoring program for practicing clinicians. *J Pain Symptom Manage*. 2020;60(3):602–612.

47. Starks H, Coats H, Paganelli T, et al. Pilot study of an interprofessional palliative care curriculum: course content and participant-reported learning gains. *Am J Hosp Palliat Care*. 2018;35(3):390–397.

48. Podgurski L, Greco C, Croom A, Arnold R, Claxton R. A brief mindfulness-based self-care curriculum for an interprofessional group of palliative care providers. *J Palliat Med*. 2019;22(5):561–565.

49. Wittenberg E, Ferrell B, Goldsmith J, Ragan SL, Paice J. Assessment of a statewide palliative care team training course: COMFORT communication for palliative care teams. *J Palliat Med*. 2016;19(7):746–752.

50. Shaw V, Davies A, Ong BN. A collaborative approach to facilitate professionals to support the breathless patient. *BMJ Support Palliat Care*. 2019;9(1):e3.

51. Gordon E, Ridley B, Boston J, Dahl E. The building bridges initiative: learning with, from and about to create an interprofessional end-of-life program. *Dynamics*. 2012;23(4):37–41.

52. Graham R, Lepage C, Boitor M, Petizian S, Fillion L, Gélinas C. Acceptability and feasibility of an interprofessional end-of-life/palliative care educational intervention in the intensive care unit: a mixed-methods study. *Intensive Crit Care Nurs*. 2018;48:75–84.

53. Campion-Smith C, Austin H, Criswick S, Dowling B, Francis G. Can sharing stories change practice? A qualitative study of an interprofessional narrative-based palliative care course. *J Interprof Care*. 2011;25(2):105–111.

54. Kortes-Miller K, Habjan S, Kelley ML, Fortier M. Development of a palliative care education program in rural long-term care facilities. *J Palliat Care*. 2007;23(3):154–162.

55. Lally KM, Ducharme CM, Roach RL, Towey C, Filinson R, Tuya Fulton A. Interprofessional training: geriatrics and palliative care principles for primary care teams in an ACO. *Gerontol Geriatr Educ*. 2019;40(1):121–131.

56. Solberg LB, Solberg LM, Carter CS. Geriatric care boot cAMP: an interprofessional education program for healthcare professionals. *J Am Geriatr Soc*. 2015;63(5):997–1001.

57. Friedrichsdorf SJ, Remke S, Hauser J, et al. Development of a pediatric palliative care curriculum and dissemination model: education in palliative and end-of-life care (EPEC) pediatrics. *J Pain Symptom Manage*. 2019;58(4):707–720.e703.

58. Nicholl H, Price J, Tracey C. An evaluation of an interprofessional master's level programme in children's palliative care: the students' evaluation. *Nurse Educ Pract*. 2016;17:60–66.

8

Interprofessional Palliative Care Education in Academic Settings

Mary Lynn McPherson and Lisa Kitko

Key Points

- Educators in academic settings need to meet multiple competencies within a curriculum, including profession-specific competencies, those set by accrediting bodies, and/or specialty area competencies.
- Critically important to assessing the attainment of curriculum objectives is first determining the level of the learner and what competencies are appropriate for each level of learning.
- Signature pedagogies, methods, and practice of teaching in professional academic programs form the character of practitioners through a 4-pronged approach of knowledge, skills, attitudes, and ethics.
- To optimize an interprofessional or transdisciplinary practice setting, it is critically important that prelicensure students learn in an interprofessional environment.
- Maintaining or advancing one's skills in palliative care necessitates a lifelong commitment to learning; a "60-year curriculum" offers a variety of learning opportunities to meet these varied needs over time.

Introduction

Everyone has heard the idea that the minute you drive a new car off the lot, it begins to depreciate. Does this concept hold true for the knowledge base of healthcare providers who graduate with their entry-level degree? Where can we turn for guidance on this issue? Perhaps Mahatma Gandhi best explained it with this quote: "Live as if you were to die tomorrow. Learn as if you were to live forever."[1] The healthcare field evolves at lightning speed, and continuing professional development is (or should be) mandatory. For some, this may be honoring a personal commitment to learning something new every day. Others may choose to select continuing education activities that meet their professional needs, including those that culminate in the award of a certificate. Some may opt to seek a graduate academic certificate or advanced degree from an accredited academic institution in their area of interest or specialization. Prelicensure health profession students are often eager to seize opportunities for advanced study or specialization, not only to increase their knowledge but also to optimize the likelihood of securing a desired residency or position. The majority of this chapter will explore facets of interprofessional palliative care education that are especially pertinent in academic settings, including competencies, leveling the learners, course design, learning structures, and pragmatics, followed by 3 aspirational topics to consider: transdisciplinary education and practice, the progression from primary and secondary to tertiary practice, and the "60-year curriculum" as applied to palliative care.

Interprofessional Education

Palliative care is defined by the World Health Organization as "an approach that improves the quality of life of patients (adults and children) and their families who are facing problems associated with life-threatening illness. It prevents and relieves suffering through the early identification, correct assessment and treatment of pain and other problems, whether physical, psychosocial or spiritual."[2] Clearly, based on this definition, the practice of palliative care is a team sport. No single healthcare professional can address all the physical, psychosocial, and spiritual needs of the unit of care, which is the patient and family. If effective palliative care requires the presence and collaboration of multiple health professionals, shouldn't we train prelicensure students and practitioners in an interprofessional environment? Interprofessional education requires educators and learners from 2 or more health professions to create and foster a learning environment. A core element of interprofessional education is embodied by the principle of "learning with, from and about each other."[3] The goal is to demonstrate interprofessional team behaviors and competence as defined by the Interprofessional Education Collaborative (IPEC).[4]

The importance of interprofessional education in general is well documented in the current literature and has been highlighted throughout this text. Interprofessional palliative care education has been shown to improve patient-centered communication, improve interprofessional team practice, and increase palliative care consultations.[5-7] Previous studies have also shown that students who learn in an interprofessional environment demonstrate improved interprofessional collaborative practice competencies as compared to students who do not learn in such an environment.[8,9]

Facets of Interprofessional Palliative Care Education Programs in Academic Settings

Interprofessional Core Competencies

Competencies have become the standard of practice for assessing outcomes in the education of professional students. IPEC, which represents 21 national health professions associations, works in collaboration with academic institutions to "promote, encourage, and support health professionals in interprofessional practice."[4(p1)] This group has developed 4 core competencies with 38 sub-competencies which guide patient care and interprofessional collaboration. They are as follows:

- Competency 1: Values/Ethics: Work with individuals of other professions to maintain a climate of mutual respect and shared values.
- Competency 2: Roles/Responsibilities: Apply knowledge of one's own role and those of other professions to appropriately assess and address the healthcare needs of patients, and to promote and advance the health of populations.
- Competency 3: Communication: Communicate with patients, families, communities, and professionals in health and other fields in a responsive and responsible manner that supports a team approach to the promotion and maintenance of health and the prevention and treatment of disease.
- Competency 4: Teamwork: Apply relationship-building values and the principles of team dynamics to perform effectively in different team roles.

This cohesive teamwork allows groups to plan, deliver, and evaluate patient/population-centered care, as well as population health programs and policies that are safe, timely, efficient, effective, and equitable.[4] The National Center for Interprofessional Practice and Education (NEXUS-IPE) maintains a comprehensive website (www.nexusipe.org) with resources designed to support educators in implementing the IPEC competencies, as well as state-of-the-art assessment and evaluation tools and opportunities to connect and engage with others who are committed to interprofessional education in health professions education. NEXUS-IPE is a public-private partnership founded in 2012 to guide the development of interprofessional education and collaborative practice within healthcare.

In addition to the IPEC core competencies, each health profession has a set of competencies that guide learning, and the majority include a competency or sub-competency that addresses the importance of interprofessional practice. These competencies are typically defined by the various accrediting bodies for the specific professional discipline. As examples, the Association of American Medical Colleges (AAMC) lists teamwork as one of the 15 core competencies for medical students.[10] Similarly, the American Association of Colleges of Nursing (AACN), one of the professional organizations that provide national accreditation for nursing programs, lists interprofessional partnerships as an essential domain.[11]

A third type of competency guiding specialty* practice focuses on the specialty's discipline (knowledge base). The National Consensus Project's (NCP) Clinical Practice Guidelines for Quality Palliative Care provide the framework for interprofessional clinicians to deliver high quality palliative care.[12] The NCP Clinical Practice Guidelines also provide guidance for the content of palliative care educational programs in academic settings. All of the available guidance and competencies that surround interprofessional, profession-specific, and palliative care discipline-specific education pose a challenge for academic educators. Interprofessional palliative care curricula need to provide content reflective of multiple competencies—IPEC, profession-specific competencies set by accrediting bodies, and/or specialty-area competencies.[9]

Educators are limited by a lack of guidance on how best to integrate competencies into curriculum design in interprofessional palliative care programs. Very few useful or practical tools are available to determine if competencies are achieved by the learner, especially in the context of palliative care.[14] Additional evidence—generated from rigorous programs that are competency-based and both profession-specific and interprofessional—is needed to provide guidance on the best mix of content for interprofessional palliative care education programs and to validate the proposed characteristics of high-quality programs.[15] Additional discussion of competencies is presented in Chapter 6, "Principles of Interprofessional Education Applied to Palliative Care."

Leveling the "Learners"

In a palliative care interprofessional education program, the learners are immersed in a competency-based curriculum that addresses the attributes embodied in the IPEC competencies, with the end goal of a collaborative practice-ready workforce.[9] Critically important to assessing the attainment of competencies is first determining the level of the learner and what competencies are appropriate for each level of learning. The "leveling of learners" is conceptually supported by the Dreyfus Model of Skill Acquisition which was popularized in nursing by Patricia Benner.[16] The idea that health professionals develop in their practice, from novice through the spectrum of advanced beginner, competent, proficient, and finally to expert level, has been applied to interprofessional clinicians.[17,18] As learners advance to the next level, they build upon the skills they developed in the earlier levels.[16] Leveling of learning experiences permits the participants to gain confidence while building

---

* Palliative care is considered to be a subspecialty within medicine and nursing, but a specialty in spiritual care and social work. For this book, we standardize the language by referring to palliative care as a specialty when referring to the team as a whole.

upon previous knowledge and skills, providing a scaffolding to build on throughout the curriculum.[19-21] In a Delphi survey related to the developmental progression of knowledge, skills, and attitudes with the Quality and Safety Education for Nurses (QSEN) competencies for prelicensure nursing students, recommended progressive development of competencies included sustained exposure and reinforcement of foundational nursing concepts across the entirety of the curriculum.[19]

Leveling of competencies within the framework of interprofessional palliative care education poses several challenges. Some learners will have extensive knowledge of a subject, while others are novices in terms of the content. A strategy for interprofessional educators is to match students who will be learning based on their level of knowledge and skill.[22]

In contrast, an argument could be made for educating learners with more advanced peers so the novice learners might benefit from the modeling of their peers, while the more advanced learners have the opportunity to solidify their knowledge.[23] Experienced health professions educators categorized the level of learners (social workers, dental hygienists, physician assistants, nurses, physicians, pharmacists, physical therapists) from Level 1 "Novice," which included mostly first-year students, to Level 4 "Expert" for practicing clinicians.[24] The level of learners was then mapped to the 38 IPEC sub-competencies through a Delphi process. The resulting document can be used to guide developmentally appropriate longitudinal interprofessional education curricula. These examples of foundational work should serve as a framework for academic educators in interprofessional palliative care programs.

Course Design

For learning to occur in any setting, teachers and learners need to play an active role in the learning process. Determining the best teaching–learning strategy (or strategies) to deliver the content is an important process. Pedagogy in the simplest definition is the art and science of teaching, which may encompass a range of teaching strategies, from readings and lectures to simulations and clinical experiences. The pedagogical strategies can be combined for use in either a traditional classroom or online environment, depending on the learning objectives and purpose of the course (see Chapter 6, "Principles of Interprofessional Education Applied to Palliative Care"). Within traditional pedagogies, the educator determines the best strategies for teaching and learning. Heutagogy is defined as self-determined learning that is directed by the students, who decides what they will learn and how they will learn. Andragogy is the teaching of adults, which can be pedagogical, heutagogical, or a combination of both.[25]

When teaching a specific area of study or in professional preparation such as interprofessional palliative care, the concept of "signature pedagogy" refers to the character formation of practitioners through a 4-pronged approach of knowledge, skills, attitudes, and ethics.[26] The development of this professional identity poses challenges to interprofessional educators whose goal is to teach collaborative practice. The pedagogies of each profession are not inherently interprofessional and may, in fact, impede interprofessional learning. Although there have been significant gains in defining interprofessional education, there is still a critical need to develop a "signature pedagogy of interprofessional palliative care collaboration" that addresses the professional identity of a specific practitioner, their role as an interprofessional clinician within the discipline of palliative care, and that encompasses the best practices of teaching and learning. This may be accomplished in several ways, such as teaching profession-specific content concurrently with interprofessional content and team learning, or, as long as the interprofessional principles are upheld, profession-specific identity can be taught separately or sequentially in other coursework.

Learning Structures

Building on the various types of pedagogies to enhance learning are physical, emotional, and pedagogical structures that can individually or collectively be utilized to enhance the student's acquisition of knowledge, skills, ethics, and attitudes.

Parallel or Community Learning

Parallel learning, also known as communities of practice, promotes learning and change within organizational structures. [27] Communities of practice are an additional informal mechanism to promote learning in a "community" with a common interest through sharing of expertise with the goal of developing knowledge and building professional practice.[28] Groups consisting of various professionals develop new ways of exchanging information and knowledge, which works in a parallel structure to the normal organizational structure.[29] Although open to any level of practitioner, communities of practice are not designed for the novice, as this builds on the cumulative knowledge of the community and brings the practice of members to a new advanced level.[30]

The benefits of a community of practice (or learning) in the context of an interprofessional palliative care program are multifactorial, including building core knowledge and competencies, diffusion of evidence-based practice more quickly, and increasing access to expertise. The majority of interprofessional palliative care programs, outlined in Table 8.1, include a clinical or practicum component which could provide the groundwork for the development of an informal community of practice.

Interactive Learning

Interprofessional education inherently creates opportunities for interactive learning across disciplines. In addition, palliative care as a model of practice is

Table 8.1 Prelicensure Interprofessional Palliative Care Education in Academic Settings

Program	Eligible Participants	Degree or Certificate	Curriculum	Method of Delivery
Post-Graduate Interprofessional Palliative Care Education in Academic Settings	Future health and healthcare workers who are enrolled as a degree-seeking student at Arizona State University	Certificate (not awarded prior to the award of an undergraduate degree). Participants may pursue this undergraduate certificate as a nondegree-seeking graduate student if they already hold an undergraduate degree.	• 12 required credits: Elements of Hospice and Palliative Care; Alzheimer's and other Dementias; Palliative Care: Managing Complex Serious Illness; Internship. • 6 elective credits (multiple options)	Face to face
University of Louisville Interdisciplinary Curriculum for Oncology Palliative Education (iCOPE), Louisville, KY http://icopeproject.org/	Students enrolled at the University of Louisville at one of the schools of medicine, nursing, social work, and clinical pastoral education	Curriculum component of medicine, nursing, social work, and clinical pastoral education	• 4 online modules to teach core concepts of palliative care: roles of interdisciplinary team members, palliative care structure and process, pain and symptom management communication, grief and loss, spiritual dimensions of care, social and cultural care, and ethics • Interdisciplinary case management experience • Clinical rotation and critical reflection paper	Hybrid (online and face to face)

(continued)

Table 8.1 Continued

Program	Eligible Participants	Degree or Certificate	Curriculum	Method of Delivery

Grand Valley State University Palliative and Hospice Care Graduate Certificate, Grand Rapids, MI https://www.gvsu. edu/acad/palliative-and-hospice-care-graduate-certificate.htm	Individuals interested in palliative care and hospice with a bachelor's degree from an accredited institution or enrolled in prelicensure program	Graduate certificate	• 12 credits of coursework including:
			  ○ Chronic and Terminal Illness: The Palliative and hospice model
			  ○ Complex Pain and Symptom Management
			  ○ Death, Grief, and Loss
			• Choice of one elective
				Hybrid (online and face to face)

Penn State College of Nursing—Primary Palliative Care Graduate Certificate Program, State College, PA https:// bulletins.psu.edu/graduate/ programs/certificates/ primary-palliative-care-graduate-credit-certificate-program/#text	Individuals with a bachelor's or higher degree in nursing or a related health discipline from an accredited institution or enrolled in prelicensure program	Graduate certificate	• 6 credits of coursework:
			  ○ Primary Palliative Care: An Interdisciplinary Approach
			  ○ Primary Palliative Care: Interdisciplinary Management of Advanced Serious Illness
			• 3 credits of practicum
			  ○ Interdisciplinary practicum of the primary palliative care role
				Completely online

Program	Audience	Credential	Coursework	Format

University of Washington Graduate Certificate in Palliative Care, Seattle, WA http://uwpctc.org	Practicing healthcare professionals from nursing, medicine, social work, spiritual care and other disciplines seeking specialty training in palliative care	Graduate certificate	• Three 5-credit quarters:
			  ○ Introduction to Person Centered and Interprofessional Palliative Care
			  ○ Advanced Topics in Person Centered and Interprofessional Palliative Care
			• Palliative Care Quality Metrics and System Integration
				Hybrid (online and face to face)

University of Colorado Denver Palliative Care Graduate Program, Aurora, CO	All healthcare providers and allied health professionals	Graduate certificate	• 12 credit coursework:
			  ○ Core Concepts, Principles & Communication Skills
			  ○ Basic Pain Assessment & Management: IDT Care
			  ○ IDT Care for Non-Pain Symptoms: Part A and Part B
			• One 3-day weekend intensive completed on the Anschutz Medical Campus
				Hybrid (online and face to face)

(continued)

Table 8.1 Continued

Program	Eligible Participants	Degree or Certificate	Curriculum	Method of Delivery
	MSPC Biomedical Track: physicians, physician assistants, registered nurses (BSN and Advanced Practice RN), and pharmacists MSPC Allied Health Professional Track: social workers, spiritual care providers, psychologists, counselors, therapists, grief specialists and medical ethicists	Master of Science (MS)	• 36 credits didactic content (see website for details) • Three 3-day on-campus weekend intensive experiences completed on the Anschutz Medical Campus	Hybrid (online and face to face)
University of Maryland Baltimore Online Master of Science, PhD and Graduate Certificates in Palliative Care, Baltimore, MD graduate.umaryland.edu/palliative	Individuals with a bachelor's degree or higher from an accredited institution	Graduate certificate in Principles and Practice of Hospice and Palliative Care.	• 12 credits of coursework for Graduate Certificate in Principles and Practice of Hospice and Palliative Care: ○ Principles and Practice of Hospice and Palliative Care	Completely online

Four additional advanced graduate certificate options are available:

- Clinical Hospice and Palliative Care
- Leadership and Administration in Hospice and Palliative Care
- Psychosocial/Spiritual Aspects of Hospice and Palliative Care
- Aging and Applied Thanatology

- Communication and Healthcare Decision-Making
- Psychosocial, Cultural, and Spiritual Care
- Symptom Management in Advanced Illness

(continued)

Table 8.1 Continued

Program	Eligible Participants	Degree or Certificate	Curriculum	Method of Delivery

	Individuals with a bachelor's degree or higher from an accredited institution	Master of Science (MS)	• 12 credits as shown in Graduate Certificate in Principles and Practice of Hospice and Palliative Care (above)
			• 12 elective credits (taking all 12 credits in one pathway results in award of an advanced graduate certificate); see website
			  ○ Clinical Hospice and Palliative Care Pathway
			  ○ Leadership and Administration in Hospice and Palliative Care Pathway
			  ○ Psychosocial/spiritual Aspects of Hospice and Palliative Care Pathway
			• 3 credits: Research and Outcomes Assessment in Hospice and Palliative Care
			• 3 credits: Advanced Team Base Palliative Care
				Completely online

	Doctor of Philosophy (PhD)		

• Master of Science in Palliative Care, or
• Master's degree or higher in a relevant field, plus 2–3 years of experience and current employment in palliative care
	Doctor of Philosophy (PhD)	• 36 credits
		  ○ Understanding the Foundation of Palliative Care: Building Blocks for the Future
		  ○ Applied Biostatistics for Palliative Care
		  ○ Critical Appraisal of Evidence in Palliative Care
		  ○ Quantitative Research in Palliative Care
		  ○ Qualitative Research in Palliative Care
		  ○ Person-Centered Outcomes Research
		  ○ Teaching Methodology in Palliative Care
		  ○ Leading Change in Palliative Care
		  ○ Dissertation (12 credits)
			Completely online

interprofessional. Based on experiential learning strategies, students who engage in interactive collaborative education activities will be more likely to bring this collaborative approach to their work as healthcare clinicians.[31]

Essential to capturing the importance of interactive learning with an interprofessional education program is designing or delivering a curriculum that adheres to the definition of interprofessional "learning with, from and about each other."[2] Interprofessional education that addresses all aspects of the WHO definition is a necessary step to prepare health professionals for interprofessional collaborative practice.[32]

Pragmatics

The benefits of palliative care interprofessional learning and practice include effects on patient outcomes and clinician well-being.[33] The "elephant in the room" is that interprofessional education is challenging to implement from a teaching and learning perspective. These challenges are multifactorial and include logistics of collaboration around busy schedules, differing academic calendars between disciplines, availability of the appropriate professional schools, and resource availability to support curriculum delivery.[34]

As many of the academic programs in interprofessional palliative care are stand-alone programs in addition to specific health profession education, the sustainability of the programs remains a challenge. Threats to sustainability include identifying enough interprofessional faculty who are able and qualified to teach in the program. Also, most academic programs are designed to be self-sustaining from a financial perspective and receive limited financial support from the home institution. Both factors are significant barriers to the development, delivery, and long-term viability of such programs.

Beyond these pragmatic issues of interprofessional education, there are more implicit challenges to education within healthcare. Attention to the work climate and culture of various healthcare settings and the impact on the learning environment[35] may also impact curriculum outcomes. Many educators and healthcare professionals do not address the relational factors that coexist with any team-based program. This lack of attention to relational factors can limit the effectiveness of interprofessional learning. The ASPIRE model (Figure 8.1) is an empirically tested theoretical framework for designing, implementing, and assessing interprofessional education while accounting for the relational factors that are so important to optimizing the work climate and culture. The model was developed by mapping the IPEC core competencies into 3 overlapping content areas: practical tools, leadership, and relational factors to guide curriculum development.[36] Utilization of the framework in a train-the-trainer delivery model demonstrated improved capabilities of learners to apply the knowledge gained to the clinical setting.[37]

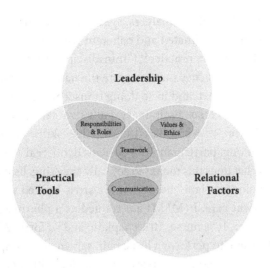

Figure 8.1. The ASPIRE model.
Reprinted from Moule P, E-learning for healthcare students: Developing the communities of practice framework. *Journal of Advanced Nursing* 2006;(54)3: . With permission from John Wiley and Sons.

The maintenance of profession-specific identity and the embedded hierarchical structure in healthcare may also impact the goal of interprofessional collaboration.[37] As students in healthcare professions acquire discipline-specific competencies, they are also socialized into the culture, roles, and values of the specific profession.[38] This professional role identity could impede the process of interprofessional education and the development of true collaborative practice (see Chapter 3). In a recent longitudinal study by Haugland and colleagues,[32] students from 7 different professional education programs involved in interprofessional education participated in focus groups. The aim of the study was to determine the impact on how interprofessional education can contribute to both professional and interprofessional identity. The authors concluded that interprofessional education improved the student's view of their own professional identity as well as their identity as a part of the interprofessional team.

Transcending Interprofessional Education and Practice: Transdisciplinary Practice

Perhaps we are a little greedy in palliative care education, but educators like to aim for even more than interprofessional education! Yes, palliative care teams are multidisciplinary ("draws on knowledge from different disciplines but stays within the boundaries of those fields")[39(p 359)] including physicians, pharmacists, nurses, advanced practice nurses, physician assistants/associates, social workers, chaplains, administrators, volunteers, grief and bereavement specialists, and more.[39,40] They

are interdisciplinary (defined as "analyzes, synthesizes and harmonizes links between disciplines into a coordinated and coherent whole")[39(p 359)] as well, but the
holy grail is a transdisciplinary practice[41] ("transdisciplinary approaches to human
health are defined as approaches that integrate the natural, social and health sciences in a humanities context, and in so doing transcend each of their traditional
boundaries").[40,42-43(p 359)] Transdisciplinary palliative care practice "transcends
disciplinary boundaries . . . with shared knowledge, skills, responsibilities, and
decision making among participants . . . focused on real-world or common
problems."[44(p 359)] What does this mean? Practically speaking, healthcare providers
do not strictly "stay in their lane" but rather are cross-trained sufficiently to provide synergistic patient care. I (MLM) am trained as a pharmacist but I believe
I am 10% social worker, 10% nurse, 10% chaplain, and so forth. All palliative care
providers should be able to perform a basic pain screen, a basic spiritual wellness
screen, and have a values and preferences conversation with a patient and family
(see Chapter 3).

Primary, Specialty, and Tertiary Palliative Care Skills

All healthcare providers should possess "primary" palliative care skills. These include basic skills such as "assessing the patient's physical and nonphysical symptoms
ensuring the patient understands his/her illness and prognosis, and establishing the
goals of medical care."[45(p 704)] It would be optimal if these skills were taught in an
interprofessional practice in professional schools of medicine, nursing, pharmacy,
social work, and so forth. Unfortunately, evidence suggests that there is insufficient
palliative care content taught in our professional curricula, that students lack confidence in primary palliative care skills, and thus professional organizations call for
additional content.[46-55]

Specialty palliative care refers to palliative care specialist clinicians and organizations that provide interprofessional palliative care on a consultative basis.[56]
These practitioners reach this level of competence either through "on-the-job
training," or increasingly, by completing postgraduate training such as a graduate certificate or degree, continuing education course, or fellowship, often
followed by board or professional organization certification. Tertiary palliative
care "refers to the academic medical centers where specialist knowledge for the
most complex cases is practiced, researched, and taught."[56(p 876-877)] Tertiary palliative care providers are usually academicians or researchers. Competence in
education and research is achieved by significant advanced training and experience. Academic institutions may provide educational experiences that train
providers in primary, specialty, and tertiary palliative care. Tertiary care includes
the complex care provided at centers with advanced clinical services such as cardiopulmonary life support (ECMO) and transplant, in addition to academic research and education.

The "60-Year Curriculum" and Examples in Interprofessional Palliative Care

Many have hypothesized that people born in the past decade, and certainly into the future, may well live to be 100 years old. This suggests that "people will have five to seven stages in their lives, not just the three traditional stages of school, work, and retirement."[57] Certainly a high school diploma is unlikely to sustain those stages of growth, and a bachelor's degree may be insufficient as well. Dr. Gary Matkin states that universities can develop and offer a "60-year curriculum" designed to assist lifelong learners in retooling throughout their career.[58] These educational offerings may be continuing professional development credit, or may result in the award of a degree, including graduate studies. Table 8.1 provides examples of palliative care educational opportunities in academic settings. See Chapter 10 for discussion of continuing education courses and Chapter 9 for more information about clinical residencies and fellowships in palliative care.

Primary Palliative Care Training Prelicensure

While not all professional schools provide adequate or comprehensive training in palliative care, some do offer additional training for eligible students. For example, in pharmacy, the University of Maryland School of Pharmacy offers several "pathways" of specialization, one of which is "Geriatrics and Palliative Care."[59] This requires Doctor of Pharmacy students to take specified didactic electives, and an experiential rotation in hospice or palliative care.[60] Arizona State University offers an interprofessional certificate in Hospice and Palliative Care to future healthcare workers who are enrolled as degree-seeking students at the college. Students at the University of Louisville can take advantage of the "iCOPE" curriculum, which accepts students from the schools of medicine, nursing, social work, and clinical pastoral education. This course consists of 4 online modules that address interprofessional palliative care. Refer to Box 8.1 for a further description of this program.

Primary Palliative Care Training Post-Graduation

There are a number of interprofessional graduate certificate options available in the United States (see Table 8.1). Examples include Arizona State University, Grand Valley State, Penn State College of Nursing, University of Washington, University of Colorado, and the University of Maryland, Baltimore. All of these graduate certificates are available for a number of healthcare disciplines and offer academic credit. A greater discussion of one example, Penn State College of Nursing, is provided in Box 8.2.

Box 8.1. The iCOPE Agenda

The Interdisciplinary Curriculum for Oncology Palliative Education (iCOPE) project was initially funded by the National Cancer Institute (1R25CA148005) to develop and implement interprofessional palliative education for medical, nursing, social work, and chaplain students.[a] The program consists of 4 on-line modules—1 on teamwork, and 3 case-based interactive modules—which teach the fundamentals of palliative oncology care and level the learners. This prepares the students for a face-to-face interactive session, the Interdisciplinary Case Management Experience (ICME), where teams of students from the various professions meet together to consider a case, evaluate the video of a family meeting, and develop an interprofessional plan of care. Learners also participate in a clinical rotation led by a practicing interprofessional team, after which they write a critical reflection based on their experience.[b]

Over 500 learners took part during the funded period, which ended in 2015. The program has continued under the leadership of the Medical Education Department. Approximately 100 medical students, 100 nursing students, 15 social work students, and 15 chaplain students have completed the mandated program annually for the past 6 years. Program evaluation demonstrates that the curriculum is successful in teaching palliative care skills and knowledge, increases the learners' self-efficacy related to interprofessional learning, and makes a positive impact on their attitudes and abilities related to the practice of team-based palliative care in oncology.[c]

[a] Head B, Schapmire T, Hermann C, et al. The Interdisciplinary Curriculum for Oncology Palliative Care Education (iCOPE): Meeting the challenge of interprofessional education. *J Palliat Med.* 2014;17(10):1107–1114. doi:10.1089/jpm.2014.0070 PMID: 24972279.

[b] Head BA, Furman CD, Lally AM, Leake K, Pfeifer MP. Medicine as it should be: Teaching team and team-work during a palliative care clerkship. *J Palliat Med.* 2018;21(5):638–643. doi:10.1089/pm.2017.0589 ISSN 1096-6218.

[c] Head B, Schapmire T, Earnshaw L, et al. Evaluation of an interdisciplinary curriculum teaching team-based palliative care integration in oncology. *J Cancer Educ.* 2016;31(2):358–365. PMID: 25708910.

Contributed by Barbara Head.

Specialty Palliative Care Training

For individuals who wish to achieve a higher degree of training in interprofessional palliative care, a Master of Science degree is available at 2 universities in the United States—the University of Colorado, and the University of Maryland, Baltimore. The Colorado program is a hybrid (mostly online) and the University of Maryland, Baltimore, program is completely online. Both offer a graduate academic certificate program, and learners may continue to earn the Master of Science degree. At the University of Maryland, Baltimore, some learners who are already working in the field enroll to gain a richer, deeper understanding of hospice and palliative care, while others obtain the degree hoping to either augment their current skill set (e.g.,

---

Box 8.2. Penn State College of Nursing

The Penn State College of Nursing is home of the Primary Palliative Care Graduate Certificate Program. The goal of the program is to prepare individuals with a bachelor's or higher degree in nursing or a related health discipline in the principles and practice of primary palliative care. The interdisciplinary program was initially developed and implemented with funding from the Macy Faculty Scholar Program.

The curriculum includes 6 credits (two 3-credit courses) of didactic content in primary palliative care and interprofessional management of advanced serious illness and one 3-credit practicum course on the interprofessional practice of the palliative care role. The practicum course involves the application of knowledge acquired in previously completed courses related to primary palliative care. The practicum builds upon and extends learners' previous experiences and fulfills objectives that have been mutually negotiated between faculty and student based on the student's identified learning needs. All courses are delivered using distance technology, and the practicum course includes interprofessional virtual simulations. The 2 didactic courses are available to health professional students independent of the certificate program as electives or as stand-alone courses.

Required Courses for the Primary Palliative Care Graduate Certificate Program
- Primary Palliative Care: An Interdisciplinary Approach: 3 credits (didactic)
- Primary Palliative Care: Interdisciplinary Management of Advanced Serious Illness: 3 credits (didactic)
- Interdisciplinary Practicum of the Primary Palliative Care Role: 3 credits (practicum)

Learning Outcomes for the Primary Palliative Care Graduate Certificate Program
1. Describe the fundamentals of primary palliative care for providing person-centered care to individuals with advanced serious illness and their family members, including pediatric, adult, and geriatric populations.
2. Describe an interprofessional approach to primary palliative care.
3. Describe the interprofessional management of persons with advanced serious illness and their family members.
4. Demonstrate evidence-based management and communication with individuals with advanced serious illness and their family members in a healthcare setting.
5. Demonstrate the ability to work effectively in an interprofessional team.

Additional Resources
- Dede CJ, Richards J, *The 60-Year Curriculum: New Models for Lifelong Learning in the Digital Economy*. Routledge; 2020.
- Interprofessional Education Collaboration, *Core Competences for Interprofessional Collaborative Practice: 2016 Update*. Interprofessional Education Collaborative; 2016.

hospitalists, critical care practitioners, etc.) or transition to a career in hospice or palliative care. See Chapter 6 for an in-depth description of the Colorado program.

Tertiary Interprofessional Palliative Care Training

The University of Maryland, Baltimore, recently received approval for an online PhD in Palliative Care, and accepted its inaugural class in Fall 2021. The program builds on a Master of Science in Palliative Care, or a master's degree or higher in a medical field plus palliative care experience. This program is interprofessional and may include chaplains, social workers, nurses, advanced practice providers, pharmacists, physicians, therapists, and others. It is anticipated that graduates of this program will assume a position in academia or leadership, and work with others to advance the field of palliative care. A PhD in Palliative Care is also available through Lancaster University in the United Kingdom. Learners attend on-site coursework for a few days at the beginning of each academic year, and participate part-time via e-learning for a total of 4–7 years to earn their doctorate.

These educational opportunities have all been developed in the past decade, and it is likely that many more will be created and offered in the future. These programs illustrate the growing ability of prelicensure professional students to acquire specialty training in palliative care, as well as post-licensure practitioners to develop primary and specialty palliative care skills.

Conclusions

Critical to any successful palliative care educational program in an academic setting is the integration of evidence-based teaching and learning strategies that promote interprofessional education and result in best principles for collaborative practice. Key concepts that are integral to this programming in palliative care include: competencies, both profession-specific and interprofessional; a clear understanding of the learners' fund of knowledge; discipline-specific learning objectives; and interprofessional group dynamics to foster the learning environment.

In this chapter, interprofessional palliative care programs in an academic setting have been described (Table 8.1) and guidance for faculty to develop a program have been detailed based on current evidence, as well as guiding principles for teaching and overcoming challenges in the learning environment. Challenges remain for educators to develop a pedagogy of interprofessional collaboration that addresses both the professional identity of a specific practitioner, their role as an interprofessional practitioner in palliative care, and best evidence-based practices for translation into academic learning environments.

Discussion Questions

1. How should academic interprofessional palliative care program educators integrate competencies into curriculum design that address both discipline-specific and professional competencies?
2. The development of a professional identity poses challenges to interprofessional educators whose goal is to teach collaborative practice. How might an educator leverage a practitioner's professional identity to enhance interprofessional learning?
3. Discuss challenges in the delivery of interprofessional palliative care education programs in the academic setting.
4. How do multidisciplinary, interdisciplinary,[†] and transdisciplinary education and practice differ?
5. How do the skill sets of primary, specialty, and tertiary palliative care providers differ?
6. What is meant by the "60-year curriculum?" How might individuals take advantage of a 60-year curriculum?

References

1. Mahatma Gandhi. Live as if you were to die tomorrow. Accessed May 30, 2021. https://www.brainyquote.com/quotes/mahatma_gandhi_133995
2. Palliative Care. Accessed May 30, 2021. https://www.who.int/news-room/fact-sheets/detail/palliative-care
3. IPE Collaborative Home. Accessed May 30, 2021. https://www.ipecollaborative.org/
4. Interprofessional Education Collaborative. *Core Competencies for Interprofessional Collaborative Practice: 2016 Update.* Interprofessional Education Collaborative; 2016.
5. Brock KE, Cohen HJ, Sourkes, BM, Good JJ, Halamek, LP. Training pediatric fellows in palliative care: A pilot comparision of simulation training and didactic education. *J Palliat Med.* 2017;20(910):1074–1084. doi:10.1089/jpm.2016.0556.

[†] Although we typically use "interprofessional," to mean the healthcare professions learning and practicing together, we have left the terminology "interdisciplinary" in this chapter since the term is so commonly used in the nomenclature of academic coursework, where the focus is knowledge as well as practice.

6. Starks H, Coats H, Paganelli T, et al. Pilot study of an interprofessional palliative care curriculum: course content and participant reported learning gains. *Am J Hosp Palliat Care.* 2018;25(3):390–397. doi10.1177/1049909117725042.

7. Wittenberg-Lyles E, Goldsmith J, Ferrell B, Burchett M. Assessment of an interprofessional online curriculum for palliative care communication training. *J Palliat Med.* 2014;17(4):400–406. doi: 10.1089/jpm.2013.0270.

8. Buring SM, Bhushan A, Brazeau G, Conway S, Hansen L, Westberg S. Keys to successful implementation of interprofessional education: Learning location, faculty development, and curricular themes. *Am J Pharm Educ.* 2009;73(4):60. doi:10.5688/aj730460.

9. Reeves S, Fletcher S, Barr H, et al. A BEME systematic review of the effects of interprofessional education: BEME guide no 39. *Med Teach.* 2016;38(7):656–658. doi:10.3109/0142159X.2016.1173663.

10. Association of American Medical Colleges (AAMC) Core Competencies for Entering Medical School. Accessed May 30, 2021. https://www.aamc.org/services/admissions-lifecycle/competencies-entering-medical-students.

11. American Association of Colleges of Nursing. The Essentials: Core Competencies for Professional Nursing Education. Published April 2021. Accessed May 30, 2021. https://www.aacnnursing.org/Portals/42/AcademicNursing/pdf/Essentials-2021.pdf.

12. National Coalition for Hospice and Palliative Care. Palliative Care Guidelines. Published 2018. Accessed May 30, 2021. https://www.nationalcoalitionhpc.org/wp-content/uploads/2020/07/NCHPC-NCPGuidelines_4thED_web_FINAL.pdf.

13. Dow AW, DiazGranados D, Mazmanian PE, Retchin SM. Applying organizational science to health care: A framework for colloborative practice. *Acad Med.* 2013;88(7):952–7. doi:10.1097/ACM.0b013e31829523d1.

14. Donesky D, de Leon K, Bailey A, et al. Excellence in postlicensure interprofessional palliative care education. *J Hosp Palliat Nurs.* 2020;22(1):17–25. doi:10.1097/NJH.0000000000000602.

15. Benner P. Using the Dreyfus model of skill acquisition to describe and interpret skill acquisition and clinical judgment in nursing practice and education. *Bull Sci Technol Soc.* 2004;24(3):188–199. doi:10.1177/0270467604265061

16. Benner, P. From novice to expert. *Am J Nurs.* 1982;82(3):402–407.

17. Wiegand DL, Cheon J, Netzer G. Seeing the patient and family through: Nurses and physicians experiences with withdrawal of life-sustaining therapy in the ICU. *Am J Hosp Palliat Med.* 2019;36(1):13–23. doi:10.1177/1049909118801011.

18. Esplen MJ, Hunter J, Maheu C, et al. De Souza interprofessional practice cancer competency framework. *Support Care Cancer.* 2020 Feb;28(2):797–808. doi:10.1007/s00520-019-04823-z. Epub 2019 May 31. PMID: 31152301.

19. Barton AJ, Armstrong G, Preheim G, Gelmon SB, Andrus LC. A national Delphi to determine developmental progression of quality and safety competencies in nursing education. *Nurs Outlook.* 2009;57:312–322.

20. van Diggele C, Roberts C, Haq I. Optimising student-led interprofessional learning across eleven health disciplines. *BMC Med Educ.* 2021;21:157.

21. Taber KS. Scaffolding learning: Principles for effective teaching and the design of classroom resources. In: Abend M, ed. *Effective Teaching and Learning: Perspectives, Strategies and Implementation.* Nova Science; 2018:1–43.

22. Poirier T, Wilhelm M. An interprofessional faculty seminar focused on interprofessional education. *Am J Pharm Educ.* 2014;78(4):80 doi:10.5688/ajpe78480.

23. Tolsgaard MG, Kulasegaram KM, Ringsted CV. Collaborative learning of clinical skills in health professions education: The why, how, when and for whom. *Med Educ.* 2016 Jan;50(1):69–78. doi:10.1111/medu.12814. PMID: 26695467.

24. Koehn ML, Charles SC. A Delphi study to determine leveling of the interprofessional core competencies for four levels of interprofessional practice. *Med Sci Edu.* 2019;29:389–398.

25. Bansal A, Jain S, Sharma L, Sharma N, Jain C, Madaan M. Students' perception regarding pedagogy, andragogy, and heutagogy as teaching-learning methods in undergraduate

medical education. *J Educ Health Promot*. 2020 Nov 26;9:301. doi:10.4103/jehp.jehp_221_20. PMID: 33426105; PMCID: PMC7774633.

26. Shulman LS. Signature pedagogies in the professions. *Daedalus*. 2005;134(3):52–59.

27. Zand DE. Collateral organization: A new change strategy. *J Appl Behav Sci.*1974;10(1):63–89.

28. Wenger E, McDermott R, Snyder WM. *Cultivating Communities of Practice: A Guide to Managing Knowledge*. Harvard Business School Press; 2002.

29. Bratianu C. *Organizational Knowledge Dynamics: Managing Knowledge Creation, Acquisition, Sharing, and Transformation*. IGI Global; 2015. doi:10.4018/978-1-4666-8318-1.ch01182(3), Chapter 9, 207–229.

30. Moule P. E-learning for healthcare students: Developing communities of practice framework. *J Adv Nurs.*2006;54(3):370–380.

31. Speakman E. Effective interprofessional education and collaborative practice in nursing education. Accessed May 30, 2021. https://www.wolterskluwer.com/en/expert-insights/effective-interprofessional-education.

32. Haughland M, Brenna SJ, Aanes MM. Interprofessional education as a contributor to professional and interprofessional identities. *I Interprof Care*. 2019 Dec;9:1–7.

33. Bogetz JF, Friebert S. Defining success in pediatric palliative care while tackling the quadruple aim. *J Palliat Med*. 2017 Feb;20(2):116–119. doi:10.1089/jpm.2016.0389. Epub 2016 Oct 19. PMID: 28085547.

34. O'Keefe M, Henderson A, Chick R. Defining a set of common interprofessional learning competencies for health profession students. *Med Teach*. 2017;39(5):463–468.

35. Gruppen LD, Irby DM, Durning SJ, Maggio LA. Interventions designed to improve the learning environment in the health professions. In: *Proceedings of a Conference Sponsored by Josiah Macy Jr., Foundation in April 2018*. Josiah Macy Jr. Foundation; 2019:57–103.

36. Brashers V, Haizlip J, Owen JA. The ASPIRE model: Grounding the IPEC core competencies for interprofessional collaborative practice within a foundational framework. *J Interprof Care*. 2020;34(1):128–132.

37. Joynes VCT. Defining and understanding the relationship between professional identity and interprofessional responsibility: Implications for educating health and social care students. *Adv Health Sci Educ Theory Pract*. 2018;23(1):133–149.

38. Lindquist I, Engardt M, Garnham L, Poland F, Richardson B. Developmental pathways in learning to be a physiotherapist. *Physiother Res Int*. 2006;11(3):129–139.

39. Choi BC, Pak AW. Multidisciplinarity, interdisciplinarity and transdisciplinarity in health research, services, education and policy: 1. Definitions, objectives, and evidence of effectiveness. *Clin Invest Med*. 2006;29(6):351–364.

40. (NSERC) Natural Sciences and Engineering Research Council of Canada. Guidelines for the Preparation and Review of Applications in Interdisciplinary Research. 2004. https://www.nserc-crsng.gc.ca/.

41. Mueller SK. Transdisciplinary coordination and delivery of care. *Semin Oncol Nurs*. 2016 May;32(2):154–63. doi:10.1016/j.soncn.2016.02.009. Epub 2016 Mar 4. PMID: 27137472.

42. Bernard-Bonnin A, Stachenko S, Bonin D, Al E. Self-management teaching programs and morbidity of pediatric asthma: A meta-analysis. *J Allergy Clin Immunol*. 1995;95:34–41.

43. Soskolne C. Transdisciplinary approaches for public health. *Epidemiology*. 2000;11:S122.

44. Van Bewer V. Transdisciplinarity in health care: A concept analysis. *Nurs Forum*. 2017;52(4):339–347. doi:10.1111/nuf.12200.

45. Ahia CL, Blais CM. Primary palliative care for the general internist: Integrating goals of care discussions into the outpatient setting. *Ochsner J*. 2014;14:704–711.

46. Boland JW, Brown MEL, Duenas A, et al. How effective is undergraduate palliative care teaching for medical students? A systematic literature review. *BMJ Open*. 2020;10:e036458. doi:10.1136/bmjopen-2019-036458.

47. Fitzpatrick D, Heah R, Patten S, et al. Palliative care in undergraduate medical education—how far have we come? *Am J Hosp Palliat Care*. 2017;34(8):762–773.

48. Denney-Koelsch EM, Horowitz R, Quill T, et al. An integrated, developmental four-year medical school curriculum in palliative care: A longitudinal content evaluation based on national competency standards. *J Palliat Med.* 2018;21(9):1221–1233.

49. Zolot J. the AACN recommends increased palliative care training in undergraduate nursing education. *AJN.* 2016;116(5):16.

50. Pieters J, Dolmans DHJM, Verstegen DML, et al. Palliative care education in the undergraduate medical curricula: Students' views on the importance of, their confidence in, and knowledge of palliative care. *BMC Palliat Care.* 2019;18:72. https://doi.org/10.1186/s12904-019-0458-x.

51. Pruskowski JA, Patel R, Nguyen K, et al. A systematic review of palliative care content in the Doctor of Pharmacy curriculum. *Am J Pharm Educ.* 2021;85(6):459–467.

52. Lippe M. Assessment of primary palliative care content within prelicensure nursing education: A multisite feasibility study. *J Hosp Palliat Nurs.* 2019;21(5):373–381.

53. Head BA, Schapmire TJ, Earnshaw L, et al. Improving medical graduates' training in palliative care: Advancing education and practice. *Adv Med Educ Pract.* 2016;7:99–113.

54. Dickinson GE. End-of-life and palliative care education in US pharmacy schools. *Am J Hosp Palliat Med.* 2012;39(6):532–535.

55. Berkman C, Stein GL. Palliative and end-of-life care in the masters of social work curriculum. *Palliat Support Care.* 2018;16(2):180–188.

56. Von gunten CF. Secondary and tertiary palliative care in US hospitals. *JAMA.* 2002;287(7):875–881.

57. Branon R. University of Washington Continuum College. 60-Year Curriculum Resource Guide: Supporting the Changing Landscape of Lifelong Learning. Accessed August 4, 2021. https://continuum.uw.edu/getmedia/8fc250b1-5bfc-4a40-bab5-41f4f02b07ae/uwc2-60-year-resource-guide.pdf.

58. Matkin G. The 60-year curriculum: What universities should do. *eCampus News.* Published January 6, 2020. Accessed August 4, 2021. https://www.ecampusnews.com/2020/01/06/the-60-year-curriculum-what-universities-should-do/2/.

59. University of Maryland School of Pharmacy. Dual degrees and pathways. Accessed August 4, 2021. https://www.pharmacy.umaryland.edu/academics/dualdegrees/.

60. Iowa College of Pharmacy. Palliative care certificate. 2021. Accessed August 4, 2021. https://pharmacy.uiowa.edu/pharmd/dual_cert/palliative.

9

Interprofessional Specialty Palliative Care Clinical Education and Training

Allison Kestenbaum, Thomas Reid, and Constance Dahlin

Key Points

- The definition of and approach to specialty palliative care education and training vary greatly among social work, medicine, chaplain, and nursing professions.
- Barriers to graduate and early career palliative care interprofessional education (IPE) are numerous and significant but not insurmountable. Transdisciplinary education, like transdisciplinary clinical work, is difficult to create but critical to the effective practice and philosophy of palliative care.
- In the context of perceived and actual interprofessional power dynamics, the ongoing process of understanding and engaging with both our own and others' professional identities and cultural norms must form the foundation of IPE. It takes repeated reinforcement and modeling to overcome existing maladaptive role assumptions.
- If the field is to truly establish interprofessional palliative care, it is essential to be educated and trained in an interprofessional manner to practice that way. That means not accepting the status quo and moving to organize institutional structures around palliative care in which the process is interprofessional from the beginning rather than "in addition to" by profession. This means being open to new models of care and not falling back on "this is the way we have always done it" or "we cannot do it that way because that is not how it is done."

Introduction

By its nature, specialty palliative care teams are composed of clinicians from multiple professions who have undergone specialist training.[1] Clinical learning opportunities are essential in the development of effective interprofessional palliative care specialist clinicians. Although palliative care is often the topic of prelicensure didactic learning experiences, as its inherently interprofessional nature lends itself well to interprofessional case studies and discussions,[2] very few of those prelicensure learning experiences incorporate an interprofessional experience in the clinical environment. Similarly upon graduation, clinicians do not have many opportunities for interprofessional palliative care specialist training in the clinical environment.

The National Consensus Project (NCP) Clinical Practice Guidelines delineate the team as composed of chaplains, physicians, registered nurses, social workers, and other professionals based on need.[1] Most of the professions listed within this chapter have defined specialist clinical competencies, but their approaches to education, training, and certification are different (see Chapter 3). The core* professions of palliative care differ widely in how they conceptualize specialization and the paths their practitioners take to attain it.

There is richness in the history of profession-specific recognition of specialty palliative practice.[3] The first discipline to acknowledge the specialty[2†] of hospice and palliative care was nursing for both registered nurses (RNs) and advanced practice registered nurses (APRNs). This occurred in 1987 with endorsement of specialty scope and standards of the American Nurses Association, followed by a specialty board certification in 1994.[4] Board certification for physicians was developed in 1997, followed by recognition as a medical specialty in 2006.[5] Social work specialty acknowledgment occurred in 2000 with the initiation of certification between the National Association of Social Workers and the National Hospice and Palliative Care Organization.[6,7] In 2019, the Social Work Hospice and Palliative Network initiated a new certification following an examination.[8] Palliative chaplaincy was recognized as specialty practice in 2010 when the Association of Professional Chaplains Board of Chaplaincy Certification first offered certification, followed by the National Association of Catholic Chaplains in 2014.[9]

The purpose of this chapter is to explore the education (theoretical learning) and training (application of skills) in the clinical setting required to develop interprofessional palliative care specialists. Specialty interprofessional palliative care clinical education builds on profession-specific palliative care competencies and palliative care curricula representing literature from all disciplines to develop clinicians with a shared expertise in palliative care in addition to their profession-specific competencies.[1,10] Because specialty interprofessional clinical education is still rare, much of this chapter is aspirational. The chapter begins with a comparison among residencies, fellowships, and clinical immersion courses as options for

---

* In this book, we use the term "core" to refer to chaplains, nurses, physicians, and social workers, who are all named as part of the interprofessional team for both the Medicare hospice guidelines and the NCP guidelines. This designation does not minimize the importance of other team members who contribute to the palliative care of patients and families

† Palliative care is considered to be a subspecialty within medicine and nursing, but a specialty in spiritual care and social work. For this book, we standardize the language by referring to palliative care as a specialty when referring to the team as a whole. We use the term "subspecialty" when referring specifically to nursing or medicine.

clinical education. It proceeds with a discussion of barriers and potential solutions for interprofessional clinical education in palliative care and concludes with caveats for faculty to consider when developing their own interprofessional program. The scope of this chapter includes: (1) the "core" palliative care professions as delineated within the NCP guidelines—medicine, nursing, social work, and spiritual care; and (2) interprofessional clinical education and training in specialty palliative care.

NCP describes many other potential clinical palliative care team members, in addition to the core professions, depending on the availability of specialist clinicians and whether the population is for adults, children, or both. This includes psychological and psychiatric professionals (e.g., psychologists, psychiatrists, and child life specialists),[11] pharmacists, physician assistants/associates (PA), rehabilitation specialists (e.g., physical therapy, occupational therapy, speech and language pathologists), expressive art therapists (e.g., music therapy, art therapy), and integrative therapists (e.g., massage, acutherapy, etc.).[1] Team members vary according to the setting where care occurs—in the acute-care setting, clinic, long-term care, or in the home. Administrative staff play key roles in interprofessional education (IPE) since these individuals serve in positions of schedulers, administrative assistants, interpreters, and the like, who support the clinical encounter. All professionals' perspectives are critically important and should be incorporated when available. Family caregivers are also critically important members of the palliative care team.

How Are Specialist Palliative Care Practitioners Educated and Trained?

Specialty palliative care clinical education and training thus far includes residencies, fellowships, and immersion courses. Residencies are profession-specific clinical training opportunities available either during the final term before graduation or immediately after licensure, depending upon the profession. Fellowship is clinical training for a particular specialty such as palliative care. Immersion courses are brief clinical opportunities designed for working professionals who are seeking additional expertise in a specific area of practice. Few programs incorporate a truly IPE approach in training palliative care specialists, and palliative care clinicians are dependent upon profession-specific residencies, fellowships, or immersion programs for their clinical education.[12,13] Often, attempts at IPE in the clinical setting have been tacked onto physician clinical fellowships with little accommodation for IPE faculty, understanding of profession-specific scope of practice, or revision of content using references from journals that reflect all professions.[12] Ideally, professions can grow together, rather than just in parallel, with interprofessional faculty collaborating together on curriculum development and learner goals to "learn about, from and with each other."[14(p 7)]

Residencies

The term "residency" is generally defined as enhanced clinical training for entry to practice, but the term is operationalized differently within various health professions. For physicians, residency is the second year of practice after graduating medical school, where physicians learn in-depth clinical knowledge within a designated graduate medical education (GME) training program under the supervision of experienced attending physicians.[19] For nursing, residency is a 6–12-month planned comprehensive program immediately after graduation, sponsored by a hospital or healthcare agency, in which a registered nurse (RN) or advanced practice registered nurse (APRN) acquires the skills and knowledge for practice.[20-22] For social work, residencies (also referred to as internships or practicums) occur during Masters of Social Work (MSW) programs and offer additional didactic content in a selected area of study prior to graduation.[23] Chaplain residencies are mentored clinical experiences that are embedded within the requirements of Clinical Pastoral Education (CPE) and/or the prerequisite Masters of Divinity or graduate-level theological education. With the exception of one chaplain residency,[24] none of the core palliative care professions offers a palliative care residency. In contrast, 31 postgraduate second-year residencies in pain and palliative care are available for pharmacists in the United States.[25,26] To our knowledge, no interprofessional palliative care residencies have been developed.

Fellowships

Fellowships are universally defined as one-year postgraduate programs in an area of specialization. Again, there may be a difference in clinical expertise upon entrance to a palliative fellowship. Physicians have several years of postgraduate training prior to fellowship. MSWs and chaplains may have clinical experience, whereas advanced practice providers (APPs, which includes both APRNs—clinical nurse specialists [CNSs] and nurse practitioners [NPs]—and PAs) may be new to their advanced practice role. Although rare, interprofessional faculty in palliative care training programs are beginning to develop interprofessional fellowship programs. A long-term interprofessional pediatric palliative fellowship in Boston, Massachusetts, has been successful in IPE collaboration, demonstrated by interprofessional peer relationships, interprofessional mentoring in spite of roles, and fulfillment of educational needs.[17] The Veterans Administration Interprofessional Fellowship in Palliative Care incorporated explicit IPE,[18] though several VA IPE fellowships are on pause and their future is unclear.

Due to federal funding through Medicare, many physician palliative care fellowships are funded under the auspices of Graduate Medical Training. Although, theoretically, monies could be allocated to IPE training, thus far this has not happened, although the Government Accounting Office has put forth recommendations to do so for PAs and NPs.[27] The result is that there are few focused, 1-year clinical fellowships for master's-prepared APRNs, master's-prepared social workers (MSWs), and chaplains. This translates to the fact that in the United States, nursing, social work, spiritual care, and pharmacy combined graduate only 5%–10% as many palliative care specialists annually as their physician counterpart programs, often due to a lack of funding outside of physician training. While fellowships are necessary in medicine for specialty palliative board certification, other professions use different criteria, including practice-hour requirements obtained through on-the-job training (see Chapter 3). Eligibility may also include other activities such as academic activities—writing, teaching, precepting, and committee work.

The imbalanced numbers of formally trained specialists mean that far more clinical mentors are typically available to physicians than to other interprofessional clinicians. As non-physician fellowships and clinical training opportunities develop, there will be a demand for palliative care certified mentors representing all the core palliative care professions. Though existing formal inter-institutional mentorship programs have begun to bridge the gap, such as through the Social Work Hospice and Palliative Network (SWHPN),[28] mentorship must still be a high priority for non-physician palliative residents and fellows. Finally, the disproportion of formal specialist training opportunities and absence of IPE fellowship opportunities demonstrates that social work, spiritual care, nursing, and other clinicians need more attention and resources to develop these programs.

Immersion Programs

The variability in residencies and fellowships, as well as the dearth of postgraduate opportunities for non-physicians, has led to palliative care immersion programs.[29,30] Immersion programs are defined as intensive programs which may offer education over days- to weeks-long education, potential for clinical observation, and clinical mentoring.[31-33] They are an affordable option for many clinicians to cultivate a deeper knowledge. Currently, there are 5 established programs that vary in length, content, cost, and eligibility, but none of them is fully interprofessional with representation from all 4 core palliative care professions in the faculty and learner cohorts.

The frequent scheduling and locality of immersion programs allow the highest ability to promote interprofessional collaborative practice. Examples are the Four Seasons Institute in North Carolina and Coleman Palliative Medicine Training Program in Illinois.[29,34,35] They are held many times during a year and are open to all professions to apply. Some courses are in-person, some are online, and others have been a hybrid. Moreover, they often have tiered fees for the various professions to better ensure parity of cost to salary. The challenge is that clinicians need to utilize educational funds or personal funds to attend them. While this may not be a problem for physicians, educational funds for non-physicians have decreased, particularly as a result of financial challenges caused by the COVID-19 pandemic. To be successful, immersion programs need highly regarded interprofessional faculty.

Barriers and Solutions

In 2013, the Institute of Medicine listed some of the challenges of IPE. They discussed curricular innovations, how to ensure that content met learning needs, and pedagogic innovations related to how and where information is presented. They also focused on cultural elements—who is being taught by whom, human resources, expansion of capacity, and metrics related to learner assessment and evaluation of educational impact.[36] Additional areas of consideration are unique to interprofessional specialty palliative care education and training because of the variation in interprofessional development of specialty practice, competencies, and certification. A survey administered through the Center to Advance Palliative Care revealed progress in specialty education and training of interprofessional residencies, fellowships, and immersion programs.[37] Specifically, the data revealed that there is a wide range of possible specialty education, including an increased number of graduate palliative care programs available to the interprofessional team, and a wide range of training for the interprofessional with a marked increase in the number of Palliative Care APRN fellowships, which are sometimes categorized as APP fellowships (for either PAs or APRNs).

This section delineates common barriers to interprofessional clinical education in palliative care, along with ideas for potential solutions. Discussion is built on existing literature, author experience in facilitating IPE palliative care education, and expert opinion derived from surveys, interviews, and communication with palliative care thought leaders. Barriers to IPE can be categorized into the broad classifications of issues related to (1) politics and resources; (2) healthcare culture; (3) curricula; (4) people; and (5) the clinical learning environment. In addition, these issues can manifest at one or more levels: (1) government and professional (macro); (2) institutional (meso); and (3) individual (micro) (see Figure 9.1).

Politics and Resources

Given the magnitude of governmental involvement in healthcare, with educational funding and health insurance benefits dependent upon congressional action, palliative care clinical education is inherently dependent on political advocacy. Resources are also dependent on leadership in government, healthcare systems, universities, professional societies, and accrediting organizations.

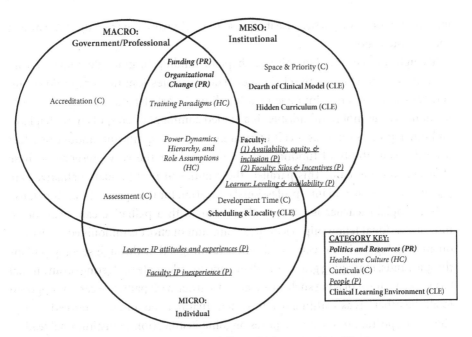

Figure 9.1. Barriers to interprofessional clinical education in palliative care.

Funding

Funding sources for graduate clinical training vary but have certain commonalities. In the current system in the United States, physician graduate medical education (GME) is the only recipient of federal and state funding through Medicare, Medicaid, the Department of Defense, the Veterans Affairs (VA) system, and the Health Resources and Services Administration (HRSA).[38] These funds are primarily directed to teaching hospitals and reach physician trainees through their GME offices. Positions funded by these sources are also implicitly funded by private insurance payments made to the teaching hospital. While the majority of GME positions are funded in this way, many hospice and palliative medicine (HPM) fellowships also receive support from philanthropy, academic departments, and divisions in schools of medicine—including clinical revenue, local hospice organizations, local hospitals, insurers, HMOs, physician groups, and grants.

Many interprofessional education and training programs seek financial support through HRSA grant funding, philanthropy, other grants, and collaborations between healthcare organizations and schools/colleges of nursing or social work. Programs may try to offset costs by having trainees bill for care such as in the case of APRNs or LCSWs (Licensed Clinical Social Workers). The ratio of such monetary support reveals the inequity of financial support to non-physicians and explains the challenge of integrating interprofessional clinical training programs. Chaplain, social work, and nursing programs sometimes also use clinical salary support that is available through streams not usually dedicated to education (e.g., clinical revenue) as well as support from professional schools. For HPM physician fellows, this form of support is illegal because it represents double dipping from the government sources listed above.

Though unique, the dynamics of chaplain funding in graduate palliative care clinical education hints at the challenges of health professions that simply do not receive any government reimbursement for clinical work, let alone postgraduate education. "We are not reimbursable" is a loaded comment often spoken by chaplains and other professionals as a call to awareness that a significant amount of effort toward sustainability of funding will be required for the very presence of these clinicians on the team. This parallels the realities in postgraduate palliative care profession-specific and interprofessional education for non-prescribing clinicians.

If a chaplain learner is consistently present with a palliative care team or an interprofessional fellowship, a significant amount of effort is undoubtedly devoted, on an ongoing basis, to secure and renew funding either through seeking philanthropic funds, managing grants, or advocating for adequate budgeting on an annual basis. The value of placing such an advanced learner with palliative care, as opposed to all the other areas within a health system that may be under-resourced in psychosocial spiritual resources, requires ongoing justification to institutional leadership. The time devoted by the palliative care chaplain administrator to protecting and justifying the chaplain learner's financial existence is not available for IPE, team support, or care for patients at the bedside.

A long-term solution for funding interprofessional palliative care clinical education will come from the macro and meso levels. At the macro level, interprofessional clinical education will need to be integrated into the federal and state funding sources currently designated for medical education. At the meso level, institutions can show their support for interprofessional palliative care education in the clinical setting by developing offices/centers of interprofessional palliative care education with a designated department focused on the clinical learning environment. Philanthropic organizations focused on palliative care and/or interprofessional collaboration could designate funding for interprofessional clinical education. With the assistance of a talented and creative administrator, palliative care teams in healthcare systems could be structured to support interprofessional clinical learning funded by professional revenue and cost savings for the institution in partnership with managed care organizations.

Organizational Change

The inherent requirement for buy-in of and cooperation among multiple high-level stakeholders leaves IPE programs vulnerable to disruptions in leadership and organizational structure. Such disruptions "can result in a loss of ownership, expertise, continuity, enthusiasm and communication between the stakeholder groups."[39(p 2)] At the meso and macro levels, wholehearted support for interprofessional collaboration will not occur until the executive leadership of professional societies, training programs, and palliative care teams represents all of the professions on a palliative care team. Until that occurs, conscious effort must be focused on developing and maintaining relationships among stakeholders and professional societies representing all professional perspectives in the interprofessional team. While individual champions are necessary to initiate an IPE program, such programs are only sustainable through changes to organizational culture that create a greater appreciation of the value of IPE.[40] Moreover, until there is more hard evidence of improved patient outcomes related to IPE, it may be difficult to make the case to support the resources necessary to create interprofessional education to effect interprofessional collaborative clinical care.[41]

Healthcare Culture

Many clinicians have a limited or incorrect understanding of the roles, skills, and styles of other professions.[42] Indeed, many students enter their professions with misunderstanding about other healthcare professionals.[43] The varying professions have a different view of the patient—biomedical versus holistic and some offer more qualitative information rather than quantitative. Scope of practice as legally and culturally understood for physicians is very broad relative to other professions. This difference in scope of practice may cause a tentativeness to learn a wider breadth of knowledge since it may not pertain to a profession. Clinicians may also hold incorrect assessments of their own potential role, especially in palliative care where transdisciplinary[‡] practice blurs role boundaries (see Chapter 3). Other professions tend to defer to physician opinions, even when the doctor exceeds their knowledge base.

Together, these assumptions may result in experienced social workers, nurses, and chaplains believing they are not qualified or not allowed to engage in transdisciplinary practice that includes responsibilities traditionally granted to physicians, even in the presence of explicit encouragement and contrary evidence.[44] Pharmacists embrace their own expertise in medications and pharmacotherapy, and physicians may in fact defer to them. Other professionals on the team may have their own profession-specific experience when growing into the role of a palliative care specialist.

While some constraints are real and even necessary, examining these assumptions is a critical first step for many clinicians to fully engage in transdisciplinary IPE. And whether in formal education or within teams, it is vital to discuss professional roles and responsibilities and how they overlap. Even seasoned clinicians have more to learn about the roles and expertise of interprofessional colleagues.[44] Furthermore,

---

[‡] The process a transdisciplinary framework is pointing to is more accurately described as transprofessional, since it illustrates the collaboration and synergy between professions rather than disciplines. However, in this chapter and throughout the book, the term "transdisciplinary" is used since it is currently the word most used in the literature to signify this form of team collaboration. When we refer to "interprofessional" it is within this framework of working at the transdisciplinary collaborative level. It is referring to an advanced level of professional synergy.

all faculty and clinicians can benefit from developing greater awareness of their biases about interprofessional care and collaboration, and how their actions may unwittingly contradict their words.

The assumptions clinicians make about themselves and each other are perhaps the most potent and most complicated barrier to both transdisciplinary practice and effective IPE (see Chapter 4). These assumptions are rooted in both histor-ical precedent and lived experience and are inculcated in trainees at every level of health professions education. Clinical assumptions and abilities are embedded, deliberately and accidentally, in nearly every aspect of nearly every health system. Professional identity also intersects with many other forms of identity, such as race, gender, socioeconomic class, ability or disability, and others. The fundamental nature of the lived experience of faculty and learners from different professions means that addressing these concerns must be at the core of any successful IPE that moves beyond a superficial level of collaboration. Palliative care's transdisciplinary aspirations only make this exploration more essential.

Power Dynamics, Hierarchy, and Role Assumptions

While imbalances in power in the healthcare system have been well described else-where,[45, 46] a few highlights may be illustrative to how the power dynamics play out in palliative care IPE, often with negative outcomes. Most acute care palliative care teams include physicians, who have received significantly more formal training than other team members. This is the opposite in community-based programs, where the non-physician team members may have more experience and contin-uing education than physicians. This disjunction may exacerbate underlying power dynamics, though the explicit incorporation of transdisciplinary principles and experiences into that training might counterbalance this effect.

Another major issue is scope of practice. The difference in scope of practice be-tween clinicians is grounded in education, licensure, and certification. APPs have a more similar palliative care practice authority to physicians, allowing them to order medications and other therapies; consequently, their scope of practice allows for re-imbursement of services and they are often referred to collectively with physicians as "providers."[§] This may cause friction with other team members.

Of all interactions between the professions, registered nurse-physician collab-oration has been best studied, and the patterns observed may serve as a template for challenges in other interprofessional relations. Historically, physicians took on a directive role and registered nurses were "expected to acquiesce to physicians and focus on patient care."[45(p 166)] Though modern curricula explicitly reject this

---

§ Concerns have been raised about the use of the term "provider" in healthcare as it suggests a commer-cial transaction rather than a relationship between clinician and patient, and it obscures the specific role and credentials of individual clinicians. The terms "clinician," "practitioner," or "healthcare professional" are suggested as preferable when an overarching term is necessary (Scarff JR, What's in a name? The problematic term "provider," *Federal Practitioner* 2021;38(10):446). For this edition, the decision was made to keep the term "provider" when it was used by chapter authors, while recognizing that this change may be necessary for future editions.

paradigm in favor of a collaborative model, cultural residue remains. In their collaboration with physicians, registered nurses most commonly desire decisional equity, input into plans of care, 2-way knowledge exchange, active listening, and respect for their opinions.[45] In many settings, physicians have the ultimate legal and professional responsibility for overseeing patient care, which shapes physician vision and expectations for collaboration or lack thereof.[47] This becomes most evident when there is a difference of opinion. In that realm, more often than not, there is not a shared decision-making process. Rather, the physician's decision trumps all other interprofessional views. Though culture is changing, a significant number of physicians still feel collaboration is most effective when they maintain control.[48] Changing the locus of control to a shared decision-making model will take dedicated time and effort.

Of the core palliative care professions, physicians are typically granted the most power and authority by the system. Physician and APP (nurse practitioners [NPs], clinical nurse specialists [CNSs] in most states, and PA) time is implicitly acknowledged as valuable through billing, while social workers, registered nurses (RNs), and chaplains typically do not generate independent revenue. Social workers with a clinical license can bill in some outpatient settings and bill for advance care planning services by direct or incident to billing. Registered nurses are also able to bill for advance care planning services by incident to billing. In spite of the range of expertise and education of all clinicians, physicians often hold the majority of leadership roles in health systems, and their perspectives are typically considered even when other professions might have more expertise. In medical care, physicians write "orders" that members of other professions are expected to carry out. This language grounds the hierarchical paradigm in interprofessional relationships because of scope of practice alone[47] (see Chapter 4 for greater discussion of interprofessional tension).

In the educational setting, faculty and students may display explicit, suppressed, or implicit biases during training. Learners may struggle with transdisciplinarity as they attempt to learn their profession-specific role. They may reject the idea that certain roles, such as screening outside of their domain or shared leadership, are within their scope of practice. When leading interprofessional education, even experienced faculty benefit from setting aside time to reflect together on their professional assumptions and talk about the impact of hierarchy on their experience. They should expect that unexamined assumptions and cultural patterns will surface and should make time and space to process them. Interprofessional coursework depends on ground rules for full faculty participation in all interprofessional curriculum development and explicit review of all content to ensure that all professional voices are reflected. Longitudinal courses can devote time to centering learners in their own professional role while educating learners about the roles of other professions. Recognizing the time, faculty development, and careful facilitation that are necessary to properly explore issues related to power dynamics, hierarchy, and role assumptions, faculty who are teaching in brief courses or single sessions may want to acknowledge the issue but not delve into topics that cannot receive the time and attention they deserve. Faculty can uncover and address biases as they surface, and model transdisciplinary work as they teach together.

Training Paradigms

The process of socialization in the various professions emphasizes different elements. Though they share many similarities, educational approaches may also vary by profession, which can lead to clashing assumptions between both instructors and learners. For example, physicians are often trained as directive leaders. They are expected to have an opinion and to assert it, as reinforced by such practices as "pimping," when a learner is subject to "a series of difficult and often intentionally unanswerable questions . . . in quick succession" with the intention "to teach, motivate, and involve the learner in clinical rounds while maintaining a dominant hierarchy and cultivating humility by ridding the learner of egotism."[49(p 2347)] They are expected to take the lead in any mixed group unless someone more senior is present.

There are some other distinctions that occur within the education of health professionals. One characteristic is the difference of care models within the professions. A biomedical care model is most often used by physicians, advanced practice providers, and pharmacists. A more person-first model of care is used by chaplains and social workers. This is further exemplified by the degree to which various individual, group, and facilitated reflective practices are utilized. Generally, reflection practices are more common in chaplain and social work than in nursing, medicine, and pharmacy. Medicine is taught from a deductive perspective, teaching the basic sciences before applying those principles to patients, while nursing is taught from an inductive perspective where they meet patients very early in their education and use the observations from their clinical work to build their scientific knowledge.

In addition, social work and chaplains often utilize a "supervision" model, where individuals meet regularly with a mentor and a peer group to discuss difficult cases in a structured manner. Overall, the professions also make very different assumptions about the importance of context.[50] Regardless of the salient differences, uncovering assumptions about how training "should" proceed is critical to building an effective IPE curriculum. When an interprofessional colleague's perspective is met with a high degree of resistance, this may be a sign of interprofessional tension related to the differences in training paradigms. These occasions can become insightful learning opportunities when embraced with curiosity.

The transdisciplinary model assumes that each team member will share overlapping professional spheres of practice, functioning as a palliative care specialist in their own profession and a generalist in all of the other core professions of palliative care (see Chapter 3). These overlapping skills include understanding of disease trajectories, communication, pain and symptom assessment, psychosocial, spiritual, and psychiatric distress assessment, and management of physical and psychiatric symptoms, as delineated in the NCP Clinical Practice Guidelines.[1,10] However, more work is needed on developing the IPE specialty palliative care clinical competencies that reflect these skills. This will take time for IPE faculty to truly collaborate to develop competencies that reflect the principles of IPE and palliative care.

Curricula

Palliative care is a relatively new specialty, competing for space in health professions curricula that have been in existence for decades or centuries. Most university and health systems administrators recognize the unique needs of patients who are seriously ill, but the practical issues of time and space often interfere with the intention to prioritize palliative care education and training.

Space and Priority

Educational program directors and faculty leaders may feel their uni-professional curriculum is "full." Clinical placements may be prioritized based on accreditation or availability. Depending on the background and experiences of faculty, they may not recognize the value of interprofessional palliative care. Palliative care IPE may therefore compete with, or be perceived as competing with, existing content for space in the curriculum.[51] While some trade-offs may be necessary, careful analysis and planning can address shared content collaboratively, enriching the experience for all health professions programs. Palliative care champions, both faculty and students, can focus on building relationships with professional leaders and developing a sense of necessity for implementing interprofessional palliative care education. Even full curricula can offer opportunities for interprofessional faculty who teach or co-teach content.

Development Time

IPE curricula often take longer to build because they require multiple individuals to coordinate the integration of several disparate professional and training cultures. Moreover, it requires time and effort to ensure representation of faculty to co-create a comprehensive curriculum with all the professions at the table to create it, reflecting IP collaboration, rather than it being created and then asking other faculty to approve it. It also necessitates the time to perform a literature search and to ensure that perspectives from all the professions reflect the unique and similar work of each profession, as well as the commonality of the work and skills. High faculty workloads may make this additional work unappealing. With the support of leadership, it is essential to plan for the extra time required to ensure that content and course structure reflect all professional perspectives.

Accreditation and Assessment

Broad-based changes in curricular values and structure such as IPE are often driven by national consensus, commonly expressed through accreditation standards.[52] The Health Professions Accreditors Collaborative (HPAC; https://healthprofess ionsaccreditors.org/) was formed in 2014 to provide accreditors representing the health professions with a forum where they could problem-solve and prepare for interprofessional collaborative practice. In palliative care, physicians currently have specific national palliative care-focused accreditation for fellowships. While those accreditation standards do include interprofessional elements, they stop short of requiring or encouraging interprofessional training with learners from different professional backgrounds. While not focused on palliative care, the National Collaborative for Improving the Clinical Learning Environment (NCICLE; https://www.ncicle.org/) is dedicated to improving educational experience, patient care outcomes, and quality of learning and patient care within the clinical learning environment.[53]

The work for specialty palliative care education and training is straightforward, that is, to integrate the characteristics of optimal interprofessional learning environments in palliative care to focus on: (1) patient centeredness—a strong attribute of palliative care; (2) continuum of learning—in which all participants involved in palliative care education are committed to lifelong learning; (3) reliable communication—this ensures patient-centered palliative care plans which anticipate differing opinions; (4) team-based care—understanding that palliative care teams thrive when they truly practice team-based care; (5) shared accountability—the constant need to evaluate and maintain an IPE approach within specialist palliative care delivery and specialty palliative care education and training; and (6) evidence-based practice centered on interprofessional care—a value that palliative care espouses.[53]

People

When developing interprofessional palliative care clinical learning opportunities, the characteristics, attitudes, and experiences of both the learners and the faculty will influence the success of the project. The influence of other stakeholders such as administrators and other decision-makers is included in the discussion on politics and resources.

Leveling and Availability of Learners

Overall, far more formal, robust palliative care specialist training programs exist for physicians than for all other core professions (see Chapter 3). Interprofessional palliative care training at a particular institution is therefore very likely to include learners with different levels of training and clinical experience, if appropriate learners can be found at all. Depending on proximity to health professions schools and hiring practices, learners representing some of the core team members may not be available at all. Physicians will likely have more formal education, which is often privileged more than other types of learning, while other team members may have more practical, employment-related, and/or personal experience. In addition to having different levels of overall experience, learners of different professions may under- or over-value both their own experience and that of learners from other professions, especially if professional or local institutional norms suggest that transdisciplinary work is out of their scope of practice.[54] Differences in professional education and background may contribute to the perception of difference in training and clinical experience between professional groups, even when the leveling is appropriate. For example, professionals who were trained or practice where questions and double-checking are valued may be seen as tentative and inexperienced, while those who have been socialized to "think on their feet" and formulate best-guess answers may be seen as arrogant and know-it-all. Faculty can prepare for the various contingencies by discussing actual and perceived experience levels of the learners in advance, facilitate appreciation and recognition of the contributions of all learners, consider inter-institutional partnerships if learners are not locally available, and adapt the curriculum to mitigate challenges experienced by minority learners.

Learners' Interprofessional Attitudes and Experiences

Though increasing, relatively little exposure to interprofessional learning occurs in healthcare. Both learners and faculty may therefore lack training and development in IPE. For faculty, even extensive experience with transdisciplinary clinical practice may not fully translate into knowledge of IPE best practices (see Chapter 10). Faculty may not have as thorough an understanding of the roles of their teammates as they believe.[55] Meanwhile, learners may undervalue interprofessional experiences, especially when they are optional or singular.[39] Faculty are encouraged to explicitly discuss learner experiences with and attitudes toward IPE whenever appropriate.

Faculty Inexperience with Interprofessional Team Collaboration

The publication of interprofessional competencies in 2011 has facilitated the development of IPE.[15] All professions are striving to meet these competencies in continuing education. In palliative care specialty education, medical education has a well-established role of medical educator, an expert attending physician whose job description includes time for both clinical practice and teaching students. This academic career path does not exist in nursing, social work, or spiritual care. Indeed, many programs do not allow their clinical non-physician staff academic time to teach or to create educational programs.

In nursing, educational faculty are doctorally prepared nurses with PhDs who work mostly in research and not in clinical sites, while nurses with DNPs (Doctorate in Nursing Practice) practice clinically and focus on quality improvement. The challenge is providing financial compensation to clinically expert nursing faculty educators. In social work, faculty educators are often former clinicians, as a joint clinical and educational role in academia is not a common model in social work education. Social work faculty often teach IPE models in healthcare-related electives, but often these electives are not required for social workers to graduate or be hired in palliative care or healthcare roles. Ideally, social workers are exposed to collaborative team experiences during required practicum courses where they work with social workers in the field. Chaplains are exposed to IPE by the nature of their work, but need role models and formal interprofessional education to obtain more expertise.

Faculty Availability, Equity, and Inclusion

Though academic physician job descriptions include the expectation of teaching and are commonly structured to "protect" at least some time for such activities, the same is rare for social work, spiritual care, and nursing at academic centers—especially if these clinicians are working at an institution without a professional school or training program of their profession. These team members may have more ability to offer both education and clinical care in the community, or they may be required to maintain continuity in the clinical service while their academic colleagues rotate on and off service.

Different institutions may have relatively more clinicians of one profession than another. This often leads to a skewed understanding of the benefits of interprofessional collaboration and abilities. Individual members of the less-represented profession(s) are then called upon to represent their profession for a variety of projects far more often than their colleagues from better-represented professions. This practice may inadvertently lead to reinforcing stereotypes, as one individual's perspective cannot represent intra-professional variability in viewpoint. These factors together can lead to fewer people doing more clinical work with less time and support—a recipe for moral injury and burnout since the literature demonstrates that all clinicians need to have a break from clinical care.[56,57]

Faculty Silos and Incentives

Although palliative care is conceptually transdisciplinary, programs at academic medical centers and elsewhere are most commonly administered by physician-led clinical service lines or academic divisions. Members of other professions may not technically report to or be funded by this group, even if they identify with it. Supervisors, often organized along professional lines or "silos," may have priorities or beliefs that are at odds with those of the palliative care team, such as requirements for non-specialist clinical coverage, unrealistic productivity targets, or an expectation of full-time clinical employment based on professional equity or union contracts. Interprofessional leadership is not encouraged or supported. Clinical team members may not have the opportunity for academic appointments within medical centers, or if they are invited to apply for an academic appointment, they may only have a volunteer appointment available. These separate professional or clinical structures can inhibit organic collaboration.

Clinical Learning Environment

Highly functional transdisciplinary clinical practice remains relatively rare. Learners notice the disjunction when clinicians talk about transdisciplinary practice but actually practice otherwise. This disconnect undermines the learning opportunities that the faculty were trying to convey. Although IPE in the clinical learning environment is currently aspirational in large part, faculty can explicitly acknowledge this fact to learners and encourage them to reflect on the gap between aspiration and reality.

Scheduling and Locality

The scheduling of residencies and fellowships is complicated. Physician residencies and fellowships run from July to June. Nursing residencies are scheduled at the convenience of the hosting organization. Unless they are administered together, existing fellowship programs likely do not have overlapping schedules. Major differences may include start and end dates, overall duration, didactic and other non-clinical requirements, and clinical sites.

While building a fully integrated IPE program from the ground up is ideal, combining existing programs is still possible if faculty and administrative leadership are willing to work collaboratively. This may mean significant compromises. IPE by its nature also requires buy-in from several high-level stakeholders, which is inherently more difficult than working within a single organizational structure.[58] It is ideal to consider shared governance or leadership. One model is having one profession take leadership in convening the others.[59] Other professions may take leadership in coordinating curriculum revision, reference revision, interprofessional palliative care mentors, and profession-specific mentors.

COVID-19-related limitations on in-person gatherings and ethical guidance about protecting learners as a vulnerable population have led to the rapid advancement of online learning for all palliative care disciplines. Although the clinical learning at the center of residencies, fellowships, and immersion courses must still be provided in person, telehealth technology has also supported team-based care for palliative patients, and interprofessional learners can be integrated into that care. The effectiveness as well as longevity of these approaches remains to be seen, particularly at a time when learners can gather together in person or onsite. But lessons from COVID-19 distance learning can be applied from online teaching pedagogy and methods; for example, synchronous virtual learning can be incorporated in online palliative care education. Team-based communications training via videoconferencing, with actors serving as virtual patients and observers watching with their video hidden, can be even more realistic than role-play in a classroom.[60]

Virtual learning boasts some undeniable advantages to overcoming scheduling and logistical challenges to palliative care IPE. One example of this includes flipped classrooms that broaden the reach of "core" material that can now be delivered to all IPE learners, with the added bonus of combating "zoom fatigue."[61]

Modeling and the Hidden Curriculum

Regardless of how the programs are constituted, the majority of existing and future clinical specialist training time is spent in direct patient care, ideally as part of a palliative care team.[62] It stands to reason, therefore, that the clinical learning environment plays a critical role in reinforcing or undermining explicit IPE curricular elements—the so-called hidden curriculum, or the norms, values, and behaviors within a learning environment.[63] Though the transdisciplinary aspirations of palliative care as a field are likely to create better clinical modeling than in other specialties, local conditions may vary. Team professional composition, expectations of collaborative teamwork, experience, interpersonal relationships, workload, practice patterns, and leadership can have a huge impact on learner experiences. Likewise, broader implicit and explicit institutional norms—which set expectations for professional roles, hierarchies, formal and informal leadership, when and how the team is involved, and other clinical interactions—can reinforce or undermine explicit teaching.

Though potential solutions presented throughout this section can seem daunting, palliative care's transdisciplinary aspirations (see Chapter 3) can serve as a vision or shared mental model[64] to argue for significant integration of interprofessional specialist training programs within an institution. However imperfect they may be in practice, palliative care teams often represent exemplars not only of transdisciplinary clinical work, but also of the continual process of shared reflection that facilitates interprofessional care. The trust and respect developed within and among palliative care colleagues from different professional backgrounds can help to surmount macro and meso cultural barriers. Conversely, the assumption that transdisciplinarity is fully realized in palliative care can lead faculty collaborators to underestimate the challenges of working together in a different context. It is critical for a new multidisciplinary faculty group to set aside time during the curricular development process to assess and reflect on their own assumptions of professional identity, interprofessional tension, and interprofessional teamwork.

Building Interprofessional Palliative Care Specialist Training

Though national standards and curricula can and should provide overall guidance, local palliative care educational programs must include basic curricular development, such as intentional learner needs assessment, curricular design, implementation, and evaluation.[65] Conversely, the local development of curricula may not, especially in some professions such as spiritual care, extend to or be coordinated at the national level—with little if any institutional, regional, or national sharing of best practices. In addition, there may be challenges to integrating both hospice and palliative care experience, resulting in a lack of understanding of the strengths and benefits of care within the community. In many cases, champions may feel lucky to have a curriculum at all, and whoever happens to be on faculty or on the clinical team representing various professions will naturally shape what is taught and how it is presented. This purely local development may result in haphazard and idiosyncratic educational content, with no true consistent baseline or specialization of knowledge/skills for professionals. Over time, it is critical to develop national standards for content and methods. In the short term, however, something is usually better than nothing. Curricula are, in any case, living systems that should be continuously updated and improved.

Because of the challenges and barriers to the development of interprofessional clinical education in palliative care, most notably the diversity of training paradigms and variability of local resources, a universal blueprint for interprofessional palliative care clinical training will be difficult to develop. A few recommendations are offered for those who would like to enhance the interprofessional clinical training they offer in palliative care: (1) convene a group of interprofessional faculty to work collaboratively from the start; (2) consider content for all learners as well as profession-specific competencies; and (3) develop a program that contributes to required clinical hours and profession-specific certification eligibility for learners from all professional backgrounds. Although a review of basic curricular design is outside of the scope of this chapter, interested readers are referred to several interprofessional resources, such as *Curriculum Development for Medical Education: A Six-Step Approach*,[66] *Keating's Curriculum Development and Evaluation in Nursing Education*,[67] and *Building Competency-Based Curriculum in Social Work*.[68]

Case Examples

This section offers several examples of palliative care interprofessional clinical curricula, focusing on how the designers of each overcame common challenges.

Vignette #1: Problem-Based Learning to Teach Palliative Care Physicians and Chaplains about Miracles

We have found that knowing how to care for and respond to patients who express "wishes and belief in miracles" is a challenge for palliative care learners of all disciplines. Even spiritual care trainees struggle with how to address this in the clinical context. Every year, HPM Fellows and Clinical Pastoral Education (CPE) students in a palliative care specialty training program engage in a series of 6 sessions facilitated by the palliative care chaplain. The aim of this series is to deepen spiritual awareness as a clinical and self-care tool and facilitate IPE.

Problem-based learning[69] presents learners with a problem that they are not fully prepared to solve, and it requires careful consideration of IPE faculty to identify a topic, such as the role of miracles in palliative care, that can be equally engaging to all disciplines of learners. In this annual 90-minute didactic, HPM Fellows and CPE students are presented with a patient case study and are paired up to come up with a strategy, including specific language to be used, to respond to a patient's professed belief in miracles. The pair works collaboratively to acquire the information they need, largely from their partner's knowledge base, to come up with and present a plan. Learners are then presented with concrete tools to address this clinical scenario.

Vignette #2: TeamTalk

Interprofessional palliative care faculty at one institution set out to use reflection and high-fidelity simulation to teach newly defined principles and practices of "team to family communication"[54] to a combined group representing 3 professions—medical fellows (HPM and Geriatrics), advanced practice registered nursing (APRN) students, and chaplain interns. Though social work faculty participated in development and teaching, the absence of an intramural school of social work proved an insuperable barrier to the inclusion of social work trainees. Direct costs comprised only several hundred dollars for simulated patient actor fees, which was provided by the medical fellowships because they were the best funded. Commitment from the leadership of the 4 training programs was secured before curricular planning started, and was facilitated by preexisting positive relationships with, or direct inclusion of, program leaders.

Scheduling of faculty and students was coordinated through a palliative care service analyst on loan. During planning, the experienced team of social work, chaplain, nursing, physician, and pharmacy faculty educators—most of whom already had preexisting working relationships—were surprised at the degree to which their own training backgrounds and expectations informed their collaboration. They spent one meeting focused on this shared professional reflection. In the final version of the 5-session curriculum, one session each was devoted to grounding students in their own professional identity and engaging in dialogue with learners from other professions about those identities. Scheduling and the integration of multiple professional viewpoints meant that curricular development was more time-consuming overall than similar single-profession curricula. Established relationships among the faculty and a high degree of buy-in facilitated development. More physician faculty were available than faculty from other professions, in part because job and organization expectations of non-physician faculty did not support time to engage in formal education.

During classroom exercises, physician fellows were somewhat more likely to respond than APRN students and chaplains. During team-based simulated encounters, faculty of all professions noted that learners tended to drift into their "expected" roles (e.g., physicians leading and doing most of the talking, chaplains confining themselves to explicitly spiritual/religious concerns, APRNs worrying that exploring patient goals might fall outside of their scope of practice), even when the prompts, scenarios, and faculty modeling explicitly suggested otherwise. APRN students with over a decade of nursing experience were perceived by the physician fellows to be at a lower relative training level, requiring faculty to continually reinforce the expected transdisciplinary approach through expert facilitation.

Vignette #3: Early and Frequent Access to Palliative Care Throughout Training

Despite great improvement in many palliative care programs over recent years, many chaplains, social workers, pharmacists and other learners continue to struggle with arranging placements with established palliative care teams. Chaplain, social worker, and pharmacist administrators seek to protect their relationship and access to collaboration with palliative care teams. They may be reluctant to place learners within palliative care teams to learn primary palliative care skills. As a result, many chaplains, social workers, and pharmacists complete training with little or no meaningful or standardized palliative care education. Some chaplain training programs have addressed this cycle by partnering with palliative care administrators and interdisciplinary caregivers in the curriculum development, placement, and mentorship of the CPE students. Non-chaplains in palliative care serve as official clinical mentors for the CPE learners. This kind of IPE investment and partnership tends to foster a greater hospitality toward non-physician learners on the team, resulting in meaningful IPE for chaplain trainees.

Discussion Questions and Activities

1. Conduct an IPE SWOT (strengths, weaknesses, opportunities, threats) analysis: From the point of view of your organizational unit (service line, educational program, division, school, unit, office, company, etc.), what strengths, resources, people, and so on, do you already have or lack? With whom do you have relationships? Who else, especially from professions other than your own, might be interested in doing this work? What barriers to IPE exist at your institution and how can you work toward overcoming them?

2. What educational topics and expertise are shared within all interprofessional palliative care colleagues that could be the focus of an IPE palliative care module in the clinical learning environment? Can IPE

be effectively integrated in curriculum about leadership development/quality improvement and clinical skills? How might integrating IPE be different in each of these aspects of post graduate palliative care specialist education?

3. How can validated tools such as pre-/post-tests and other "objective" tools help with leveling learners?[70]

4. Given that "respect" is a cornerstone of interprofessional education, what does respect specifically look like and mean to you? How can you facilitate conversations about respect with interprofessional faculty and learners? What forums would you use and who would be present? How could you revisit this discussion throughout the training?

5. Think about your own professional training. What do you understand in retrospect about enculturation and hidden curriculum? How would you explain your insights to current trainees from your own and other disciplines?

6. Reflect on the unique aspects of this stage of training (i.e., postgraduate specialty palliative care clinical education and training). How can some of the relative freedoms of this stage foster deeper IPE?

7. Building relationships with key stakeholders in training programs and securing commitments is key to palliative care IPE. What relationships do you need to build? What compromises do you or others need to make?

8. Time limitations and lack of planning pose challenges and result in palliative care disciplines training and working separately. How can you overcome some of these challenges?

9. How do you observe resistance to the concept of palliative care specialist practice and interprofessional education in your profession?

10. How do we ensure that palliative care education reflects all the settings where palliative care occurs to assure respect for and understanding for care outside academic institutions where resources may differ—clinics, home, long-term care, community centers, and other settings?

11. How do you assure quality based on shared IPE specialty palliative care delivery?

References

1. National Consensus Project for Quality Palliative Care. *Clinical Practice Guidelines for Quality Palliative Care.* 4th ed. National Hospice and Palliative Care Coalition; 2018.
2. Head BA, Furman CD, Lally AM, Leake K, Pfeifer M. Medicine as it should be: teaching team and teamwork during a palliative care clerkship. *J Palliat Med.* 2018;21(5):638–644.
3. Dahlin C. Palliative Care Models. In: Boltz M, Capezuti E, Fulmer T, Zwicker D, eds. *Evidence-Based Geriatric Nursing Protocols for Best Practice.* 6th ed. Springer; 2021:825–846.
4. Dahlin C. *Palliative Nursing: Scope and Standards of Practice.* 6th ed. Hospice and Palliative Nurses Association; 2021.

5. American Academy of Hospice and Palliative Medicine. History of AAHPM. AAHPM. Published 2022. Accessed September 18, 2023. http://aahpm.org/about/history.
6. National Association of Social Workers. Advanced Certified Hospice and Palliative Social Worker (ACHP-SW). NASW. Published 2022. Accessed September 18, 2023. https://www.socialworkers.org/careers/credentials-certifications/apply-for-nasw-social-work-cred entials/advanced-certified-hospice-and-palliative-social-worker.
7. National Association of Social Workers. Certified Hospice and Palliative Social Work (CHP-SW) National Association of Social Workers. Published 2022. Accessed September 18, 2023. https://www.socialworkers.org/careers/credentials-certifications/apply-for-nasw-social-work-credentials/certified-hospice-and-palliative-social-worker.
8. Social Worker Hospice and Palliative Network. Announcing the APHSW-C Certifcation Program. Published 2022. Accessed September 18, 2023. https://www.swhpn.org/index.php?option=com_dailyplanetblog&view=entry&year=2018&month=05&day=30&id=23:announcing-the-aphsw-c-certification-program.
9. Dahlin C, Coyne P, Goldberg J, Vaughn L. Palliative care leadership. *J Palliat Care.* 2018;34(1):21–28.
10. Wu DS, Mehta AK, Brewer CB, et al. Defining clinical excellence for palliative care specialists: a concept whose time has come. *Am J Hosp Palliat Care.* 2022;39(12):1377–1382. doi:10.1177/10499091211073968
11. Weaver MS, Wichman C. Implementation of a competency-based, interdisciplinary pediatric palliative care curriculum using content and format preferred by pediatric residents. *Children (Basel).* 2018 Nov;5(12):156. doi:10.3390/children5120156.
12. Reville B, Foxwell AM. Blueprint for a palliative advanced practice registered nurse fellowship. *J Palliat Med.* 2021;24(10):1436–1442.
13. Thiel M, Mattison D, Goudie E, Licata S, Brewster J, Montagnini M. Social work training in palliative care: addressing the gap. *Am J Hosp Palliat Med.* 2021;38(8):893–898.
14. World Health Organization. *Framework for Action on Interprofessional Education and Collaborative Practice.* WHO; 2010. Accessed September 18, 2023. https://www.who.int/publications/i/item/framework-for-action-on-interprofessional-education-collaborative-practice
15. Interprofessional Education Collaborative. Core Competencies for Interprofessional Collaborative Practice: 2023 Update. Accessed September 18, 2023. https://www.ipecollaborative.org/assets/core-competencies/IPEC_Core_Competencies_2023_Prelim_Draft_Revisions%20(2023-04-12).pdf
16. Thiel M, Harden K, Brazier LJ, Marks A, Smith M. Improving the interdisciplinary clinical education of a palliative care program through quality improvement initiatives. *Palliat Med Rep* 2020;1(1):270–279.
17. Liaw SN, Sullivan A, Snaman J, Joselow M, Duncan J, Wolfe J. "We're performing improvisational jazz": interprofessional pediatric palliative care fellowship prepares trainees for team-based collaborative practice. *J Pain Symptom Manage.* 2021;62(4):768–777.
18. Weller R, Healy J, Hettler DL, et al. VA interprofessional fellowship in palliative care: 15 years of training excellence. *J Soc Work End Life Palliat Care.* 2019;15(2–3):85–98.
19. American College of Emergency Physicians. Definition of Emergency Medicine Residency. Published 2021. Accessed September 18, 2023. https://www.acep.org/patient-care/policy-statements/definition-of-emergency-medicine-residency/.
20. American Nurses Credentialing Center. Practice Transition Accreditation Program® (PTAP). Published 2022. September 18, 2023. https://www.nursingworld.org/organizational-progr ams/accreditation/ptap/.
21. Lee SM, Coakley EE, Dahlin C, Carleton PF. An evidence-based nurse residency program in geropalliative care. *J Cont Educ Nurs.* 2009;40(12):536–542.
22. Lysaght Hurley S, Welsh DM, Roy KM, Godzik C. Bridging the gap: a hospice nurse residency program. *J Cont Educ Nurs.* 2020;51(8):371–376.
23. Social Work Guide. How to Become a Social Worker: A Quick Guide. Red Ventures Company. Accessed September 18, 2023. https://www.socialworkguide.org.

24. Jackson-Jordan E, Stafford C, Stratton SV, Vilagos TT, Janssen Keenan A, Hathaway G. Evaluation of a chaplain residency program and its partnership with an in-patient palliative care team. *J Health Care Chaplain.* 2018;24(1):20–29.

25. American Society of Hospital Pharmacy. Overview of PGY2 Pain Management and Palliative Care Pharmacy Residencies. Published 2009. Accessed September 18, 2023. https://www.ashp.org/-/media/assets/professional-development/residencies/docs/pgy2-pain-managem ent-palliative-care.ashx.

26. American Society of Hospital Pharmacy. Residency Directory. Published 2022. Accessed September 18, 2023 https://accreditation.ashp.org/directory/#/program/residency.

27. US Governmental Accountability Office. *Health Care Workforce: Views on Expanding Medicare Graduate Medical Education Funding to Nurse Practitioners and Physician Assistants.* GAO; 2019. Accessed September 18, 2023. https://www.gao.gov/products/gao-20-162

28. Social Work Hospice and Palliative Care Network. SWHPN Mentorship Program. Accessed September 18, 2023. https://www.swhpn.org/swhpn-mentorship-program.

29. Dahlin C, Coyne PJ, Cassel JB. The advanced practice registered nurses palliative care externship: a model for primary palliative care education. *J Palliat Med.* 2016;19(7):753–759.

30. Gentry JH, Dahlin C. The evaluation of a palliative care advanced practice nursing externship. *J Hosp Palliat Nurs.* 2020;22(3):172–179.

31. Clevenger C, Pugliese K, O'Mahony S, Levine S, Fitchett G. Study of shadowing experiences among chaplains in the Coleman Palliative Medicine Fellowship. *J Health Care Chaplaincy.* 2021;27(1):24–42.

32. Levine S, O'Mahony S, Baron A, et al. Training the workforce: description of a longitudinal interdisciplinary education and mentoring program in palliative care. *J Pain Symptom Manage.* 2017;53(4):728–737.

33. O'Mahony S, Baron A, Ansari A, et al. Expanding the interdisciplinary palliative medicine workforce: a longitudinal education and mentoring program for practicing clinicians. *J Pain Symptom Manage.* 2020;60(3):602–612.

34. Ansari A, Baron A, Nelson-Becker H, et al. Practice improvement projects in an interdisciplinary palliative care training program. *Am J Hosp Palliat Med.* 2022;39(7):831–837.

35. Bull J, Kamal AH, Harker M, et al. Standardization and scaling of a community-based palliative care model. *J Palliat Med.* 2017;20(11):1237–1243.

36. Global Forum on Innovation in Health Professional Education, Board on Global Health. *Interprofessional Education for Collaboration: Learning How to Improve Health from Interprofessional Models across the Continuum of Education to Practice: Workshop Summary.* National Academies Press; 2013.

37. Dahlin C. Interprofessional specialty palliative care education and training. *Curr Geriatr Rep.* 2023;12(4):1–10. doi:10.1007/s13670-023-00381-9

38. Schuster BL. Funding of graduate medical education in a market-based healthcare system. *Am J Med Sci.* 2017;353(2):119–125.

39. Lawlis TR, Anson J, Greenfield D. Barriers and enablers that influence sustainable interprofessional education: a literature review. *J Interprof Care.* 2014;28(4):305–310.

40. McNair R, Brown R, Stone N, Sims J. Rural interprofessional education: promoting teamwork in primary health care education and practice. *Aust J Rural Health.* 2001;9(Suppl 1):S19–S26.

41. Cox M, Cuff P, Brandt B, Reeves S, Zierler B. Measuring the impact of interprofessional education on collaborative practice and patient outcomes. *J Interprof Care.* 2016;30(1):1–3.

42. Supper I, Catala O, Lustman M, Chemla C, Bourgueil Y, Letrilliart L. Interprofessional collaboration in primary health care: a review of facilitators and barriers perceived by involved actors. *J Public Health (Oxf).* 2016;37(4):716–727.

43. Tunstall-Pedoe S, Rink E, Hilton S. Student attitudes to undergraduate interprofessional education. *J Interprof Care.* 2003;17(2):161–172.

44. Donesky D, de Leon K, Bailey A, et al. Excellence in postlicensure interprofessional palliative care education: consensus through a Delphi survey. *J Hosp Palliat Nurs.* 2020;22(1):17–25.

45. House S, Havens D. Nurses' and physicians' perceptions of nurse-physician collaboration: a systematic review. *JONA.* 2017;47(3):165–171.

46. Stevens EL, Hulme A, Salmon PM. The impact of power on health care team performance and patient safety: a review of the literature. *Ergonomics*. 2021;64(8):1072–1090.

47. Lancaster G, Kolakowsky-Hayner S, Kovacich J, Greer-Williams N. Interdisciplinary communication and collaboration among physicians, nurses, and unlicensed assistive personnel. *J Nurs Scholarsh*. 2015;47(3):275–284.

48. Gergerich E, Boland D, Scott MA. Hierarchies in interprofessional training. *J Interprof Care*. 2019;33(5):526–535.

49. McCarthy CP, McEvoy JW. Pimping in medical education: lacking evidence and under threat. *JAMA Health Forum*. 2015;12(22):2347–2348.

50. Hallenbeck J. High context illness and dying in a low context medical world. *Am J Hosp Palliat Care*. 2006;23(2):113–118.

51. Curran V, Hollett A, Casimiro LM, et al. Development and validation of the interprofessional collaborator assessment rubric (ICAR). *J Interprof Care*. 2011;25(5):339–344.

52. Smith KM, Scott DR, Barner JC, Dehart RM, Scott JD, Martin SJ. Interprofessional education in six US colleges of pharmacy. *Am J Pharm Educ*. 2009;73(4):61.

53. Weiss KB Passiment M, Riordan L, Wagner R. National Collaborative for Improving the Clinical Learning Environment IP-CLE Report Work Group; Achieving the optimal interprofessional clinical learning environment: Proceedings from an NCICLE symposium; 2019. Accessed September 18, 2023. http://ncicle.org. Published January 18, 2019. doi:10.33385/NCICLE.0002

54. Donesky D, Anderson WG, Joseph RD, Sumser B, Reid T. TeamTalk: Interprofessional team development and communication skills training. *J Palliat Med*. 2020;23(1):40–47.

55. Damen A, Labuschagne D, Fosler L, O'Mahony S, Levine S, Fitchett G. What do chaplains do: the views of palliative care physicians, nurses, and social workers. *Am J Hosp Palliat Care*. 2019;36(5):396–401.

56. National Academies of Sciences, Engineering, and Medicine; National Academy of Medicine; Committee on Systems Approaches to Improve Patient Care by Supporting Clinician Well-Being. *Taking Action Against Clinician Burnout: A Systems Approach to Professional Well-Being*. Washington (DC): National Academies Press (US); October 23, 2019.

57. Perlo J, Balik B, Swensen S, Kabcenell A, Landsman J, Feeley D. IHI framework for improving joy in work. IHI White Paper. Institute for Healthcare Improvement; 2017.

58. Barnsteiner JH, Disch JM, Hall L, Mayer D, Moore SM. Promoting interprofessional education. *Nurs Outlook*. 2007;55(3):144–150.

59. Lumague M, Morgan A, Mak D, et al. Interprofessional education: the student perspective. *J Interprof Care*. 2006;20(3):246–253.

60. Ito K, Uemura T, Yuasa M, et al. The feasibility of virtual VitalTalk workshops in Japanese: can faculty members in the US effectively teach communication skills virtually to learners in Japan? *Am J Hosp Palliat Med*. 2022;39(7):785–790.

61. Periyakoil VS, Basaviah P. The flipped classroom paradigm for teaching palliative care skills. *Virtual Mentor*. 2013;15(2):1034–1037. doi:10.1001/virtualmentor.2013.15.12.medu1-1312.

62. Berzoff J, Lucas G, Deluca. Clinical social work education in palliative and end-of-life care: relational approaches for advanced practitioners. *J Soc Work End Life Palliat Care*. 2006;2(2):45–62.

63. Enders FT, Golembiewski EH, Orellana M, Silvano CJ, Sloan J, Balls-Berry J. The hidden curriculum in health care academia: an exploratory study for the development of an action plan for the inclusion of diverse trainees. *J Clin Transl Sci*. 2021;5(1):e203. doi:doi:10.1017/cts.2021.867. Published 2021 Oct 8.

64. Floren LC, Donesky D, Whitaker E, Irby DM, Ten Cate O, O'Brien BC. Are we on the same page? Shared mental models to support clinical teamwork among health professions learners: A scoping review. *Acad Med*. 2018;93(3):498–509.

65. Ury WA, Arnold RM, Tulsky J. Palliative care curriculum development: a model for a content and process-based approach. *J Palliat Med*. 2002;5(4):539–548.

66. Thomas PA, Kern DE, Hughes MT, Tackett SA, Chen BY. *Curriculum Development for Medical Education: A Six-Step Approach*. JHU Press; 2022.

67. DeBoor SS. *Keating's Curriculum Development and Evaluation in Nursing Education.* Springer; 2021.
68. Bracy W. Building a competency-based curriculum in social work education. *J Teaching Social Work.* 2018;38(1):1–7.
69. McKee N, D'Eon M, Trinder K. Problem-based learning for interprofessional education: evidence from an inter-professional PBL module on palliative care. *Can Med Educ J.* 2013;4(1):e35–e48.
70. Starks H, Coats H, Paganelli T, et al. Pilot study of an interprofessional palliative care curriculum: course content and participant-reported learning gains. *Am J Hosp Palliat Care.* 2018;35(3):390–397.

10

Interprofessional Continuing Education

Myra Glajchen and Karen Richards

Key Points

- CE programs should be interprofessional throughout—from planning through implementation and evaluation. Marketing and enrollment should also ensure a mix of learners from each profession.
- Many promising interprofessional CE courses are led by clinicians without protected time for scholarship, so these programs are not consistently evident in the peer-reviewed literature. Many published CE courses are supported by grant funding but do not continue after the conclusion of the grant.
- Instructional designers and education technology specialists are important members of the team. They ensure the use of best evidence to translate content to online learning platforms, and support knowledge and skills transfer, learner engagement, and ease of use.
- Evaluation of interprofessional CE programs includes measurement of learner satisfaction, learning outcomes related to both palliative care content and interprofessional collaboration, practice change, and impact.

Introduction

Lifelong learning for clinicians is supplemented by continuing education (CE) that is designed to provide updates and transfer or reinforce knowledge, skills, and attitudes, thereby influencing practice change and leading to improved patient outcomes.[1] Each year, millions of dollars are spent on CE activities across all professions. CE is considered to be an essential part of professional development for physicians, nurses, social workers, chaplains, and other professions; mandatory to maintain licensure or certification in most states; essential for accreditation of healthcare organizations; and reassuring to patients, families, and employers that clinicians are staying current with advances in their professions.[2] The imperative for CE has always emanated from multiple sources simultaneously: individual (work to the top of one's license), institutional (incentives, recognition, promotion), statewide (maintain licensure, meet regulatory requirements), and national (certification requirements) sources.

Although CE is prevalent across multiple professions, continuing medical education (CME) has been studied more than CE in other professions. In the 1970s and

1980s, there was a move from measuring knowledge, attitudes, and skills to measuring physician performance and patient health outcomes. Specifically, CME was measured at three levels: competence, performance, and patient health status.[3] Later, the focus shifted as educators sought to identify explanatory factors for why some teaching methods worked better than others. They found that interactive educational formats had greater effects than didactic formats; multifaceted interventions had greater effects than single interventions; and active learning was superior to passive learning.[4]

Interprofessional education is designed to prepare healthcare professionals for interprofessional practice in the real world. Interprofessional education focused on teamwork, communication, and use of best practices has been shown to change practice and improve patient outcomes such as morbidity and mortality, but methodological limitations hamper generalization of results.[5] An Institute of Medicine review on the impact of interprofessional education on healthcare delivery outcomes[6] concluded that research on interprofessional education is improving, but study designs continue to be weak.

Both interprofessional education and high-quality palliative care focus on collaboration among health professionals, communication, and teamwork to enhance patient care.[6] In spite of the growing interest in collaboration among different professions, most CE courses tend to be profession-specific and do not prepare clinicians to work in interprofessional teams. Relatively few interprofessional palliative care CE training programs are available in the United States.[7] Existing interprofessional programs may not include participants representative of the core* professions of a palliative care team, and as such, are not reflective of best practice according to the National Consensus Project palliative care guidelines (see below). These gaps, combined with limited access to basic specialty-level training for some professions, and the intense demand for palliative care across the United States, mean that palliative care services are often delivered by clinicians who lack education or expertise and who practice within a wide and diverse range of knowledge in palliative care or teamwork. This chapter will describe best practices in adult learning as applied to interprofessional CE, evaluate exemplar interprofessional palliative care CE programs using a consensus framework for quality, explore the role of the instructional designer on the team, especially in relation to designing online educational products, and examine challenges and solutions to engage a wide range of professions together in interprofessional palliative care CE.

Best Practices for Adult Learning in an Interprofessional Context

Ideally, interprofessional CE in palliative care begins with an interprofessional faculty team to guide the curriculum-development process with equal representation,

---

* In this book, we use the term "core" to refer to chaplains, nurses, physicians, and social workers, who are all named as part of the interprofessional team for both the Medicare hospice guidelines and the NCP guidelines. This designation does not minimize the importance of other team members who contribute to the palliative care of patients and families.

resulting in synergy of all professional perspectives. According to Kern's six-step approach, curriculum development should follow the same six steps every time: (1) problem identification and general needs assessment, (2) targeted needs assessment, (3) goals and objectives, (4) educational strategies, (5) implementation, and (6) evaluation and feedback.[8-10] Problems and gaps can be identified from the literature, professional associations, expert faculty, and other CE meetings. A targeted needs assessment can be done using the learners likely to be targeted by the program. Ideally, goals and objectives should be feasible and measurable, and educational strategies should be clear, deliberate, and transparent. Once CE programs are implemented, programs can integrate feedback from learners and solicit their interests to inform future planning.[9]

A hallmark of successful CE programs is support from leadership. Such support can ensure adequate resources to develop the program, dedicated or protected time for staff, faculty, and learners to participate in programs, administrative support, accountability, and oversight for the program. Ideally, initiatives should identify or acquire resources prior to launching new CE programs, including space, budget, and technology. Programs may be funded by philanthropy, operations, or learner fees. To ensure sustainability and an ample flow of learners, course directors may consider developing collaborative or affiliation agreements with healthcare systems. Ideally, faculty are compensated for their time and recognized for their participation in terms of promotion and tenure.

To be effective, interprofessional CE should be based on best practices in adult learning and in andragogy, the methods and practice of teaching adults. Adult learning is unique in that learners feel the imperative to acquire additional knowledge, learning is self-directed, learners build upon their prior experiences, and learners demonstrate readiness, motivation, and an orientation toward learning before they begin.[11] When developing educational programs for practicing clinicians, the most effective curricula synthesize the core principles from various theories[12] (see Chapter 5). For example, programs may use simulated cases and case scenarios and provide opportunities for learners to make decisions that lead to consequences, while also providing supplementary material for additional learning, remediation, coaching, reflection, and application of the learning points to various contexts and perspectives. CE is typically offered at educational meetings for practicing clinicians, and includes courses, conferences, lectures, workshops, seminars, and symposia. These meetings are generally designed to improve professional practice and, thereby, patient outcomes. The format of educational meetings varies in terms of content, audience size, type of interaction, length, frequency, and specific practices.[12]

A Cochrane Review of 81 trials concluded that educational meetings alone or combined with other interventions could improve professional practice and the achievement of treatment goals. However, the effect on professional practice tended to be small and varied between studies, and the effect on patient outcomes was generally lower. In attempting to explain the observed differences, the reviewers concluded that higher attendance at meetings was associated with greater effects, that mixed interactive and didactic education was more effective than either alone, and the effect size was smaller for more complex behaviors.[13] In addition, interprofessional palliative care education has been shown to increase palliative care consultations.[14,15] However, a systematic review of an international body of literature concluded that standards of evaluation are integral to improving palliative care education and practice, and palliative care and interprofessional education tend to utilize nonvalidated tools and methods of evaluation.[16]

CE for palliative care professionals ideally includes the knowledge, skills, and attitudes required for effective interprofessional team participation, and effectiveness depends on support for that education within the practice setting.[17] Such attitudes include openness to professional development, commitment to palliative care practices including teamwork and open communication, ongoing commitment to the integration of palliative care skills into practice, and commitment to train colleagues to do the same.[17] Six key characteristics have been proposed as indicators of quality for interprofessional palliative care educational programs. Ideally, programs teach specific competencies, content is evidence-based, educational strategies incorporate a variety of teaching methodologies, interprofessional faculty and learners teach and learn together from all the represented professions, the program includes a robust evaluation process, and systems integration is represented across settings.[8] These characteristics will be used to evaluate the published exemplar interprofessional palliative care CE courses in the following sections.

Exemplar Interprofessional Palliative Care CE Programs

As palliative care programs have proliferated across the United States, so have CE programs. Some are profession-specific, others are interprofessional. The landscape is characterized by a wide range of educational offerings that differs with respect to target audience, content, format, funding, and outcomes. Carroll and colleagues have published a list of primary palliative care educational programs, including a subset of programs that are taught from an interprofessional perspective.[7] However, new programs may have been developed since Carroll's review, and many promising interprofessional CE courses are led by clinicians without protected time for scholarship, so programs may not be well-represented in the peer-reviewed literature.

The following criteria were used for selection of the CE programs discussed in this chapter. All programs are US-based; all offer CE credits for more than one profession; the programs are developed and taught by faculty representing multiple professions; and, in keeping with the World Health Organization's definition of interprofessional education, the intention of these programs is for interprofessional learners to interact and to learn "about, from, and with each other."[18] The list of programs is not exhaustive, and readers are encouraged to review additional programs on their own.

Interprofessional CE courses in palliative care can be categorized according to the level of interprofessional integration in the program. Many interprofessional palliative care CE courses were initially designed by and for one professional group, and then subsequently broadened as other professionals were invited to attend. Some CE courses are provided to learners from a single professional background, but courses specific to other professions are available from the same organization. Several universities that offer an interprofessional Master's Degree in Palliative Care make their courses available as an academic certificate program (see Chapter 8). Although the programs listed in Table 10.1 do not meet the inclusion criteria for this chapter, they are worthwhile programs that offer varying degrees of interprofessional interaction in their coursework.

Of the exemplar programs described below, some programs are designed for teams of practicing clinicians or are integrated into the clinical setting. Other courses are designed by interprofessional teams and are specifically focused on interprofessional interaction. One innovative program adapted interprofessional palliative care education for faculty development. Another model of education is a presentation-focused series where learners can select training sessions from a series or à la carte menu. These programs are described in the following sections using the published criteria for excellence in interprofessional palliative care education.[19]

CE for Teams of Practicing Clinicians

The Interprofessional Communication Curriculum (ICC) is an interprofessional training program developed by the founders of the End-of-Life Nursing Education Consortium (ELNEC) that uses a similar curriculum model to ELNEC. Development was funded by the National Cancer Institute, and the course focuses on interprofessional communication training specific to the oncology setting. Organized by the eight domains of the National Consensus Project Guidelines for Quality Palliative Care,[20] ICC is a train-the-trainer course for interprofessional teams to prepare them to provide communication skills training at their home institutions. The course is designed for teams of two clinicians consisting of nurses, chaplains, or social workers who work in adult oncology. The two team members must be from different professions (e.g., a nurse and a social worker). All ICC courses include didactics, skill-building exercises, and interactive discussions to assist participants in integrating communication training into their clinical settings. In addition, the course identifies and reinforces specific skills in interprofessional communication and collaboration in the didactic, video, and experiential components of the course. Each team develops three institutional goals for providing communication skills training to others. Starting in January 2021, ICC courses have been, and will continue to be held, once a year for 5 years.[21]

The ICC course is evidence-based, the faculty and participants are interprofessional, training is delivered through a variety of formats, and both

Table 10.1 Courses in Palliative Care for Practicing Clinicians

Continuing Education Designed by and for One Professional Group but Others May Attend	Continuing Education Courses for All Professions Available Separately, Not Interprofessionally	Academic Degree/ Program in Palliative Care (see Chapter 8)	Palliative Care Interprofessional Team Consultation
End-of-Life Nursing Education Consortium (ELNEC)	Shiley Haynes Institute of Palliative Care	University of Washington	Palliative Care Leadership Center sponsored by CAPC
Harvard University's Palliative Care Education and Practice (PCEP)	Center to Advance Palliative Care (CAPC)	University of Colorado	Four Seasons Consulting Group
Vitaltalk		University of Maryland	
Ariadne Labs: Serious Illness Communication			
Education in Palliative and End-of-Life-Care (EPEC)			
Four Seasons Consulting Group's Palliative Care Immersion Course			
Utah Certificate of Palliative Education (UCoPE)			
Educating Social Workers in Palliative and End-of-Life Care (ESPEC)			

Sources: ELNEC, https://www.aacnnursing.org/ELNEC
Shiley Haynes Institute for Palliative Care, https://www.csusm.edu/palliativecare/
University of Washington, https://www.pce.uw.edu/certificates/palliative-care
CAPC, https://www.capc.org
University of Colorado, https://www.cuanschutz.edu/graduate-programs/palliative-care/home
Four Seasons Consulting Group, https://fourseasonsconsulting.teleioscn.org
Vital Talk, https://www.vitaltalk.org
University of Maryland, https://graduate.umaryland.edu/palliative/
Ariadne Labs, https://www.ariadnelabs.org/serious-illness-care/
EPEC, https://www.bioethics.northwestern.edu/programs/epec/
UCoPE, https://medicine.utah.edu/pediatrics/palliative-care/ucope/
ESPEC, www.socialworkers.org/ESPEC.

short- and long-term outcomes are measured. In addition, prior to workshop acceptance, participants are required to submit letters of support from their oncology supervisors and to identify three written goals for implementing communication skills training in their institutions. Post-course follow-up is conducted at 6 and 12 months to determine barriers, successes, and solutions to problems that arise. In addition, the ICC program develops a network among course participants through monthly webinars between courses. Half of each monthly session is devoted to CE, and the other half is spent on open discussion as participants share their progress and connect with one another. The developers of the ICC course have a successful track record in providing interprofessional palliative care communication courses, including the COMFORT curriculum[15] and ELNEC communication.[22]

Puchalski and colleagues designed a course on interprofessional spiritual care, using the curriculum model developed by ELNEC with identification of goals during the application process, clinician-dyads who attend the training together, online modules to be completed prior to the in-person workshop, a two-and-a-half-day train-the-trainer course, and 1 year of mentorship with evaluation based on goals identified during the application process at 6 and 12 months post-course.[23]

CE Integrated into the Clinical Setting

The Coleman Palliative Medicine Training Program (CPMTP) was developed by a group of interprofessional palliative care experts from multiple institutions who received a grant from the Coleman Foundation to address the palliative care workforce shortage in Chicago.[17] This grant-funded program was designed to prepare practicing physicians, advanced practice providers, chaplains, and social workers for primary palliative care practice. The program is geared to primary palliative care rather than specialty palliative care. The curriculum covers palliative care topics, communication skills, and program development, supplemented with clinical shadowing, individualized mentoring, resiliency training, and institutional change projects. The model integrates the six key characteristics of interprofessional palliative care education outlined above.[8] Specifically, the course comprises four main components: (1) live interprofessional conferences; (2) self-directed online learning; (3) direct observation of a mentor's clinical practice; and (4) development, implementation, and evaluation of a performance improvement plan. It centers on 29 essential adult and pediatric palliative care clinical and program development skills that were identified through an iterative process by the Collective, a group composed of local experts representing nonprofit hospices, academic medical centers, safety-net hospitals, and community-based hospitals. The content of the coursework is based on the National Consensus Project guidelines.[20]

The founding faculty includes physicians, nurses, a social worker, and a chaplain who develop and co-teach the coursework. Learners interact interprofessionally during hands-on simulated patient encounters, shadowing of experts, and best practices in interprofessional perspectives through live case-based discussions. In addition, interprofessional learners participate in a profession-focused seminar series, expand their professional networks, and develop a supportive interprofessional community of practice through their learning cohorts.

Palliative care and program-development skills are assessed before and after training. Trainees report significant increases in confidence across 12 skills that are common to all palliative care professions, and significantly increased frequency in performing 11 of 12 skills. These skills include explaining hospice and palliative care to patients and families; assessing and treating anxiety and depression; providing support to family members of actively dying patients; participating in advance care planning with patients and families; leading a discussion on communicating bad news; managing spiritual distress; navigating common legal and ethical issues in palliative care; delivering teaching sessions in palliative care; leading an interdisciplinary team; and giving bad news to children of different ages. Qualitative evaluation identified program strengths in implementation of change projects, evidence of the "systems integration" characteristic, and sense of belonging to a professional network.[17] Although the CPMPT program shows promising results in development of knowledge, skills, mentorship, and team resilience, it does not assess more complex interprofessional competencies.[24]

Project ECHO (Extension for Community Healthcare Outcomes) for Hospice and Palliative Medicine uses telehealth to provide primary care providers from underserved areas with training and specialist guidance in delivering best-practice care for patients with complex health conditions. Project ECHO is a tele-mentoring program designed to create virtual communities of learners by bringing together healthcare providers and subject-matter experts using videoconference technology, brief lecture presentations, and case-based learning, fostering an "all learn, all teach" approach. In addition to hospice and palliative medicine,[25-27] Project ECHO has been implemented in multiple specialty areas including rheumatology,[28] rural primary care,[29] diabetes care,[30] and hepatology.[31] Participants engage in a virtual knowledge network by sharing clinical challenges and learning from experts and peers. The heart of the model is its hub-and-spoke knowledge-sharing networks, led by expert teams who use multipoint videoconferencing to conduct virtual clinics with community providers. Case-based learning presentations and review by peers and subject-matter experts create an environment for learning exchange, performance improvement, and identification of best practices.

At each site, ECHO teams include a lead clinician (a physician, nurse practitioner, or physician's assistant) and a nurse or medical assistant, who help manage patient care. These teams participate in weekly video or teleconference clinics, called "knowledge networks." Providers present their cases by sharing patients' medical histories, laboratory results, treatment plans, and individual challenges. Specialists provide advice and clinical mentoring for managing patient care according to evidence-based protocols. These case-based discussions are supplemented with short didactic presentations by interdisciplinary† experts to improve content knowledge. This case-based approach creates a "learning loop", in which knowledge is imparted, skills are taught, and self-efficacy is encouraged. Longitudinal co-management of illnesses with specialists allows community providers to practice

---

†   Although often used interchangeably, "discipline" refers to a branch of knowledge, while "profession" refers to an occupation that requires special education and/ or prolonged training and a formal qualification. In this book, we have attempted to standardize the use of the term "profession" when referring to occupations such as chaplaincy, medicine, nursing, and social work, but occasionally the term "discipline" is used, especially when focused on the theory and knowledge development of the professions.

their expanded knowledge and skills in a manner that builds self-efficacy in handling real-world situations with their patients while ensuring that they follow best practices as they learn. Learning from other community-based providers who face similar clinical challenges is facilitated through shared decision-making. In the Case-Based Learning Exchange, case studies are presented using the SBAR format,[32] a tool used to improve the effectiveness of communication between individuals using the following rubric:

S = Situation (a concise statement of the problem)
B = Background (pertinent and brief information related to the situation)
A = Assessment (analysis and considerations of options—what you found/think)
R = Recommendation (action requested/recommended—what you want).

Outcomes from Project ECHO include both professional and patient outcomes. Participants of the ECHO program report improvements in knowledge, skills, and medical case management while participants' patients show reduced symptom burden and improved clinical outcomes.[31] The ECHO program is innovative in that it represents a change from the conventional approaches in which specialized care and expertise are available only at academic medical centers in urban areas.

Designed by Interprofessional Team and Focused on Interprofessional Interaction

The UCSF Interprofessional Palliative Care Continuing Education Course (Practice-PC) was created in 2015 to address a workforce shortage limiting the dissemination of palliative care in the community. The 50-hour curriculum taught one Friday per month for 9 months includes modules focused on holistic assessment, pain and symptom management, interprofessional practice, advance care planning, ethics, last hours of life, bereavement, and palliative care practice within the health system (see Figure 10.1). This program was developed to meet the needs of working professionals from a range of professions and work settings across the greater San Francisco Bay Area. Extensive focus groups with potential learners, students, and local employers supported the emphasis on interprofessional communication and teamwork. All professionals are encouraged to apply, especially nurses, physicians, chaplains, and social workers, as well as community-based clergy, pharmacists, nursing aides, case managers, psychologists, rehabilitation therapists, family support coordinators, and interpreters. Marketing and enrollment processes ensure a balance of learners across each profession. Tuition discounts are based on ability to pay, with efforts made to ensure that no qualified applicant is turned away because of financial challenges. The faculty is sensitive to exploring systemic barriers that interfere with fully integrated interprofessional practice. Faculty are paid equally for their contribution, regardless of professional background or base pay. All sessions are planned and taught with all faculty present, consistent with the holistic

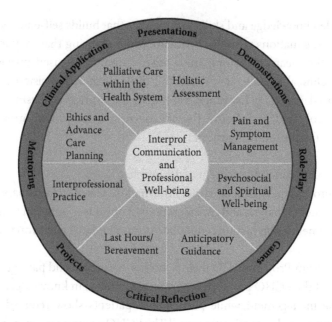

Figure 10.1. The UCSF Interprofessional Palliative Care Continuing Education Course (Practice-PC) curriculum uses a variety of educational strategies to present palliative care topics that were selected by the interprofessional faculty, with special emphasis on interprofessional communication and professional well-being.

palliative care philosophy. Because the interprofessional faculty worked together on curriculum development from the inception of the curriculum, psycho-social-spiritual topics are featured prominently in the course content. The format is designed to maximize interaction between students and faculty and among students themselves, to promote integration of new learning into clinical practice, and to support the development of a palliative care community of practice throughout Northern California. More information can be obtained at the program's website: https://palliativemedicine.ucsf.edu/practice-pc.

Interprofessional Faculty Development

The Interprofessional Education Exchange (iPEX) program at the University of Louisville, Kentucky, is designed to provide training and resources for interprofessional faculty teams and to facilitate the creation and implementation of evidence-based interprofessional education curricula in palliative oncology education.[33] Individuals apply to the program as interprofessional teams of 3–5 members (representing three or more professions) with a common objective: enhance their knowledge and skills related to interprofessional education in order to improve interprofessional palliative care education in their home institution. Participants include chaplains, ethicists, music therapists, nurses, optometrists, pharmacists, physicians, physical therapists, psychologists, public health professionals, and social workers.

Program components include two webinars and three interactive online modules teaching palliative care in oncology and basic skills for interprofessional teaching; evidence-based education including model curricula and other resources; a two-and-a-half-day workshop focused on hands-on skill development; team time for planning, program development, and exchange of ideas with the other teams and project faculty; ongoing support and mentorship from an experienced liaison; and presentation of their plan to the other teams and project faculty for feedback. The teams receive ongoing support as needed for 2 years post-program completion and are asked to report on the outcomes of their projects.

The iPEX program is a model program for several reasons. It is evidence-based, education is delivered in multiple formats, and the program is interprofessional from development through implementation across faculty and teams. The focus on team building, team dynamics, team culture, and team hierarchy is unique. In addition, the requirement for project development and implementation is a feasible and measurable outcome. iPEX is funded by the National Cancer Institute (R25 CA203637). More information can be found on the project's website: https://www. ipexproject.org.[34,35]

Presentation-Focused Series

The MJHS (previously Metropolitan Jewish Health System) Interprofessional Webinar Series in Palliative Care is an online CE program developed by the MJHS Institute for Innovation in Palliative Care, New York City, in September 2015. The curriculum is composed of didactic online webinars developed as CE for physicians, nurse practitioners, registered nurses, social workers, and chaplains, with selected courses for case managers and music therapists. A curriculum planning committee includes representatives from medicine, nursing, social work, hospice, instructional design, and development; spiritual care is not represented on the planning committee. Together, the clinicians identify learning and training gaps from the peer-reviewed literature and from the needs of the MJHS organization and staff in their respective disciplines, as well as appropriate faculty to function as expert presenters. The most popular subjects for the live broadcasts have been professional caregiver burnout, hospice and palliative care during COVID-19, the impact of trauma on Holocaust survivors, LGBTQ inclusion, the multifaceted nature of pain, and COPD.

The CE program includes webinars for hospice and palliative care professionals from different disciplines; recently, interactive multimedia modules were added. Webinars are offered at no charge to organization staff members, while free and fee-based options are extramurally promoted to other healthcare professionals. Learners are able to view webinars and online events individually or as interprofessional groups, which can stimulate team discussion and minimize learning in isolation—one of the drawbacks of online learning. The webinar series is presented live, with at least 15 minutes of audience participation in question-and-answer sessions. Clinicians can access webinars and online courses from computers, tablets, or smartphones. Including a smartphone option via an app is important because many hospice and palliative care clinicians provide community-based patient care, and participate in webinars while in transit.

An instructional designer (ID) contributes to team efforts by reviewing webinar goals, learning objectives, and posttests submitted by the faculty. The ID works with graphic designers to develop the branding and messaging for each series, which includes slide template design and promotional materials. Once the branding is in place, the ID reviews each submission from the faculty to ensure consistent formatting and readability relative to font style, font size, and images. The ID promotes live (real-time) and on-demand (asynchronous) webinars, provides customer support, and manages the operation of the learning-management system, the platform for learner self-enrollment and administration of CE credit.

Webinars and online courses are evaluated using the Kirkpatrick model of training evaluation.[36] Kirkpatrick Level 1 measures the learner's reaction to training. Were the stated learning objectives met? Was the speaker engaging? Was the training relevant to practice? Kirkpatrick Level 2 measures knowledge and skills transfer, as well as attitude, confidence, and self-reported commitment to practice change. Knowledge transfer is evaluated for the webinars using multiple-choice posttests. Mandatory CME/CE evaluations (approved by the CE accreditors for physicians, nurses, social workers, case managers, and music therapists) are required prior to enabling the printing of CME/CE certificates. The entire webinar system has been automated using Web programming to support self-registration and attendance tracking, enabling learners to print their own CME/CE certificates. Members of the healthcare team who are not physicians, nurses, or social workers are offered their choice of either CME or attendance certificates.

Lessons learned from the MJHS program are these: dedicated staff who can focus on the technical details and production of an online interprofessional education curriculum are important interprofessional team members; an interprofessional focus is maintained by including faculty from different professions in all parts of the process (i.e., planning, accreditation, evaluation); online course participants require technical support; immediate learner feedback is important for identifying learning gaps and new topics and refining registration and distribution processes; independent fundraising is necessary, so courses can be provided to learners free of charge; adding new topics as the specialty evolves is crucial to growing the program; and future improvements are dependent on effective faculty feedback. Feedback from learners highlights satisfaction with the content, the speakers, the convenience of online learning, and the community of practice with learners from other professional backgrounds. Of note, the course directors noticed an increase in live webinar attendance and on-demand course completions in the 18 months after the onset of the COVID-19 pandemic. However, development of robust methods to support interprofessional participants in learning "with, from and about" each other[18] during asynchronous webinars are necessary before interprofessional CE seminar series can move completely online.

The Instructional Designer as Part of the Interprofessional Education Team

As content experts and frontline clinicians, healthcare educators may collaborate with instructional designers (IDs) as part of course- or curriculum-design teams when they need expertise in adult-learning theory, educational technology design and development, and evaluating learning outcomes. IDs can also serve as the liaison between content experts and software development teams. The demand for IDs continues to evolve in medical education,[37] especially since the COVID-19 pandemic, when not only academia but also corporate training transitioned from in-person classrooms to mostly online learning.[38]

Online CE Design

Scheduling conflicts and logistics are an ongoing challenge in interprofessional education. That becomes even more true with CE courses where learners may work in multiple locations. Studies suggest that online learning in healthcare education can be an effective modality for clinical skills transfer, as good as—and in some cases superior to—traditional teaching methods, and can improve clinical practice,[39,40] although few published studies report changes in clinician behavior and patient outcomes. Methods grounded in adult-learning and best-evidence principles to deliver effective online learning for healthcare provider CE include construction of realistic clinical cases with elements relevant to an interprofessional audience; use of instructional design principles to guide the lesson flow, learner feedback, and remediation; development of interactivity and selection of relevant multimedia to support knowledge and skills; construction of learning assessments to measure outcomes; and learner acceptance and usability (ease of use) testing.[41,42]

Online learning presents many opportunities for CE in terms of presentation quality and delivery modalities outside of traditional lectures. These include simulations and interactive multimedia modules designed for experiential and scenario-based learning, which support interprofessional team learning and knowledge sharing as learners navigate real-world patient cases and can view the clinician's role from multiple perspectives as the case evolves. With minimal technical skills, learners can access cost-effective CME/CE-accredited programming anytime and anywhere. They can pursue lifelong, self-directed learning, thereby helping to maintain licensure or workplace compliance while keeping abreast of current research.[42]

User-Experience Design

Designing how the user interfaces or interacts with software systems is underpinned by learning theory and research. Goal-based learner activities within an online learning environment are an example of applied activity theory, which suggests that conscious learning occurs through learner activity or task-based performance. Activity theory has propelled advances in human-computer interaction and interaction design, enabling skill sets that support the design of software used in online learning.[43] In designing online courses that engage learners and help them achieve instructional goals, many designers employ the "Eight Golden Rules of Interface Design."[44] These rules affect (1) *consistency* through the product design and interactions; (2) designing *usability* for the range of learners; (3) giving *informative feedback*; (4) giving learners a feeling of accomplishment and *closure*; (5) preventing them from making *errors* that cause software malfunctions or offering ways to recover (e.g., *undo* buttons); (6) allowing learners to *reverse* their actions in the course (e.g., *clear* or *back* buttons); (7) making the interface responsive and giving users a sense of *control*; and (8) reducing the *cognitive load* (learner's mental effort while performing required tasks) within screens and navigation.[44]

The Future of Online Learning

Deployment and uptake of online learning modalities has accelerated during the COVID-19 pandemic, allowing clinicians to access healthcare provider CE at an unprecedented rate. Online learning options, such as webinars and virtual conferences, are expected to continue in tandem with in-person events in hybrid formats. Time will tell if the desire to network will draw clinicians to large in-person venues for post-pandemic CE.[45] Several technologies are currently utilized in healthcare provider education and show promise for wider penetration in the online learning space. These include webinars, mobile learning, simulation, and artificial intelligence.

Webinars

A recent meta-analysis examining differences in learning and learner satisfaction among webinars, face-to-face instruction, and asynchronous instruction suggests that webinars may be equally effective for learning, and learner satisfaction with webinars may equal face-to-face and asynchronous (on-demand) online instruction.[46] Webinars provide a suitable and cost-effective alternative to in-person instruction when the content needs to be delivered at a distance and accommodate diverse learner schedules. Organizations can find helpful webinar software reviews by experts on technology websites,[47,48] and information technology departments can assist with any telecommunications requirements.

Mobile Learning

Best practices involving the design of mobile learning for healthcare professionals have been identified. Successful designs enable microlearning (small chunks of instruction) and access to educational resources anytime and anywhere to supplement classroom instruction, enable contextual learning with problem-solving and critical-thinking interactions, and support positive user experience, learner engagement, and autonomy while permitting team communication and collaboration.[49,50] Areas for suggested future research include learning outcomes, instructional methods, learning theories (including psychological theories of learning), and learner motivation.[51]

Simulation

Simulation is defined as "a technique that creates a situation or environment to allow persons to experience a representation of a real event for the purpose of practice, learning, evaluation, testing, or to gain understanding of systems or human actions."[52(p 15)] Pedagogical foundations of simulations in healthcare professional education have been developed to prevent medical errors and increase workforce efficiency. These involve sequencing the flow (i.e., briefing or orienting the learner, enacting the scenario, and debriefing the learner).[53]

The use of simulations has been studied in palliative care.[54] Most of these studies have been designed for physicians and nurses, with a small percentage designed for social workers and chaplains. Only 16% of the studies involved learner collaboration, and most studies used the standardized patient encounter (68%). The most commonly taught skills were eliciting treatment preferences and communication (i.e., delivering bad news and empathy). Symptom management amounted to 13% and team communication skills to 6%. On evaluation, only 17% of the studies assessed skill improvement, and only three studies assessed patient outcomes. The authors recommend including a wider range of clinicians from specialties involved in palliative care, building interprofessional skills, and conducting more rigorous evaluation with an emphasis on patient outcomes.[54]

Artificial Intelligence

Artificial intelligence (AI) describes technologies that use computer algorithms to perform tasks that would normally be done by humans. AI is being used in

healthcare for diagnosis, reduction of medical errors and mortality rates, and reduction of costs, among other tasks.[55] Though AI is not without its challenges,
healthcare providers need to focus on the more personal or patient-centered
aspects of care while understanding AI inputs, algorithms, and diagnoses to ensure
that no errors are made. Clinicians will need a grasp of basic AI methodology, data
mining, and the ethical and legal challenges involved in AI use. This training will
be provided by educators from the computer sciences, mathematics, and combined
disciplines. These opportunities are currently being provided at several conferences
focused on AI in healthcare. Coupled with the increasing body of scientific knowledge, AI promises to complement the clinical decision-making process and enable
health-provider efficiency and efficacy.[55]

Challenges in Interprofessional Education

Detailed descriptions of resources necessary to develop and implement
programs are often lacking, which makes replication difficult. The medical model
predominates in both interprofessional practice and education; this hinders the integration of professionals trained outside this model in interprofessional CE activities. Most CE faculty are full-time clinicians who lack sufficient time to devote to
teaching and program evaluation. Most CE programs rely heavily on faculty who
hold clinical, research, and teaching positions, and who generally need an hono-
rarium for their time. Similarly, learners may lack funding and time for CE courses,
and they may lack support from employers or managers. These lead to difficulties
in balancing clinical responsibilities with protected time for education to improve
learning and development of new skills.[18]

Much variation exists in the measurement of outcomes used for interprofessional
education, with no consensus on best practices.[18] Assessment strategies are variable and include qualitative or quantitative assessments with few quality metrics.
Assessment tends to target knowledge, skills, attitudes, perceptions, satisfaction,
and readiness, but these do not necessarily translate into improved clinical practice. Some commonly used assessment tools include participant reflections, the
Readiness for Interprofessional Learning Scale,[56] the Interdisciplinary Education
Perception Scale,[57] the Team Skills Self-Assessment Tool,[58] and the Interprofessional
Facilitation Skills Scale.[59] Some additional challenges are that merely learning together does not automatically create understanding between professional or collaborative teamwork in palliative practice since issues related to trust, professional
identity and power, and learners coming from diverse training backgrounds are not
simple things to address, although they must be included in the curriculum to start
to build collaborative learning environments.

Solutions

Looking ahead, both live and on-demand (archived) educational offerings, learner-centered online courses, and alternatives to live offerings are necessary to provide CE programs for learners, especially during unexpected challenges, such as the COVID-19 pandemic. Such courses should be built according to how adults learn, using versatile learning platforms, a combination of instructor-led and self-directed learning, and learner-engagement techniques. We recommend selecting an interprofessional faculty to develop the course curriculum and review the content to ensure that all learning activities are interprofessional, thereby addressing learning objectives necessary for the various professions to function as a collaborative team. This helps address the systemic hierarchies and biases common among professions in healthcare. To overcome profession-related cultural differences between learners and faculty, the content should be reviewed by educators with different professional backgrounds and subject-matter experts. We believe there is a place for combining both interprofessional and profession-specific learning as long as they have clear and measurable objectives to measure content, knowledge base, and competencies.[18] We expect that adaptation in palliative care CE will continue to increase and influence how clinicians learn.

Conclusion

A variety of methods can be used to present the ever-increasing corpus of knowledge, skills, and attitudes to clinicians who pursue lifelong interprofessional learning in palliative care. Medical research in CE needs to be supplemented by research from the core clinical professions (e.g., nursing, social work, spiritual care, and others) to enable interprofessional learning with its unique supports for all members of the palliative care interprofessional team. Many promising interprofessional CE courses are led by clinicians without protected time for scholarship, so peer-reviewed literature does not always reflect current program options, and published programs do not always continue after the conclusion of grant funding. With the exception of the National Cancer Institute, funding for interprofessional palliative care educational initiatives is scarce. More research needs to be conducted into which techniques—in-person, online, or a hybrid or blended approach—are superior in helping palliative care professionals learn to effectively interact with one another and provide patient care informed by the synergy of the entire team, as well as achieve their personal learning goals and enhance clinical practice, leading to superior patient outcomes.

Discussion Questions

1. How can CE programs ensure that their participants are truly representative of palliative care teams and reflective of the real-world environment?
2. What principles from the exemplar interprofessional CE programs can be disseminated and implemented in other settings?
3. How can CE courses provide basic specialty-level training and meet the intense demand for palliative care across the United States?
4. What are the unique curricular aspects that train interprofessional post-licensure learners for collaborative practice in palliative care?
5. Does profession-based learning supersede interprofessional learning, and can both be accommodated in the same program?

References

1. Institute of Medicine (IOM). *Redesigning Continuing Education in the Health Professions.* National Academies Press; 2010.
2. Peck C, McCall M, McLaren B, Rotem T. Continuing medical education and continuing professional development: international comparisons. *BMJ.* 2000;320(7232):432–435. doi:10.1136/bmj.320.7232.432.
3. Mansouri M, Lockyer J. A meta-analysis of continuing medical education effectiveness. *J Contin Educ Health Prof.* 2007;27(1):6–15. doi:10.1002/chp.88.
4. Marinopoulos SS, Dorman T, Ratanawongsa N, et al. Effectiveness of continuing medical education. *Evid Rep Technol Assess (Full Rep).* 2007;149:1–69.
5. Reeves S, Perrier L, Goldman J, Freeth D, Zwarenstein M. Interprofessional education: effects on professional practice and healthcare outcomes (update). *Cochrane Database Syst Rev.* 2013 Mar 28;2013(3):CD002213. doi:10.1002/14651858.CD002213.pub3.
6. Institute of Medicine (IOM). *Measuring the Impact of Interprofessional Education on Collaborative Practice and Patient Outcomes.* National Academies Press; 2015. https://doi.org/10.17226/21726.
7. Carroll T, El-Sourady M, Karlekar M, Richeson A. Primary palliative care education programs: review and characterization. *Am J Hosp Palliat Care.* 2019;36(6):546–549. https://doi.org/10.1177/1049909118809947.
8. Thomas PA, Kern DE, Hughes MT, Chen BY. *Curriculum Development for Medical Education: A Six-Step Approach.* 3rd ed. Johns Hopkins University Press; 2016.
9. Sweet LR, Palazzi DL. Application of Kern's six-step approach to curriculum development by global health residents. *Educ Health (Abingdon, England).* 2015;28(2):138–141. https://doi.org/10.4103/1357-6283.170124.
10. Robertson AC, Fowler LC, Niconchuk J, et al. Application of Kern's 6-step approach in the development of a novel anesthesiology curriculum for perioperative code status and goals of care discussions. *J Educ Periop Med.* 2019;21(1):E634.
11. Knowles M, Horton E, Swanson R. *The Adult Learner: The Definitive Classic in Adult Education and Human Resource Development.* Elsevier; 2005.
12. Health Professions Accreditors Collaborative. *Guidance on Developing Quality Interprofessional Education for the Health Professions.* Health Professions Accreditors Collaborative; 2019.

13. Jamtvedt G, Young JM, Kristoffersen DT, O'Brien MA, Oxman AD. Audit and feedback: effects on professional practice and health care outcomes. *Cochrane Database Syst Rev.* 2006 Apr 19;(2):CD000259. doi:10.1002/14651858.CD000259.pub2.

14. Starks H, Coats H, Paganelli T, et al. Pilot study of an interprofessional palliative care curriculum: course content and participant-reported learning gains. *Am J Hosp Palliat Med.* 2017;35(3):390–397.

15. Wittenberg E, Goldsmith J, Ferrell B, Buller H, Mendoza Y, Ragan SL. Palliative care communication: outcomes from COMFORT, a train-the-trainer course for providers. *Clin J Oncol Nurs.* 2020;24(1):E1–E6. doi:10.1188/20.CJON.E1-E6.

16. van Riet Paap J, Vernooij-Dassen M, Sommerbakk R, et al. Implementation of improvement strategies in palliative care: an integrative review. *Implement Sci.* 2015 Jul 26;10:103. doi:10.1186/s13012-015-0293-2.

17. Levine S, O'Mahony S, Baron A, et al. Training the workforce: description of a longitudinal interdisciplinary education and mentoring program in palliative care. *J Pain Symptom Manage.* 2017;53(4):728–737.

18. World Health Organization. Framework for action on interprofessional education & collaborative practice (WHO/HRH/HPN/10.3). 2010 Sept 1. Accessed October 6, 2021. https://www.who.int/publications/i/item/framework-for-action-on-interprofessional-education-collaborative-practice.

19. Donesky, D, De Leon, K, Bailey, A, et al. Excellence in post licensure interprofessional palliative care education: consensus through a Delphi study. *J Hosp Palliat Nurs.* 2020;22:17e25.

20. Ferrell BR, Twaddle ML, Melnick A, Meier DE. National Consensus Project clinical practice guidelines for quality palliative care guidelines, 4th ed. *J Palliat Med.* 2018 Dec;21(12):1684–1689. doi: 10.1089/jpm.2018.0431.

21. Buller H, Ferrell BR, Paice JA, Glajchen M, Haythorn T. Advancing interprofessional education in communication. *Palliat Support Care.* 2021;19(6):1–6. https://doi.org/10.1017/S1478951521000663

22. Ferrell B, Buller H, Paice J, Anderson W, Donesky D. End-of-Life Nursing and Education Consortium Communication Curriculum for interdisciplinary palliative care teams. *J Palliat Med.* 2019;22(9):1082–1091. https://doi.org/10.1089/jpm.2018.0645.

23. Puchalski C, Jafari N, Buller H, Haythorn T, Jacobs C Ferrell B. Interprofessional Spiritual Care Education Curriculum: a milestone toward the provision of spiritual care. *J Palliat Med.* 2020 May 29;23(6):777–784. http://doi.org/10.1089/jpm.2019.0375.

24. O'Mahony S, Baron A, Ansari A, et al. Expanding the interdisciplinary palliative medicine workforce: a longitudinal education and mentoring program for practicing clinicians. *J Pain Symptom Manage.* 2020;60(3):602–612. https://doi.org/10.1016/j.jpainsymman.2020.03.036.

25. Lalloo C, Osei-Twum JA, Rapoport A, et al. Pediatric Project ECHO®: a virtual community of practice to improve palliative care knowledge and self-efficacy among interprofessional health care providers. *J Palliat Med.* 2021 Jul;24(7):1036–1044. doi: 10.1089/jpm.2020.0496. Epub 2020 Dec 16. PMID: 33326309; PMCID: PMC8215401.

26. Arora, S, Smith, T, Snead, J, et al. Project ECHO: an effective means of increasing palliative care capacity. *Am J Managed Care.* 2017;23(7 Spec No.):SP267–SP271. PMID: 28882048.

27. De Witt Jansen B, Brazil K, Passmore P, et al. Evaluation of the impact of telementoring using ECHO© technology on healthcare professionals' knowledge and self-efficacy in assessing and managing pain for people with advanced dementia nearing the end of life. *BMC Health Serv Res.* 2018;18(1):228. https://doi.org/10.1186/s12913-018-3032-y.

28. Lewiecki EM, Rochelle R. Project ECHO: telehealth to expand capacity to deliver best practice medical care. *Rheum Dis Clin North Am.* 2019 May;45(2):303–314. doi: 10.1016/j.rdc.2019.01.003. Epub 2019 Mar 8. PMID: 30952400.

29. McDonnell MM, Elder NC, Stock R, Wolf M, Steeves-Reece A, Graham T. Project ECHO integrated within the Oregon Rural Practice-based Research Network (ORPRN). *J Am Board Fam Med.* 2020 Sep-Oct;33(5):789–795. doi: 10.3122/ jabfm. 2020.05. 200051. PMID: 32989075.

30. Cuttriss N, Bouchonville MF, Maahs DM, Walker AF. Tele-rounds and case-based training: Project ECHO Telementoring Model applied to complex diabetes care. *Pediatr Clin North Am*. 2020 Aug;67(4):759–772. doi: 10.1016/j.pcl.2020.04.017. Epub 2020 Jun 19. PMID: 32650871.

31. Page K, Qeadan F, Qualls C, Thornton K, Arora S. Project ECHO revisited: propensity score analysis and HCV treatment outcomes. *Hepat Med*. 2019 Oct 7;11:149–152. doi: 10.2147/HMER.S212855. PMID: 31632162; PMCID: PMC6789170.

32. Thomas CM, Bertram E, Johnson D. The SBAR communication technique: teaching nursing students professional communication skills. *Nurse eEduc*. 2009;34(4):176–180. https://doi.org/10.1097/NNE.0b013e3181aaba5.

33. Schapmire TJ, Head BA, Pfeifer M. The interprofessional educational exchange (iPEX) program: preparing faculty to develop interprofessional education in palliative oncology. *Psycho-Oncol*. 2020;29:66–117. https://doi.org/10.1002/pon.5328.

34. Head B, Schapmire T, Jones C, et al. "Opening eyes to real interprofessional education": results of a national faculty development initiative focused on interprofessional education in oncology palliative care. *J Interprof Care*. 2022;36(5):698–705. doi:10.1080/13561820.2021.1965102.

35. Schapmire TJ, Head BA, Furman CD, et al. The Interprofessional Education Exchange: the impact of a faculty development program in interprofessional palliative oncology education on trainee competencies, skills, and satisfaction. *Palliat Medi Rep*. 2021;2(1):296–304. https://doi.org/10.1089/pmr.2021.0045.

36. Kirkpatrick JD, Kirkpatrick WK. *Kirkpatrick's Four Levels of Training Evaluation*. ATD Press; 2016.

37. Love LM, Anderson MC, Haggar FL. Strategically integrating instructional designers in medical education. *Acad Med*. 2019;94(1):146.

38. Decherney P, Levander C. The hottest job in higher education: instructional designer: the Sherpas of online learning teams, more than ever in the COVID-19 era. Insider Higher Ed Digital Learning Blog. 2020 April 24. Accessed October 6, 2021.https://www.insidehighered.com/digital-learning/blogs/education-time-corona/hottest-job-higher-education-instructional-designer.

39. Phelan JE. The use of E-learning in social work education. *Social Work*. 2015;60(3):257–264.

40. O'Dunn-Orto A, Hartling L, Campbell S, Oswald AE. Teaching musculoskeletal clinical skills to medical trainees and physicians: a Best Evidence in Medical Education systematic review of strategies and their effectiveness: BEME Guide No. 18. *Med Teach*. 2012;34:93–102.

41. Bonevski B, Magin P, Horton G, Bryant J, Randella M, Kimlin MG. An internet based approach to improve general practitioners' knowledge and practices: the development and pilot testing of the "ABC's of vitamin D" program. *Int J Med Inform*. 2015;84(6):413–422.

42. Curran V, Gustafson D, Simmons K, et al. Adult learners' perceptions of self-directed learning and digital technology usage in continuing professional education: an update for the digital age. *J Adult Cont Educ*. 2019;25(1):74–93.

43. Kaptelinin V. Activity theory. In: Soegaard M, Friis Dam R, eds. *The Encyclopedia of Human-Computer Interaction*. 2nd ed. Interaction Design Foundation; 2014. Accessed September 7, 2023. https://www.interaction-design.org/literature/book/the-encyclopedia-of-human-computer-interaction-2nd-ed/activity-theory.

44. Shneiderman B, Plaisant C, Cohen M, Jacobs S, Elmqvist N, Diakopoulos N. *Designing the User Interface: Strategies for Effective Human-Computer Interaction*. 6th ed. Pearson Education; 2017.

45. Shah S, Diwan S, Kohan L, et al. The technological impact of COVID-19 on the future of education and health care delivery. *Pain Physician*. 2020;23:S367–S380.

46. Ebner A, Gegenfurtner E. Webinars in higher education and professional training: a meta-analysis and systematic review of randomized controlled trials. *Educ Res Rev*. 2019;28:100293. https://doi.org/10.1016/j.edurev.2019.100293.

47. Pickavance M, Turner B. Best webinar software of 2021. *TechRadar*. 2021, June 15. Accessed October 7, 2021. https://www.techradar.com/best/best-webinar-software.

48. SoftwareWorld. 10+ best webinar software & platforms of 2021 (free & paid). 2021. Accessed October 7, 2021. https://www.softwareworld.co/webinar-software/.

49. Kellam, H. Developing interactive mobile learning experiences for healthcare professionals: content and community of practice recommendations. *Int J Mobile Human Comput Interact*. 2020 April–June;12(2):40–52.

50. Bernacki ML, Crompton H, Green JA. Towards convergence of mobile and psychological theories of learning. *Contemp Educ Psychol*. 2020;60:101828.

51. Mayer, RE. Where is the learning in mobile technologies for learning? *Contemp Educ Psychol*. 2020;20:101824.

52. Lopreiato JO, ed. *Healthcare Simulation Dictionary*. Agency for Healthcare Research and Quality; 2016 October. AHRQ Publication No. 16(17)-0043. Accessed October 7, 2021. https://www.ahrq.gov/sites/default/files/publications/files/sim-dictionary.pdf.

53. Nyström S, Dahlberg J, Edelbring S, Hult H, Dahlgren A. Continuing professional development: pedagogical practices of interprofessional simulation in health care. *Studies Cont Educ*. 2017;39(3):303–319. doi:10.1080/0158037X.2017.1333981.

54. Kozhevnikov D, Morrison LJ, Ellman MS. Simulation training in palliative care: state of the art and future directions. *Adv Med Educ Pract*. 2018;9:915–924. https://doi.org/10.2147/AMEP.S153630.

55. Paranjape K, Schinkel M, Nannan Panday R, Car J, Nanayakkara P. Introducing artificial intelligence training in medical education. *JMIR Med Educ*. 2019 Jul–Dec;5(2):e16048. Accessed October 6, 2021. https://www.ncbi.nlm.nih.gov/pmc/articles/PMC6918207/.

56. Reid R, Bruce D, Allstaff K, McLernon D. Validating the Readiness for Interprofessional Learning Scale (RIPLS) in the postgraduate context: are health care professionals ready for IPL? *Med Educ*. 2006;40(5):415–422. https://doi.org/10.1111/j.1365-2929.2006.02442.x.

57. McFadyen AK, Maclaren WM, Webster VS. The Interdisciplinary Education Perception Scale (IEPS): an alternative remodelled sub-scale structure and its reliability. *J Interprof Care*. 2007;21(4):433–443. https://doi.org/10.1080/13561820701352531.

58. Roper L, Shulruf B, Jorm C, Currie J, Gordon CJ. Validation of the self-assessment teamwork tool (SATT) in a cohort of nursing and medical students. *Med Teach*. 2018;40(10):1072–1075. https://doi.org/10.1080/0142159X.2017.141884.

59. Sargeant J, Hill T, Breau L. Development and testing of a scale to assess interprofessional education (IPE) facilitation skills. *J Cont Educ Health Prof*. 2010;30(2):126–131. https://doi.org/10.1002/chp.20069.

11

Hospice

The Origins of Interprofessional Palliative Care

Dona J. Reese and Amy Ruth Bolton

Introduction

The conceptualization of palliative care, as originally developed in England, was a holistic care model for terminally ill patients, which included physical, emotional, social, and spiritual aspects of care. When hospice care developed in the United States, it was provided by an interprofessional team, including professionals who were educated to address all of these aspects of care, with trained volunteers and family members playing significant roles in patient care. Medicare coverage was developed for hospice care, which was provided when a doctor determined that a patient is terminally ill and has 6 months or less to live. The field of palliative care subsequently developed in the United States based on these concepts, providing holistic care to patients who are seriously or terminally ill. The National Association of Social Workers defines palliative care as an approach that focuses on quality of life through prevention and relief of suffering on physical, psychosocial, and spiritual levels, when no cure is possible. Hospice is a form of palliative care that is offered specifically in terminal illness.[1] This chapter discusses the development of hospice as the origin of interprofessional palliative care, the unique role of each interprofessional member of a hospice team, and benefits and challenges of interprofessional collaboration specific to the hospice setting.

A Brief History of Hospice as the Beginning of Palliative Care

The palliative care and hospice movement began in England in the 1960s. Dame Cicely Saunders was inspired by her training as a nurse, physician, and social worker to develop a holistic care model for terminally ill patients, known in England as palliative care.[2,3] Although it was originally recognized in England as non-curative care specifically for terminally ill patients in hospice, the term "palliative care" was later used in the United States to refer to non-curative comfort care for seriously ill patients.

From the beginning, the care espoused by Dame Saunders was interprofessional, addressing the physical, psychological, social, and spiritual concerns of patients and their loved ones. Dame Saunders pioneered this interprofessional approach by establishing an inpatient hospice, St. Christopher's, in London in 1967. Volunteers played a significant role from the beginning of the hospice movement, in both England and in the United States.[2] In addition, family members played significant roles in care for the patient in home hospice care in the United States. Saunders's treatment model was focused not on *curative treatment* or *disease-directed therapy*, with the goal of curing the patient's disease, but on *palliative care*, aimed at promoting quality of life during death and dying. She accomplished this by establishing interprofessional care to promote aggressive symptom management of not only physical distress, but also emotional and spiritual distress. She promoted a new value of empowerment of the patient and family; this movement resulted in the Patient Bill of Rights in 1972, requiring patient consent for treatment, the right to all comfort measures, and the right to know one's prognosis.[3]

In addition, through hospice care, the family became the unit of care. In referring to the concept of family, hospice clinicians use the concept "familiness",[4] which may include blood relatives, but can also refer to a family of choice, including other loved ones, and in some cases a paid caregiver who in some situations may interact as family. Under Medicare, hospice considers the patient and family together as the unit of care. The concept of "familiness" emphasizes this unique community of caregivers who are needed to provide holistic care for a person day and night and are identified as an integral part of the interprofessional care team. Trained volunteers are members of the community who also provide care and support to the patient and family unit. Support may include visiting patients, running errands, reading to patients, assisting families in respite care, childcare assistance, and bereavement support programs. Some volunteers may have additional special skills, such as musicians. Specific programs are designed to train volunteers to be present and support a patient when family cannot be present during the dying process. One program for this support, including some volunteers, is called "No One Dies Alone," or NODA[5] (see also https://www.peacehealth.org/sacred-heart-riverbend/no-one-dies-alone).

In the United States, Saunders first introduced the concept of palliative care at Yale University in 1963. Inspired after interning at St. Christopher's, in the early 1970s nurse Lillian Wald, former dean of the Yale School of Nursing, founded the Connecticut Hospice to provide in-home hospice care, along with registered nurse (RN) Katherine Klaus, pediatrician Dr. Morris Wessel, oncologic surgeon Dr. Ira Goldenberg, the Rev. Dr. Edward F. Dobihal, Jr., and Father Canny—an interprofessional team from the start. In 1974, Connecticut Hospice opened the country's first in-patient hospice center. At the government policy level, during these same years physician Elisabeth Kübler-Ross testified in front of the Senate to promote the hospice model of care.

Early U.S. hospice workers usually helped families to care for dying patients in their own homes. Hospice was a countercultural approach, not covered by health insurance. Patients were cared for free of charge by professionals volunteering their time, with daily care provided by volunteers and family members. The hospice movement advocated for a new set of values about end-of-life care, referred to as "hospice philosophy." This philosophy focused not on length of life, but on quality of life during death and dying. Dame Cicely Saunders referred to this as "to live until you die." Patient self-determination is a focus, as well as a right to information about the prognosis.[3] This movement gained support, and home hospice eventually became attractive to the government because of the reduced expense as compared to institutional care. Home hospice became common in the United States, and in-patient hospice programs were also developed for patients who did not have anyone to care for them in the home. Additional settings for hospice care include assisted living, long-term care facilities, and acute care hospitals.

Advocacy with the federal government, documenting that home hospice was less expensive than institutional care, led to Medicare reimbursement for hospice under the Tax Equity and Fiscal Responsibility Act in 1982.[3] The Medicare Hospice Benefit transformed hospice philosophy into federal regulation, requiring an interprofessional approach that included a bereavement counselor, home health aide, nurse, physician, social worker, and "pastoral care or other counselor." Note that the role of "pastoral care or other counselor" has a multiplicity of titles depending on the specific setting or organization, including "chaplain," "spiritual counselor," and "spiritual care provider." Within the field of professional chaplaincy itself, there remains debate over which is most appropriate, in part due to the challenges of articulating and concretizing outcomes in the spiritual realm.[6,7] We have chosen to use "spiritual counselor" for this chapter, as to these authors it best reflects the unique and inclusive expertise of these professionals in the hospice setting.

To be eligible for the hospice benefit, a patient must be certified by a hospice physician and by their own physician as "terminally ill," with an expected prognosis of 6 months or less if the illness runs its normal course. Since a focus of the Medicare Hospice Benefit was to save money, eligibility limitations were imposed, and a patient enrolled in hospice had to agree to forgo curative or life-sustaining treatments. In 1986, states were given the option to include a hospice benefit within Medicaid programs, and today are required to provide this benefit, though there are state differences in how "terminally ill" is defined.[8] Thus, hospice care became available for nursing home residents whose care is paid through Medicaid. In 1995, the military began offering hospice benefits to family members. Most commercial insurances have now followed suit. Today, in some circumstances, patients can receive "open-access" hospice, in which hospice care services are concurrent with disease-directed therapy.[9]

Hospice care in the United States has moved from the fringe to the mainstream. At the same time, as an insurance designation, hospice care is limited by policy, terms/definitions, and other changes in Medicare/Medicaid, which continue to impact reimbursement, staffing, and the structure and roles of the care team. A recent example is the role of telehealth in hospice care, and how it will impact care delivery in both hospice and palliative care in the years to come.[10] During the COVID-19 pandemic, most hospices like other healthcare settings moved to telehealth for any services that could be appropriately provided virtually, either through video or phone visits. This included routine nursing, social work, and spiritual care support. During the Public Health Emergency of 2020–2022, the U.S. Centers for Medicare and Medicaid Services (CMS) introduced temporary regulatory waivers and rules allowing this flexibility in healthcare delivery, including regulations that hospices may provide services via telehealth as long as it is "feasible and appropriate."[11] As of this writing, it is still unclear how many of these will become permanent, or how they will impact the financial future of hospice and palliative care in the United States.[12]

Following the expansion of the hospice movement in the United States, in the 1980s the need for palliative care for patients suffering with chronic incurable illness was recognized. Many people who live with chronic illness are not terminally ill, but do require ongoing symptom management, and benefit from care that is holistic, interprofessional, and aligned with their personal values and quality-of-life concerns. Today in the United States, palliative care is provided at hospitals as a consult service or in designated inpatient units, and on an outpatient basis in medical offices and patients' homes. This movement has continued to grow, with health insurance companies advocating for palliative care as a less expensive and preferable option than inappropriate attempts at curative care, or as concurrent care with disease-directed therapy. The exponential increase in palliative care options and settings in the United States can all be traced back to the original work of Dame Cicely Saunders, Lillian Wald, and the other pioneers of hospice care.

Transition of Palliative Care Philosophy from Home-Based Hospice into Hospitals: An Interprofessional Team Approach

Holistic, interprofessional care, as promoted and developed by the hospice movement, has become the gold standard not only for home-based hospice, but also for palliative care in hospitals. It is natural that the beginnings of hospital palliative care in North America came from the world of oncology, where healthcare providers encountered patients daily who were suffering from debilitating "total pain"—a term coined by Dame Cicely Saunders, referring to physical, emotional, and spiritual pain.[13] Canadian oncologist Dr. Balfour Mount began to introduce hospice care innovations into hospital settings in 1975, drawing upon not only his work as a physician treating terminally ill cancer patients, but also his personal experience as a cancer survivor. He referred to this care as "palliative care," which he said means caring for the whole person—body, mind, and spirit. Like Lillian Wald, Dr. Mount had traveled to the United Kingdom to visit St. Christopher's and learn from "Hurricane Saunders"—his affectionate nickname for Cicely Saunders.[14] In 1987, British-trained oncologist Declan Walsh founded the first palliative care program in the United States at the Cleveland Clinic Cancer Center in Ohio, which became the training site of the first U.S. palliative care clinical and research fellowship, as well as the first acute pain and palliative care inpatient unit.[15]

The interprofessional focus in palliative care brings an increased attentiveness and accountability to each respective discipline's care, thus benefiting the patient. The specialty-based care in modern hospitals can feel fragmented, with a lack of communication, and a sense that it is every specialty for themselves. This is not so in inpatient palliative care settings, where patients and families can have access to care providers from multiple disciplines in one physical location.

Roles of the Hospice Team Members

The collaborative functioning of the interprofessional team is the cornerstone of hospice care. Patients and their loved ones are best cared for when the members of the team work together to promote physical, emotional, and spiritual support and comfort. This is accomplished through provision of physician services, nursing services, medical social services, and counseling services. The interprofessional team provides comprehensive treatment of total pain and addresses the needs of the whole family unit.[16] The Centers for Medicare and Medicaid Services (CMS) and the National Hospice and Palliative Care Organization (NHPCO) identify the core hospice team professionals as follows (in alphabetical order)[17,18]: bereavement counselor, nursing team (with at least one registered nurse), pastoral or other counselor, physician (may be the medical director of the hospice), and social worker. Hospices are also mandated to provide access to home health aides, trained volunteers, physical and speech therapists, and dieticians if needed.

In its 2018 Guidelines, NHPCO states, "the hospice interdisciplinary team, in partnership with the patient, family, caregiver and other individuals identified by the patient, develops, coordinates, and implements a care-directed, individualized and safe plan of palliative care."[19(np)] The essential characteristics of the professional team include collaboration, adaptability, and flexibility. Patient conditions can change very rapidly, and family situations can be volatile. Another key characteristic is cultural sensitivity—the ability to work with people across the socioeconomic spectrum, from a variety of religious, ethnic, and cultural backgrounds. Team members must be able to respond appropriately as they are called to provide care in vastly divergent settings with respect to family dynamics, socioeconomic status, and cultural norms.

The list of interventions comprising each hospice discipline's* role, based on current research and policy statements in the hospice field, is discussed below.

---

* Although often used interchangeably, "discipline" refers to a branch of knowledge, while "profession" refers to an occupation that requires special education and/or prolonged training and a formal qualification. In this book, we have attempted to standardize the use of the term "profession" when referring to occupations such as chaplaincy, medicine, nursing, and social work, but occasionally the term "discipline" is used, especially when focused on the theory and knowledge development of the professions.

(Note: we have listed them in alphabetical order, so as to avoid any appearance of promoting the importance of one discipline over another.) The term "interprofessional team," as is used throughout this work, emphasizes the collaboration between professionals of different fields of expertise, which is essential to the provision of holistic, compassionate, and culturally sensitive care. (For additional information on roles of the interprofessional team members in palliative care, see Chapter 3.)

In our experience, when a hospice patient or significant other raises a concern, it is important to respond promptly, as time may be of the essence. Although all team members may respond to any issues of concern, each team member is responsible for discussing client issues with the entire interprofessional team, allowing the individual with the most appropriate expertise to follow up. The expertise of each discipline is summarized below.

Bereavement Counselor

Hospice care, by mandate, provides bereavement services post-death to families and loved ones for 13 months, to assist with issues related to grief, loss, and adjustment.[20] This may include individual counseling, groups, periodic phone and mail check-ins, newsletters, and annual memorial services. Though some groups and services may be open to the larger community, the primary role of the bereavement counselor is to support the loved ones of those who died under the care of their hospice. Sometimes the bereavement counselor may be called in prior to a patient's death, especially when young children are involved, to provide age-appropriate tools and resources for grief support as the patient transitions through the dying process.

Hospice bereavement professionals must have appropriate mental health and bereavement training to conduct ongoing risk assessments and counseling, and to address complicated grief and potential suicidal risk. Most bereavement counselors have a master's degree in a related field, including social work, counseling, thanatology (the study of death and dying), and even art therapy. The hospice may require one of a variety of certifications for the bereavement counselor, with the Certification in Thanatology (CT) from the Association of Death Education and Counseling (ADEC) being the gold standard. Some professionals may opt to pursue ADEC's highest level of certification, Fellow in Thanatology (FT). Several alternative credentialing organizations, such as the American Academy of Grief Counseling, provide additional training. The bereavement program is not expected to operate as a mental health agency, and bereavement counselors refer clients to appropriate therapeutic and community resources when needed.

Home Health Aide

The home health aide is supervised by the registered nurse on the team. The Certified Hospice and Palliative Nursing Assistant (CHPNA) examination is designed for experienced hospice and palliative nursing assistants. Home health aides may support patient care in the following ways, depending on the person's individual care needs: (1) helping with basic activities of daily living (ADLs), including bathing, toileting, dressing, eating, and personal grooming; (2) reporting health concerns to the team nurse; (3) measuring vital signs; (4) housekeeping for the patient; and (5) tending to overall patient care needs, such as repositioning to prevent skin breakdown, and assisting with wound care under the supervision of the nurse.

Nurse

In the home hospice model, registered nurses (RNs), with the support of licensed practical/vocational nurses (LPN/LVNs) and nurse practitioners (NPs), provide the direct clinical care to patients and serve as a patient advocate, care coordinator, and patient and family educator. Often called a "coordinator of care," the nurse oversees the patient's holistic care in collaboration with the team physician. Advanced practice registered nurses (including Nurse Practitioners—NPs), who hold a graduate degree at either the master's or Doctor of Nursing Practice (DNP) level in addition to nursing licensure, expand the capacity to deliver direct patient care.[21] Nurses provide regular assessment and treatment of patients' symptoms and collaborate with other hospice team members to optimize patients' comfort and families' understanding of and adaptation to the dying process.[22] RNs do not provide the ongoing daily care of a patient; rather, they instruct family members or other caregivers on how to provide the care.[18] As individuals decline, the nurse adjusts the plan of care accordingly in consultation with the team physician, engages in supportive discussions with families around death and dying, and monitors for signs the person is entering the dying process. These may include changes in breathing patterns, cessation of intake, "seeing" deceased family and friends, and increased agitation. Nurses collaborate with the interprofessional team, to ensure that a patient and family are receiving not only the physical, but also the emotional and spiritual support they need.[22]

Specialty certifications are available from the Hospice and Palliative Credentialing Center (HPCC) for hospice nurses who wish to advance their education. These include the Advanced Certified Hospice and Palliative Nurse (ACHPN) for advanced practice nurses, the Certified Hospice and Palliative Nurse (CHPN) or the Certified Hospice and Palliative Pediatric Nurse (CHPPN) for registered nurses, and the Certified Hospice and Palliative Licensed Nurse (CHPLN) credential.

Hospice Physician

The hospice physician oversees the patient's medical care and is often the primary physician for hospice patients. An individual's personal physician or physician specialist must make a terminal prognosis for the patient to be eligible for hospice. Once a patient transitions to hospice, the hospice physician often becomes their "primary physician." The hospice physician supports the nurse's ongoing assessment and medical care of the patient. The main role of the physician is to ensure continuous implementation and review of the patient's plan of care, with the goal of alleviation of symptoms.

Hospice physicians offer phone, video, and in-person consults with patients and/or their loved ones, as requested either by them or by other team members. They oversee the prescription of medications and other symptom-relieving treatments and are responsible for determining eligibility of patients for re-certification and any changes in level of hospice care (for example, moving to GIP [general inpatient level of care] from RHC [routine home care]). They may also refer patients to other services, including short-term physical and/or speech therapy when appropriate. In cases where patients remain under the oversight of their personal physician, the hospice physician coordinates with the patient's physician as needed.

Hospice and Palliative Medicine has been officially recognized as a subspecialty by the American Board of Medical Specialties and American Osteopathic Association since 2008. Physicians interested in working in hospice or palliative care now must complete the Hospice and Palliative Care Medicine Fellowship and pass a board certification exam.

Social Worker

The social work role in hospice has been traditionally misunderstood, although social workers were included in the first hospice teams in England and the United States. The main reason social workers were included on the hospice team following Medicare reimbursement is because it was required by policy for the reimbursement to occur. Twenty-four interventions considered by social workers to represent their role in hospice are listed in Table 11.1. These interventions are based on Kulys and Davis's study,[23] in which they found that only 2 interventions were considered by other disciplines to be part of the social work role, as well as on subsequent research regarding the social work role in hospice.[24] The interventions reflect Reese's model of psychosocial and spiritual variables that predict hospice outcomes,[25] as well as the Social Work Assessment Tool.[26] Including these interventions was justified by existing evidence that social workers address these issues in the field, and in most cases address them more often than nurses.[27] The items are consistent with NASW's *Standards for Social Work Practice in Palliative and End of Life Care*,[28] and

Table 11.1 Roles Recognized by Social Workers in Hospice

Primary Roles Recognized by Hospice Social Workers	Social Work Roles Recognized by Other Disciplines in Kulys and Davis Study (1986)	Social Work Roles Recognized by Other Disciplines in Reese (2011) Study
Financial counseling	X	X
Referrals		X
Assessment of emotional and social problems		X
Counseling about suicide		X
Facilitating social support		X
Counseling about denial of terminality		X
Promoting cultural competence		X
Community outreach		X
Counseling regarding anticipatory grief		X
Crisis intervention		X
Bereavement counseling		X
Counseling about death anxiety		X
Intake interview		
Civil and legal assistance	X	
On-call responsibilities		
Counseling about safety issues		
Supervising hospice workers		
Directing the hospice		
Discharge planning		
Upholding preferences about the environment for patient/family		
Advocacy for patient and family		
Supporting direct spiritual experience		
Discussing meaning of life		
Ensuring culturally competent end-of-life decisions		

NHPCO's *Guidelines for Social Work in Hospice*.[19] The most recent evidence has shown that 12 of the 24 roles recognized by hospice social workers as primary roles that they fill are now recognized by other professions in hospice.[24]

Hospice social workers provide assessment and counseling to patients and families, addressing emotional concerns such as desire for suicide or to hasten death, denial of terminality, anticipatory grief, and death anxiety. They facilitate social support and provide counseling about safety issues and crisis intervention counseling. Social workers also support the patient in direct spiritual experience, and spiritual questions such as discussing the meaning of life. Hospice social workers provide bereavement counseling after the patient's death.

Social workers also facilitate cultural competence on the team, support patients' end-of-life decisions according to their religious and cultural perspectives, uphold their preferences about the environment, and advocate for their preferences in general. They also connect patients and significant others to outside resources—providing financial counseling such as assisting with Medicaid applications, referral to resources, civil and legal assistance, and discharge planning. Social workers are skilled in community outreach, and public information efforts. Social work interventions may include leading outreach into the community to increase access for diverse cultural groups.[21] For example, a hospice connected with the Black community in partnership with a school of social work provided public information sessions in a local church and assigned racially diverse field interns to serve Black patients.[29] This is a unique role of social workers, who are trained in community intervention and social action. Finally, research has found better patient and organization outcomes when the social worker participates in the intake interview and supervision of social workers.[30]

CMS requires that hospice social workers possess a bachelor of social work (BSW) degree, or a related degree. Most hospice social workers, however, have a master of social work (MSW) degree.[30] Some social workers have a licensed clinical social worker (LCSW) license, which is a state certification, and for which the title may vary between states. A social worker may choose to pursue the Advanced Certified Hospice and Palliative Social Worker (ACHP-SW) certification from the National Association of Social Workers, which requires an MSW. There is also the Advanced Palliative and Hospice Social Work Certification (APHSW-C) from the Social Work Hospice and Palliative Care Network (see Chapter 3 for more information).

Spiritual Counselor

The importance of counseling from a spiritual perspective has always been recognized in hospice. Spiritual counselors assess and address the spiritual orientation, needs, and well-being of patients and their loved ones. This may include a connection to a specific religious tradition; however, the role of a spiritual counselor is more expansive than providing religious support: "Spirituality is a dynamic and intrinsic aspect of humanity through which persons seek ultimate meaning, purpose, and transcendence, and experience relationship to self, family, others, community, society, nature, and the significant or sacred. Spirituality is expressed through beliefs, values, traditions, and practices."[31(p 646)] Using evidence-based spiritual care assessments and interventions, the spiritual counselor helps patients and their loved ones identify and connect with sources of meaning in their lives, in order to help them navigate their end-of-life journey (see, e.g., the work of George Fitchett, DMin, PhD).[32]

Spiritual counselors guide individuals as they explore and express their hopes, beliefs, and fears in facing terminal illness and mortality, including the afterlife, closure with family members, and life review. With patients or loved ones who are connected to a specific spiritual tradition, a spiritual counselor may facilitate prayer, scriptural readings, and rituals, and collaborate with their religious community and clergy/spiritual leader as requested. Spiritual counselors also facilitate communication and understanding between patients, loved ones, and other hospice team members. Additionally, the spiritual counselor plays an important role in supporting the other interprofessional team members, formally and informally. Physicians, nurses, social workers, and others often view the spiritual counselor as a confidential sounding board. The spiritual counselor offers support to the interprofessional team as a whole, such as offering weekly spiritual reflections and facilitating staff debriefs and support groups.

Hospice spiritual counselors are often, though not always, ordained clergy or a recognized spiritual leader in their tradition. In the United States, standards for professional practice training for spiritual counselors include 4 units of Clinical Pastoral Education (CPE) from an accredited center with board certification, preferred through one of the 5 organizations in North America that certify chaplains based on the "Common Qualifications and Competencies for Professional Chaplains" adopted by the Board of Chaplaincy Certification.[33] Some spiritual counselors have a master of divinity degree, or additional training in areas including grief counseling, nonpharmacological therapies for pain and anxiety, or medical ethics. A hospice service may also recruit clergy members from the community who volunteer to provide specific religious support when requested by patients, significant others, or caregivers, though this model is not ideal in promoting ongoing interprofessional collaboration.

Volunteer Coordinator and Trained Volunteers

Since hospice began as a volunteer effort in the United States, it is only fitting that Medicare today requires trained volunteers as part of the interprofessional team. NHPCO describes the volunteer role as "providing companionship to a person in the final months and weeks of life, offering support to family members and caregivers, or helping with community outreach and fundraising."[34(np)] Volunteers provide much-needed additional social-emotional support to patients and families. Some volunteers are loved ones of patients who died in hospice. As outlined by the Hospice Foundation of America, volunteer activities are diverse and can include both direct patient/family support and administrative help. Volunteers enrich patient and family support through friendly visits, taking them on walks, providing massage, music, and/or other therapies if certified, and pet therapy. Volunteers may also provide support to the hospice through administrative work like sending holiday or bereavement cards, fundraising, and other specialty areas based on their professional and personal expertise.

Volunteers participate in regular trainings provided by their respective hospice organizations, both to promote their ongoing education in working with hospice patients, and to make sure they are informed regarding policies and procedures. Volunteers may periodically communicate with the other interprofessional team members, either directly or through a volunteer coordinator or manager.

Teamwork in Hospice Foundations of Interprofessional Collaboration

The key to successful interprofessional collaboration is building trust and personal relationships within the interprofessional team. Strong relationships between hospice team members are foundational to providing the best comprehensive hospice care to patients and their loved ones, as team members are more open to learning from each other and respecting a multiplicity of voices regarding patient plans of care. It is important for professionals to get to know each other as people, versus simply as representatives of a particular discipline. Team members also provide important care and support of each other, which is vital to resisting compassion fatigue and burnout as they care for the dying and grieving.

Professionals from the various disciplines must work consciously and intentionally in order to maintain consistent collaboration. In home hospice especially, team members often make home visits independently of each other. The most effective and caring hospice teams are those that are in regular touch with each other outside of the required "official" collaboration channels, mainly the official legal medical record in which all disciplines chart, and the weekly interprofessional team meetings. Organizing joint visits, bringing multiple disciplines into family meetings, and committing to regular phone and email contact between visits to share observations and concerns about patients all foster better communication and knowledge sharing, which translates into better patient outcomes.[35]

The setting in which palliative or hospice care is provided also has a significant impact on how the interprofessional team functions. Since hospice is a philosophy versus a place of care, it is provided wherever someone resides, including a private home, hospital, skilled nursing facility, assisted living, hospice residence, even a shelter. Each of these settings provides both opportunities and challenges for the interprofessional team.

Best Practices for Interprofessional Collaboration

The more people you have working together, the more chance there is for conflict and disagreement to arise. Working as part of an interprofessional team requires from each professional a high level of respect, maturity, balance of confidence and humility, and willingness to listen to and learn from multiple perspectives. Barriers within the interprofessional team to full utilization of all disciplines include (1) role blurring; (2) lack of knowledge of the expertise of other professions; (3) conflicts arising from differences between professions in values and theoretical base; (4) negative team norms; (5) client stereotyping; and (6) administrative barriers.[3] These barriers, with suggested solutions to address them, will be discussed below.

Role Blurring

When a social worker first began practice in hospice, one of her first patients asked her, "Why would God do this to me?" Having had no training in addressing spirituality with clients, she said, "Let me refer you to the spiritual counselor." She called the spiritual counselor, and he said, "Sure, I'll be there on Tuesday"; the patient died before the spiritual counselor could get there. This experience made the social worker realize that a team member cannot delay responding to the concerns of a terminally ill patient, and that teamwork requires advocacy and clear communication from each discipline.

Studies have found that the majority of issues discussed by hospice clients with social workers were spiritual issues,[27] and that social workers who do address spiritual issues with hospice clients achieve better patient outcomes,[36] including better spiritual outcomes.[26] Therefore, it is the responsibility of each team member to obtain continuing education training in addressing issues that may arise (see Chapter 10 for more information on continuing education). One pitfall to this approach of cross-role education, however, is role blurring. Team members may become offended when another discipline addresses patient issues that they consider to be within their domain, thus creating competition and decreased quality of services, if not managed. Often expertise and services provided may be similar between professions, and it may not be clear who will address which issue in a certain case. For example, a spiritual counselor in hospice told the social worker that he had spent an hour counseling a patient regarding her feelings of guilt during a home visit. He learned later that the social worker had left a few minutes earlier, and she had also spent an hour counseling the patient regarding guilt feelings. The spiritual counselor and the social worker were using conflicting approaches, however, with the result of leaving the patient exhausted and confused. Role blurring may also be defined as overlapping function of team members and may have a more positive connotation. For more information on role blurring and additional use of this term, see the Glossary and Chapter 3.

Suggested Solutions
Administrative procedures may be developed by the team which call for automatic referrals to specific team members in certain case situations.[37] In this model, although all team members may respond to any issue that arises, it is each team member's responsibility to discuss client issues with the entire interprofessional

team, and bring in the discipline with the most appropriate expertise to follow up. A clear plan of care should be developed during the team meeting which clearly assigns tasks for each team member, utilizing the unique strengths of each.[38]

Lack of Knowledge of the Expertise of Other Professions

Poor interprofessional collaboration also occurs when team members are inadequately educated on the various roles and expertise of other disciplines. This lack of awareness can lead to resistance against other all team members on cases.[24] Spearheaded by volunteer physicians and nurses in the early days, the hospice movement has always espoused a holistic philosophy, but psychosocial care was provided mainly by the medical staff until the Medicare requirement for social work services in 1983. Nurses and physicians may not understand the necessity of including spiritual counselors or social workers on every case. For example, they too often tend to view the social work role as provision of concrete services, versus honoring social workers' multiplicity of roles and how they can help patients in other ways.[24]

Spiritual counselors may be assigned to cases even less often than social workers. Nurses, physicians, and social workers often believe that spiritual counselors can only serve a religious function, and thus are of no use with non-religious patients and families. Other team members may ask, "Would you like to see a chaplain?" in their assessment, which does not appropriately identify spiritual, religious, and existential needs. When restricted to this question, patients may just respond no, without understanding the role of the spiritual counselor. In reality, spiritual care can be just as beneficial to proclaimed atheists. Spirituality can be defined as a separate concept from religion. Most everyone seeks some kind of meaning when facing one's imminent mortality. And some other common end-of-life spiritual concerns are not religious in nature.[39]

Suggested Solutions
A variety of ways to address the expertise of each team member has been described and includes orientation to the role of each profession for new as well as current staff,[40] regular joint home visits including staff of multiple disciplines to observe what each profession contributes,[41] and the Role Clarification Exercise,[42] in which each discipline shares its expertise and training during a team meeting.

Conflicts Arising from Differences between Professions in Values and Theoretical Base

Contrasts exist between values and theory underlying the perspectives of professionals on the interprofessional team.[38] Each profession has a unique culture which adheres to certain values and codes of ethics, and differs between professions.

For example, social work intervention is based on theories of human behavior underlying the intervention models; this is different from other professions' approaches to working with patients and significant others. Members may be un-aware that the other disciplines have been trained in these values and theoretical approaches; each member may see the difference, rather, in terms of a character flaw or cognitive limitation of the other team member.[43]

Examples of value differences are in the areas of patient self-determination versus doctor's orders, reporting child maltreatment versus confidentiality of confession, professional boundaries versus personal relationships with clients. Supervisors should promote understanding of the values of the other professions and orient the team toward commitment to the organization as a whole and its transcendent goals which take priority over individual professions' perspectives.[44]

Regarding theoretical differences, both social workers and professional spiritual counselors are trained to base their interventions on theoretical perspectives which form the foundation of evidenced-based care. A social worker might use counseling methods from the trans-egoic model, based on transpersonal theory, or therapy focused on spirituality, to help a patient accept terminality.[45] Spiritual counselors base their interventions on one or more Spiritual Assessment models, for ex-ample Spiritual AIM, FICA or HOPE.[46-48] These differing theoretical perspectives can lead to conflicts between social workers and spiritual counselors regarding interventions.

Suggested Solutions

Ways to address these differences include acknowledging conflict sources openly, through discussing differences and accepting them nonjudgmentally, and holding a culturally sensitive perspective toward the other professions.[49] A way to achieve this is having each profession present to the other disciplines about their own values, theoretical perspectives, and roles on the team.[50] Professions may eventually come to value the strength of the others in certain areas, and experience growth in their perspectives after learning new concepts from each other.

Negative Team Norms

It is possible for negative group norms to develop on the interprofessional team. Negative group norms are standards for behavior in team interaction which hinder the group's purpose.[51] This may include lack of commitment to the team process, lack of willingness to share equally in the work of the team, scapegoating, and power differentials on the team.

Suggested Solutions

Solutions include teaching positive group norms to the team.[41] Positive group norms are standards for behavior that promote cooperation and accomplishment by the team. Examples are establishing a plan of action in which all team members share responsibility,[52] participate fully in discussions, and play an active part on the team. A way to do this is to create small teams including one member of each profession to handle each case, in order to create opportunity for more involvement for each. The team can examine how it is performing,[53] and establish equality between team members, using a collaborative or consensus model of team functioning, emphasizing egalitarianism, cohesion, and group problem-solving.[52] A way to transcend turf issues within the team is to embrace the concept of the *transdisciplinary* team,[54] in which each team member receives core training in addressing the primary biopsychosocial-spiritual needs, is expected to be ready to address all needs, while recognizing the training, expertise, and role of each discipline,[55] and making sure to refer the client to the team member with the required expertise. Collaboration is key, to ensure that interventions are not repeated, and that the patient and significant others' personal spiritual leader is included when desired. Until we can achieve equality of status, a fully holistic approach to patient care is impossible, thereby reducing the quality of service to clients.[56]

Client Stereotyping

An additional barrier to full utilization of all members of the interprofessional team sometimes stems from patients and families themselves. Clients may be unwilling to agree to sessions with certain team members—often social workers or spiritual counselors—due to stereotypes or misperceptions about these professions. Patients and significant others may think social workers only visit to qualify them for welfare payments, to conduct a protective services investigation, or help obtain home health aide hours, while in reality they can provide much needed emotional support. They may think spiritual counselors play a strictly religious role, while in reality they help patients and their loved ones approach spiritual or existential questions from their own respective points of view.

Suggested Solutions
Educate intake and admission staff, and patients and their loved ones, on the roles of the interprofessional team members, starting from the beginning of the admissions process.[57] Research has found that conducting intake interviews using an interprofessional approach leads to better client outcomes.[30]

Administrative Barriers

In order to reduce costs, providers traditionally have engaged in downsizing and cutting services.[58] This is particularly true for non-medical care, especially if it has less insurance coverage.[59] Also, if the administrator is from a medical discipline, (s)he may not have a clear understanding of the non-medical discipline's role and why it is needed.[24] For example, some hospices rely heavily on per-diem spiritual counselors, who do not participate in regular collaboration with the other team members.

Suggested Solutions

Make sure that administrators know that non-medical disciplines reduce hospice costs in a number of ways.[30] Social workers link patients with health insurance, increasing payments. Social workers and spiritual counselors help resolve psychosocial and spiritual issues which could lead to more frequent hospitalizations, greater need for pain medication, and other negative hospice outcomes, which mean added expenses for the hospice. Spiritual counselors are able to provide regular support to high-need, distressed patients and family members who frequently reach out to their nurse for emotional-spiritual support, thus freeing up the nurses to attend to cases which require their nursing expertise versus only their supportive expertise. Along with providing such interventions, it is important to document the cost savings through collecting and analyzing program data, perhaps in cooperation with local university researchers.

The workflow from the time of the initial intake is ideally structured toward holistic care, so that all core team members can screen, make assessment, and care for the patient and caregivers, rather than a nurse serving as a gatekeeper for the other professions. For example, when a nurse uses an incorrect screening technique during the intake interview by asking, "would you like to see a chaplain?" Or, "would you like to see a social worker?" the patient may say "no" based on stereotypes or a lack of understanding of the services the professional can provide. In that case, the patient doesn't get spiritual, existential, religious, or psychosocial needs fully met.

Additional Challenges

Some challenges still remain to be addressed in the field of hospice care. One challenge is the low referral rate or late referral to hospice where a patient and family may not receive all of the supportive benefits of hospice care. Numerous barriers have been described, including physician concerns about shifting care goals and maintaining a commitment to curing illness. A provider may find it difficult to accept that there is no possibility of a cure for a patient with chronic illness, and might see this as failure on their own part. Even a physician who does accept the incurability of an illness may not have the communication skills to advise the patient of this prognosis.[60] This results in a lack of hospice care for terminally ill patients. Other members of an interprofessional team may be able to help in cases like this; social workers and spiritual counselors have extensive training in communication with the patient and family. Patient and family expectations and understanding of prognosis may also lead to a delay in hospice services.

Conclusion

While each interprofessional team member has his or her own area of expertise and training, multiple disciplines may engage in providing similar services on the hospice team. For example, a nurse may help a patient with his fear of dying, and a spiritual counselor may express concern over a patient being left alone at night. It is essential that team members consistently collaborate with each other and maximize each other's skills and training to provide the most comprehensive interprofessional care possible to patients and their loved ones. Palliative care is based on this vision and can benefit from what we have learned in the hospice field so far.

Case Presentations

Sarah

Sarah[†] was a 62-year-old wife, mother, and grandmother, living with brain cancer. After a year and a half of attempted treatments, she was enrolled in home hospice. At that point, she required assistance with toileting, eating, and transferring from her bed to a chair. She was minimally verbal, although her eyes seemed to indicate that she understood more than we might have thought. She was cared for by her devoted, loving husband Benjamin. They also had good support from their 5 adult children and enjoyed spending time with their 7 grandchildren. Sarah and her family were Orthodox Jews; her husband regularly attended synagogue and was very learned in Jewish text and Jewish law, having studied at a prestigious institution for several years. Two of their sons lived in a very traditional, insular community.

The hospice nurse, social worker, and spiritual counselor were all very involved; Benjamin welcomed all support as he grappled with losing his relatively young wife. As Sarah drew nearer to the end of her life, she stopped eating and drinking, as was to be expected with her illness course. According to a strict traditional interpretation of Jewish law, some rabbinic authorities argue that one must provide IV nutrition and hydration when someone can no longer eat for themselves, based on the mandate to preserve life at all costs. Though there is a multiplicity of views on this issue in the Jewish community, the sons held this belief. Benjamin, on the other hand, understood that Sarah's body had simply stopped being able to process any food or drink, and saw it as the natural progression of her illness and the dying process. He also understood, based on the education provided to him by the hospice team, that providing IV hydration would most likely cause Sarah more suffering rather than alleviate any symptoms, due to fluid overload. The family was at an impasse, and in danger of being torn apart over what they viewed as a religious

---

[†] Names have been changed in all case studies for the purpose of confidentiality.

dispute. The husband and sons were dealing with their anticipatory grief in different ways.

The spiritual counselor on the team was Jewish, and due to her close relationship and collaboration with the nurse on the team, the nurse was well-informed about these religious issues. She came up with a creative solution, one that would both ease the family's pain and preserve Sarah's comfort. With the hospice physician's approval, she initiated subcutaneous hydration, carefully titrated to prevent fluid overload. Sarah died at home the following week, comfortable, and surrounded by her loving family. Her husband and children were able to be relatively at peace with her death, and with each other, due to the strong work of the interprofessional team.

Mr. Jones

Mr. Jones, 79 years old, suffered from lung cancer that had metastasized beyond the possibility of treatment. He lived with his partner and was also supported and visited daily by his daughter (from a previous relationship). Mr. Jones had always "marched to his own drummer" according to his family. He was a professor, a spiritual seeker, a cultured intellectual. He loved to talk about poetry and his experience learning the ways of shamanism by following a famous shaman. When he was first admitted to hospice, he was alert, oriented, and ambulatory. By his partner's report, he became very agitated at night, and expressed a deep fear of dying. In conversations with the spiritual counselor, he tried to present himself as strong. The nurse adjusted his medications several times, but nothing eased his agitation. The nurse asked both the social worker and spiritual counselor to try to encourage him to talk about his fears.

On one of the last visits while Mr. Jones was still coherent, he expressed some fear and unease over whether or not he believed in an afterlife. Through gentle questioning, the spiritual counselor was able to encourage him to explore this question further. Mr. Jones shared that he believed—or at least, wanted to believe—that when he died, after being cremated (his desire) and his ashes scattered, that his ashes, and thus his spirit, would find their way into becoming part of another person. He was comforted by this. The spiritual counselor reminded him of this on future visits, and Mr. Jones seemed to find some solace in this idea, and it somewhat eased his fear of the unknown. At the same time, his agitation never fully resolved until just before death. The nurse, social worker, and spiritual counselor together were able to provide education to his loved ones in clinical, emotional, and spiritual terms about the fact that some people do struggle as they leave this life. Given his feisty personality, it is not surprising that Mr. Jones was one of these people. The team provided reassurance to the family that even when we cannot make this anxiety go away, they had a critical role to play in being present with him, letting him know that he did not need to suffer alone. This eased his loved ones' suffering by allowing them to feel less helpless. He died soon after that visit.

Profession-Specific Implications within the Hospice Team:
Pearls and Pitfalls

Although these pearls and pitfalls come from hospice practice, they are applicable to palliative care across the life span and in many other settings.

Pearls: Overall Interprofessional Care

- Collaborative interprofessional care = best care for patient.
- One discipline may discover unique, important information; sharing this with other team members may enhance holistic care.
- More eyes on patients mean more collaborative care.
- Team members can support each other in emotionally difficult cases, or when ethics questions arise, thus providing enhanced support and shared decision-making.

Pitfalls: Overall

- Collaboration takes time and energy—both are at a premium in today's overtaxed medical system.
- Collaboration takes time for processing, and team members may need to process in different ways, which requires tolerance of multiple communication styles and willingness to bring each other into their respective disciplines (e.g., educate enough that everyone can be on the same page).

Discussion Questions

Sarah

1. How might the outcome of care planning and symptom management for this patient have been different had the spiritual counselor not been involved in this case? How might it have impacted the family's experience of their loved one's final weeks?

2. How does true interprofessional collaboration foster creativity in developing appropriate plans of care for patients? How might this impact overall approaches to care planning in palliative care and hospice?

Mr. Jones

3. What are the unique ways that each interprofessional team member approaches a patient's fear of dying, and their loved ones' reactions to this fear? How might these approaches either complement or conflict with each other, depending on the team?

4. How might the experience of Mr. Jones and his loved ones have been different without an interprofessional approach to his agitation and fear?

References

1. Reith M, Payne M. *Social Work in End-of-Life and Palliative Care*. Lyceum; 2009.

2. Tapp A, Nancarrow C, Morey Y, Warren S, Bowtell N, Verne J. Public responses to volunteer community care: propositions for old age and end of life. *PLoS ONE*. 2019;14(7):e0218597. https://doi.org/10.1371/journal.pone.0218597.

3. Reese D. *Hospice Social Work*. Columbia University Press; 2013.

4. Schriver JM. (2010). *Human Behavior and the Social Environment: Shifting Paradigms in Essential Knowledge for Social Work Practice*. 5th ed. Allyn & Bacon; 2010.

5. DePolo M, Kennedy TR. No one dies alone: a unique volunteer program. *J Christian Nurs*. 2023, Jan-Mar 01;40(1):59–61. doi:10.1097/CNJ.0000000000000912.

6. Harding SR, Flannelly KJ, Galek K, Tannenbaum HP. Spiritual care, pastoral care, and chaplains: trends in the health care literature. *J Health Care Chaplaincy*. 2008;14(2):99–117. doi:10.1080/08854720802129067. PMID: 18697354.

7. Health Care Chaplaincy Network and Spiritual Care Association. The Chaplaincy Taxonomy: Standardizing Spiritual Care Terminology. January 2019. chaplaincy_taxonomy_standardizing_spiritual_care_terminology_r1.pdf (spiritualcareassociation.org).

8. Centers for Medicare and Medicaid Services. Hospice Toolkit: An Overview of the Medicaid Hospice Benefit. 2016. https://www.cms.gov/Medicare-Medicaid-Coordination/Fraud-Prevention/Medicaid-Integrity-Education/Downloads/hospice-overviewbooklet.pdf.

9. Harrison KL, Connor SR. First Medicare demonstration of concurrent provision of curative and hospice services for end-of-life care. *Am J Public Health*. 2016;106(8):1405–1408. doi:10.2105/AJPH.2016.303238.

10. Parker, J. Top hospice trends to watch in 2021. *Hospice News*. 2021. https://hospicenews.com/2021/01/01/top-hospice-trends-to-watch-in-2021/

11. Centers for Medicare and Medicaid Services. CMS Guidelines. 2020. https://www.cms.gov/Regulations-anGuidance/Guidance/Manuals/downloads/som107ap_m_hospice.pdf.

12. Webb M, Lysaght Hurley S, Gentry J, Brown M, Ayoub C. Best practices for using telehealth in hospice and palliative care. *J Hosp Palliat Nurs*. 2021;23(3):277–285.

13. Massachusetts Medical Society. (2020). Brief history of palliative care. 2020. https://resident360.nejm.org/content_items/history-of-palliative-care.

14. Cicely Saunders International. Dame Cicely Saunders: a brother's story. 2021. https://cicelysaundersinternational.org/dame-cicely-saunders-a-brothers-story/really-happening/.

15. LeGrand SB, Walsh D, Nelson KA, Davis MP. A syllabus for fellowship education in palliative medicine. *Am J Hops Palliat Care*. 2003;20(4):279–289.

16. Albers A, Bonsignore L, Webb M. A team-based approach to delivering person centered care at the end of life. *NC Med J*. 2018;79(4):256–258.

17. Centers for Medicare & Medicaid Services. Interim Final Rule (IFC), CMS-3401-IFC. 2020. https://www.cms.gov/medicareprovider-enrollment-and-certificationsurveycertificationge ninfopolicy-and-memos-states-and/interim-final-rule-ifc-cms-3401-ifc-additional-policy-and-regulatory-revisions-response-covid-19.

18. National Hospice and Palliative Care Organization. The hospice team. 2020. https://www.nhpco.org/patients-and-caregivers/about-hospice-care/the-hospice-team/.

19. National Hospice and Palliative Care Organization. NHPCO Guidelines. 2018. https://www.nhpco.org/wp-content/uploads/2019/04/Standards_Hospice_2018.pdf.

20. Centers for Medicare & Medicaid Services. Medicare and Medicaid programs: hospice conditions of participation. Final rule. *Federal Register*, 2008;73(109):32087–32220.

21. National Consensus Project for Quality Palliative Care. *Clinical Practice Guidelines for Quality Palliative Care*. 4th ed. National Coalition for Hospice and Palliative Care; 2018. https://www.nationalcoalitionhpc.org/ncp.

22. American Nurses Association, Center for Ethics & Human Rights. Position statement: Nurses' roles and responsibilities in providing care and support at the end of life. 2016. https://www.nursingworld.org/~4af078/globalassets/docs/ana/ethics/endoflife-positionst atement.pdf.

23. Kulys R, Davis M. An analysis of social services in hospice. *Soc Work*. 1986;11(6):448–454.

24. Reese, D. Interdisciplinary perceptions of the social work role in hospice: building upon the classic Kulys and Davis study. *J Soc Work End Life Palliat Care*. 2011;7(4):383–406.

25. Reese, D (formerly Ita D). Testing of a causal model: acceptance of death in hospice patients. *Omega*. 1995–1996;32(2):81–92.

26. Reese D, Raymer M, Orloff S, et al. The Social Work Assessment Tool (SWAT). *J Soc Work End Life Palliat Care*. 2006;2(2):65–95.

27. Reese D, Brown D. Psychosocial and spiritual care in hospice: differences between nursing, social work, and clergy. *Hospice J*. 1997;12(1):29–41.

28. National Association of Social Workers. *NASW Standards for Social Work Practice in Palliative and End of Life Care*. NASW; 2011.

29. Reese D, Buila S, Cox S, Davis J, Olsen M, Jurkowski E. University-community-hospice partnership to address organizational barriers to cultural competence. *Am J Hosp Palliat Med*. 2017;34(1):64–78.

30. Reese D, Raymer M. Relationships between social work services and hospice outcomes: results of the National Hospice Social Work Survey. *Soc Work*. 2004;49(3):415–422.

31. Puchalski CM, Vitillo R, Hull SK, Reller N. Improving the spiritual dimension of whole person care: reaching national and international consensus. *J Palliat Med*. 2014;17(6), 642–656.

32. Peng-Keller S. George Fitchett, Steve Nolan (Hg.) (2018) Case studies in spiritual care. Healthcare chaplaincy assessments, interventions & outcomes. London: Jessica Kingsley Publishers. ISBN 978-1785927836. *Spiritual Care*. 2021;10(2):188–188. https://doi.org/10.1515/spircare-2020-0129

33. Board of Chaplaincy Certification. Common qualifications and competencies for professional chaplains. 2017. https://www.professionalchaplains.org/files/2017%20Com mon%20Qualifications%20and%20Competencies%20for%20Professional%20Chapla ins.pdf.

34. National Hospice and Palliative Care Organization. Hospice volunteers. 2020. https://www.nhpco.org/patients-and-caregivers/about-hospice-care/volunteering-for-hospice/.

35. Joseph R, Brown-Manhertz D, Ikwuazom S, Santomassino M, Singleton J. The effectiveness of structured interdisciplinary collaboration for adult home hospice patients on patient satisfaction and hospital admissions and re-admission: a systematic review protocol. *JBI Evid Synthesis*. 2014;12(7):148–163.

36. Reese D. Addressing spirituality in hospice: current practices and a proposed role for transpersonal social work. *Soc Thought: J Relig Soc Serv*. 2001;20(1–2):135–161.

37. Reese D (formerly Ita D), Nelson B. The medical social work role on the multidisciplinary team: barriers, solutions, and directions for the future. 1996, April. Paper presented at the 50th Anniversary Symposium, School of Social Work, University of Illinois, Urbana.

38. Reese D, Sontag M-A. Barriers and solutions for successful inter-professional collaboration on the hospice team. *Health Soc Work*. 2001;26(3):167–175.

39. Reese D. Addressing spirituality in end-of-life care. 2021, June. Paper presented at the New Beginnings Conference, Society for Spirituality and Social Work, virtual conference.

40. Kovacs P, Bronstein L. Preparation for oncology settings: what hospice social workers say they need. *Health Soc Work*. 1999;24(1):57–65.

41. Roberts C. Conflicting professional values in social work and medicine. *Health Soc Work*. 1989;14(3):211–218.

42. Sontag M. Making it happen: Interdisciplinary collaboration in hospices. 1995, August. Paper presented at the meeting of the National Hospice Organization, San Francisco, CA.

43. Mizrahi T, Abramson J. Sources of strain between physicians and social workers: implications for social workers in health care settings. *Soc Work Health Care*. 1985;(3):33–51.

44. Abramson J. Orienting social work employees in interdisciplinary settings: shaping professional and organizational perspectives. *Soc Work*. 1993;38(2):121–240.

45. Smith E. Addressing the psychospiritual distress of death as reality: a transpersonal approach. *Soc Work*. 1995;40(3):402–413.

46. Shields M, Kestenbaum A, Dunn LB. Spiritual AIM and the work of the chaplain: a model for assessing spiritual needs and outcomes in relationship. *Palliat Support Care*. 2015 Feb;13(1):75–89. doi:10.1017/S1478951513001120

47. Puchalski, C. FAST FACTS AND CONCEPTS# 274 THE FICA SPIRITUAL HISTORY TOOL.

48. Anandarajah G, Hight E. Spirituality and medical practice: using the HOPE questions as a practical tool for spiritual assessment. *Am Fam Physician*. 2001;63(1):87.

49. Mailick M, Jordon P. A multimodel approach to collaborative practice in health settings. *Soc Work Health Care*. 1977;2(4):445–454.

50. Davis, K. *Understanding the Importance of the Interdisciplinary Team in Pediatric Hospice and Palliative Care*. National Hospice and Palliative Care Organization; 2018. https://www.nhpco.org/wp-content/uploads/2019/04/PALLIATIVECARE_Understanding IDT.pdf.

51. Health Resources and Services Administration. *Interdisciplinary Development of Health Professionals to Maximize Health Provider Resources in Rural Areas*. HRSA; 1993.

52. Sands R, Stafford J, McClelland M. "I beg to differ": conflict in the interdisciplinary team. *Social Work in Health Care*. 1990;14(3):55–72.

53. Lowe J, Herranen M. Conflict in teamwork: understanding roles and relationships. *Soc Work Health Care*. 1987;3(3):323–330.

54. Egan KA, Labyak MJ. Hospice care: a model for quality end-of-life care. In: Ferrell BR, Coyle N, eds. *Textbook of Palliative Nursing*. Oxford University Press; 2001:7–26.

55. Wittenberg-Lyles E, Parker Oliver D, Demiris G, Regehr K. Interdisciplinary collaboration in hospice team meetings. *J Interprof Care*. 2010;24(3):264–273.

56. Davidson K. Role blurring and the hospital social worker's search for a clear domain. *Health Soc Work*. 1990;15(2):228–234.

57. Soroka JT, Collins LA, Creech G, Kutcher GR, Menne KR, Petzel BL. Spiritual care at the end of life: does educational intervention focused on a broad definition of spirituality increase utilization of chaplain spiritual support in hospice? *J Palliat Med*. 2019;22(8):939–944.

58. Cottrell K. A study of the impact of organizational restructuring due to managed care and the effects on the survivor workforce as it relates to the quality of care (doctoral dissertation, California School of Professional Psychology). *Dissertation Abstracts International*, 1996;57(4-B):2918.

59. Mahoney J. Hospice and managed care. *Hospice J*. 1997;12(2):81–84.

60. Reese D. Unpublished data collected during dissertation. 1994.

12

More than the Sum of Its Parts

Interprofessional Palliative Care in the Hospital Setting

Jaime Goldberg and Paul Galchutt

Key Points

- Effective palliative care teams require buy-in and ongoing investment from all team members across professions, as well as administrative/institutional leadership.
- Palliative care consultation teams have been shown to improve patient outcomes and practitioner satisfaction.
- Transdisciplinary skills are necessary for all palliative care team members to possess; profession-specific roles and expertise are important to respect and garner.
- Best practices for palliative care consultation teams start with impeccable communication, trust, and respect among team members and expand to include various administrative, education, and clinical practices.
- Effective interprofessional palliative care teamwork leads to optimal patient and family care along with team functioning and wellness.
- The true best practice for interprofessional palliative care teams in the hospital setting is being continually attuned to patient/family and team needs and adjusting accordingly.

Introduction

Considered the foundation of the palliative care approach, the interprofessional team functions as a collaborative partnership to provide person-centered, family-focused, culturally congruent care throughout the illness trajectory. In fact, the team approach is reinforced in key definitions, guidelines, and documents of preferred palliative care practices.[1-4] Ideally, members of the interprofessional team are trained, certified, and experienced in palliative care; embrace collaborative work; and view their colleagues' expertise with respect and humility.[5,6] This expertise includes impeccable communication and interpersonal skills with patients, families, and colleagues, which enhance patient care and team cohesion. Palliative care teams at their best are "characterized by self-awareness, cohesiveness and shared decision making, trust, respect, accountability, mutual support, self-care, positive work environment, recognition of a job well done, and attention to retention and job satisfaction."[5(p677)] This chapter explores the interprofessional palliative care team in the hospital setting. It addresses team composition and functioning, challenges and strengths inherent in the team approach to care in this environment, and the evidence-based best practices that ensure optimal patient and family care as well as team wellness.

History of the Interprofessional Team in the Inpatient Setting

Palliative care philosophy challenges the traditional bio-medical, cure-focused, physician-dominant culture of healthcare that often excludes the person who is ill from being at the center of care.[2,4,5] The emergence of the hospital-based interprofessional palliative care team is traced to the landmark work of Dr. Cicely Saunders at St. Christopher's Hospice in London.[7,8] Saunders' work was documented in Elisabeth Kübler Ross's foundational volume, *On Death and Dying*.[9] Motivated by this text, Dr. Balfour Mount, a Canadian physician at Royal Victoria Hospital in Montreal, Quebec, was mentored by Dr. Saunders.[10] After his hands-on formation at St. Christopher's Hospice, Dr. Mount brought such concepts as total pain and the necessity of an interprofessional hospital-based team back to North America, where he developed the first hospital-based palliative care service in 1975.[10] The Cleveland Clinic Taussig Cancer Center in Ohio became the site of the first palliative care program in the United States in 1987 under the leadership of Declan Walsh.[11] This program expanded to include the first palliative medicine clinical and research fellowship, as well as the opportunity to care for patients on the first acute pain and palliative care inpatient unit.[11] With advocacy and support from the Robert Wood Johnson Foundation and the Open Society Institute, palliative care teams in the United States expanded significantly in the 1990s.[12]

Palliative care prevalence in hospitals in the United States has shown a steady increase over the past 2 decades, from a quarter of hospitals with more than 50 beds reporting the presence of a palliative care program in 2000 to three-quarters of such hospitals in 2017.[13] Hospital-based palliative care consultation services have been the most common and developed mechanism for palliative care service delivery since its inception, but recent trends have included the creation of inpatient palliative care units, outpatient consultation clinics or integration into specialty clinics (see Chapter 14), home- and long-term care-based programs (see Chapter 15), and the expansion of primary palliative care skills (see Chapter 16).[14,15]

Palliative Care Consultation Teams

The palliative care consultation service in the hospital setting is a referral-based holistic specialty* that is called on by the primary medical team (or others, depending on hospital protocol and culture) to share expertise regarding pain/symptom management; assist with complex communication; facilitate ongoing decision-making deliberation to discern patient/family goals, values, and preferences; and respond to patient/family psychosocial, spiritual, and emotional distress. A palliative care service may be a part of a hospital's general medicine, family medicine, critical care, psychiatry, or other department, or may constitute a separate department unto itself.

Two practice models are typically seen for inpatient palliative care teams,[16] though a variety of team and practice constellations exist based largely on needs and available resources. The first is the "solo practitioner" model, in which a lone palliative care clinician, most often a physician or advanced practice nurse, works in conjunction with the primary medical team. The benefits of this model are lower cost and less potential to overwhelm or disrupt the central role of the primary team. Disadvantages include the absence of holistic care delivered by specialty psychosocial-spiritual clinicians and lack of opportunities to process the substance and meaning of complex situations with interprofessional team members in real time. Given that palliative care is by definition a team specialty, the goal of the solo practitioner model is to develop into a specialty team.

The second model is the "full team" model, in which the palliative care advanced practice nurse, chaplain, physician, registered nurse, social worker, and other professions collaborate as a team. While each team has its own practices, policies, and workflows for day-to-day activities, some common threads are seen with this model. Once a consultation is received by the team, a triage process takes place to decide which team member(s) will complete the initial consult, based on availability, role, reason for consultation, and team/institutional norms. Initial palliative care consults are often completed by a physician or nurse practitioner, although best practice is to include social worker- or chaplain-driven initial assessments and interventions for psychosocially or spiritually oriented referrals.[17] Once the initial consultation is complete, continuous open communication among team members is needed, respectfully negotiating who will continue to see this patient/family and how often. Ideally, team members come together for routine rounds to discuss care plans and interventions, as well as any follow-up needs after transition from the hospital, including bereavement follow-up as needed. Communication with team members during formal rounds and informally throughout the day can help to maintain consistency in patient care and connections among team members.

---

* Palliative care is considered to be a subspecialty within medicine and nursing, but a specialty in spiritual care and social work. For this book, we standardize the language by referring to palliative care as a specialty when referring to the team as a whole. We use the term "subspecialty" when referring specifically to nursing or medicine.

Obvious advantages to this model are increased interprofessional input and expertise and the ability to see a higher volume of patients. A primary challenge, however, is the extra cost that may come with including all the core[†] team members, especially those who do not bill for services in a way that helps to offset their salary.[18] Leaders charged with building a palliative care team are challenged to be sensitive to the unique contributions of each profession. Chaplains, who are nationally acknowledged as core members of the team but are most often not hired as full-time members, are especially vulnerable to role-marginalization and exclusion when funding is limited.[19] Though the team model is strongly recommended,[1-4] resource limitations may impede a larger team model, especially at the beginning phases of creation of a palliative care consultation service. Perhaps the most common scenario is when the team involves one or more team members in any given consult based on the particular patient care needs and team member availability.

Interprofessional Education and the Hospital-Based Palliative Care Team

Participation in interprofessional education increases exposure to and understanding of various professional colleagues, offers opportunities for practicing interprofessional communication, and fosters positive attitudes toward healthcare teamwork.[20] Though the Institute of Medicine (IOM)[21] and World Health Organization (WHO)[22] recommend that all healthcare professionals receive education in interprofessional teamwork, the learned skill of effectively working on an interprofessional team is not readily taught or modeled in healthcare education.[23] To overcome this, interprofessional palliative care education opportunities are emerging. To facilitate effective team and family meetings, interprofessional teams need to be expert in group facilitation, information dissemination, and tending to emotions. Necessary skills for each of these roles have been identified and can be taught and practiced during interprofessional educational opportunities.[24] Members of the palliative care team can seek interprofessional palliative care education through university-based academic programs (see Chapter 8), clinical specialist training in palliative care (Chapter 9), or continuing education in interprofessional palliative care (Chapter 10).

[†] In this book, we use the term "core" to refer to chaplains, nurses, physicians, and social workers who are all named as part of the interprofessional team for both the Medicare hospice guidelines and the NCP guidelines. This designation does not minimize the importance of other team members who contribute to the palliative care of patients and families.

Roles of Each Team Member

All professions that specialize in palliative care bring a unique history, ethical base, culture, training, vocabulary, and theoretical perspective to team participation. Yet, palliative care specialists also develop core skills regardless of their professional background and unite in the mission to ease the burden of serious illness and improve quality of life. Table 12.1 delineates essential interprofessional knowledge and skills that all team members need to hone to optimize patient/family care in the hospital setting (see Chapter 6 for a list of proposed interprofessional

Table 12.1 Palliative Care Interprofessional Knowledge and Skills

Basic Palliative Care Knowledge
- Define and introduce palliative care philosophy/goals
- Understand palliative care referral process and criteria
- Knowledge of hospital policies/procedures related to palliative care
- Familiarity with palliative care education tools (e.g., all team members take CAPC pain assessment and communication courses)
- Identify, assess, intervene, or refer as appropriate for physical, psychosocial, emotional, spiritual distress and crises
- Basic pain/symptom assessment
- Knowledge of bioethics and discuss/apply concepts/refer appropriately
- Discuss hospice philosophy and practicalities of care with patients/families/staff and intervene/ educate as needed

Advance Care Planning
- Propose, explore, and elicit patient values/ goals/preferences throughout illness trajectory; discuss with team members and ensure ongoing documentation
- Understand options for advance directive documents (e.g., hospital-specific, state-specific, values-based documents) and assist with completion as appropriate
- Understand state-specific Physician or Portable Orders for Life Sustaining Treatment (POLST)/ Medical Orders for Life Sustaining Treatment (MOLST)/equivalent document; provide education to patients/families/colleagues

Patient Care Conferences
- Goal for at least 2 professions present at each meeting
- Skillfully facilitate patient care conferences
- Elicit patient/family's understanding of health condition and prognosis
- Elicit and investigate information about patient/family personality, dynamics, support system, coping, needs
- Actively engage with patient, family, and team before/during/after meeting; respond to distress, questions, nonverbal cues
- Coordinate with other team members within and outside palliative care

Surrogate Decision-Making
- Articulate differences between surrogate decision maker/healthcare agent and Durable Power of Attorney for Healthcare and use the appropriate terminology in all communication
- Familiarity with state regulations regarding hierarchy for surrogate decision-making
- Facilitate conversation to determine decision-making structure/agent within individual family
- Identify when there is conflict among family members about decision-making and facilitate problem-solving in collaboration with team members.
- Identify and document healthcare agent in appropriate places in medical record, with contact information
- Educate other healthcare providers about designated healthcare agent

Adapted with permission from MemorialCare Long Beach Medical Center Palliative Care Team.

palliative care competencies). In ideal palliative care practice, team members work interdependently, and all team members are involved in both clinical and non-clinical aspects of care.[25] In addition to the clinical roles described, all team members are ideally encouraged to be involved in education, leadership, and systems-level work to optimize palliative care integration in the hospital setting.[26] The current reality is, however, that professional background, job descriptions, biases, and expectations of some team members and institutions can lead to certain clinicians being more involved in education, leadership, and systems-level work than others.

Hospital-based palliative care teams are typically composed of several core team members—advanced practice nurse, chaplain, physician, registered nurse, social worker—though team members representing many additional disciplines[‡] contribute to the palliative care of patients in the hospital setting. Paramount to the palliative approach, the patient/family must always remain at the center of the care team. The core professions will be discussed in alphabetical order below, underscoring aspects of each role that are unique to the hospital setting, and the lateral, as opposed to hierarchical, team structure to which palliative care teams aspire (see Chapter 3 for complete discussion of education, licensure, and certification requirements for each palliative care team member).

Advanced Practice Registered Nurse (APRN)

Advanced practice registered nurses' (APRNs) training and expertise, holistic approach to care, and expanded scope of practice that integrates both medical and advanced nursing functions enable them to effectively address the complex needs of patients with serious illness and their families.[27] Expertise in communication and decision-making, pain/symptom management, patient/family education, and coordination of care are paramount for advanced practice nurses.[27,28] APRNs have prescriptive authority, as well as the ability to order treatment interventions to varying degrees in many states.[28] Often leaders on palliative care consultation services, APRNs serve as a bridge between the medical and nursing professions.[27,28] In an exploratory qualitative study of patients' perceptions of their oncology or palliative care nurse practitioner, patients highlight that nurse practitioners in these specialties are particularly empathic, helpful, supportive, and give patients a sense of empowerment and control over their disease-related choices.[29]

[‡] Although often used interchangeably, "discipline" refers to a branch of knowledge, while "profession" refers to an occupation that requires special education and/or prolonged training and a formal qualification. In this book, we have attempted to standardize the use of the term "profession" when referring to occupations such as chaplaincy, medicine, nursing, and social work, but occasionally the term "discipline" is used, especially when focused on the theory and knowledge development of the professions.

Chaplain

As a core member of the inpatient palliative care team, chaplains are clinical spiritual care specialists who are most responsible for direct assessment and care within religious, spiritual, cultural, and existential realms.[30,31] Though chaplains may personally practice a specific religious or spiritual tradition, as clinicians, they are trained to address the needs, hopes, and resources of all patients/caregivers independent of any particular belief system.[32] In a national survey of hospital-based chaplains who spent at least 15% of their time working on a palliative care team, participants identified building relationships with patients/families, caring for those experiencing active dying/death, and helping patients/families with decision-making processes as their primary foci.[33] Palliative care chaplains companion with patients/caregivers and create space for spiritual reflection and address moral distress and legacy building.[30] Palliative care physicians, nurses, and social workers value the team chaplain's role to provide support for them as well as the larger hospital community.[31] Chaplains contribute to the care of palliative care team members and colleagues through informal check-ins or by facilitating more intentional events, such as debrief sessions with staff after a difficult situation, or professional resiliency and well-being programs. Chaplains offer emotional care and spiritual support, explore patient and caregivers' religion and spirituality, address existential distress, manage illness-related and end-of-life rituals, and are equipped to adapt to each serious illness circumstance and the values-informed coping of each patient/family.[30]

Physician

While standard physician training emphasizes general health or treatment of pathology, specialist palliative care physicians focus on the prevention and alleviation of suffering and improvement to quality of life.[34] Palliative care physicians understand and communicate about illness and prognosis; explore treatment options and assist with decision-making; craft person-centered plans of care; and manage pain and symptoms.[35] On a consultation service, palliative care physicians work collaboratively with the primary and other specialty teams, especially in complex situations. In specialist inpatient units, however, the palliative care physician is typically responsible for the medical management of the patient. As the palliative care approach remains countercultural in many hospitals, palliative physicians can also serve in a liaison role; they represent the medical profession while also exemplifying palliative care tenets among colleagues.

Registered Nurse

A registered nurse on an inpatient palliative care consultation service may have different roles based on patient/caregiver and team needs. One role may be as a case manager who coordinates complex care; another may be in a triage capacity as the first person to assess consultation requests and interface with referral teams. Palliative nurses may also complete physical assessments and health histories, provide education, administer medications and treatments, perform wound care, and manage pain and symptoms.[36] These specialized nurses have adapted their practice from a focus on specific tasks such as measuring vital signs, to one centered on symptom management, comfort, and support.[36] The bedside nurses provide primary palliative care, and as such, are important team members (see Box 12.1).

Box 12.1. Bedside Nurses as Palliative Care Resource Nurses

Susan Barbour, APRN

The palliative care team at our academic medical center has a well-established Hospice and Palliative Medicine fellowship program for physician trainees and the occasional social work and chaplain trainees. The palliative care advanced practice registered nurse (APRN) has a liaison role with the Department of Nursing and the consultative palliative care team. Many bedside nurses have a strong interest in palliative care, are eager to learn more communication skills, and to engage more deeply with patients, families, and the interprofessional palliative care team. Bedside nurses trained as Palliative Care Resource Nurses (PCRN) support other nurses on their units with the palliative care needs of their patients in real time, often on the shifts with less support (nights and weekends).

Beginning in 2011 as an initiative of the Chief Nursing Officer (CNO), the PCRN program supported 2 nurses from each unit to become palliative care resource nurse champions. The 16-hour training on key palliative care concepts is now offered 1 to 3 times per year. Initially much of the training was provided by the palliative care team physicians, social workers, and chaplains. As time went on, however, bedside nurses who were strong nursing leaders and passionate about palliative care became the backbone of this training. The nursing-led education also includes other palliative care–focused workshops, such as withdrawal of life-sustaining measures and palliative care communication.

The PCRN program received a $10,000/year endowment from a retired palliative care social worker in recognition of the critical role of nursing in the delivery of palliative care. The palliative care APRN manages the endowment in consultation with the PCRNs. Together, they have chosen to use this funding for special projects specific to nurses, such as assistance with palliative care nursing board certification, support for PCRN training needs (booklets, supplies, refreshments), lanyards that identify the PCRNs, and palliative care reference pocket cards for nurses. Since the endowment does not pay for PCRN salaries, each unit manager uses staff development funds for salary reimbursement to participate in palliative care activities, and the total investment depends on the priorities of the unit and unit manager.

PCRNs participate in 3 major activities to support nursing staff:

1. *Palliative care education for bedside nurses*: The PCRN training is offered to any inpatient nurse interested in palliative care or assigned to care for patients at end of life in the comfort care (palliative care/hospice) suites. Topics include an introduction to palliative care and hospice, symptom management with a focus on pain and nausea, comfort care, spiritual care, advance directives, expectations at end of life, and a panel discussion by PCRNs. In addition, an interprofessional team developed the Integrating Multidisciplinary Palliative Care in the ICU (IMPACT-ICU) nurses communication course and disseminated this workshop to all 7 academic medical centers affiliated with University of California.[a,b] A nurse/physician team from each medical center serves as IMPACT-ICU facilitators, using a 70-page handbook for course fidelity.

2. *Bimonthly PCRN Committee meeting*: The APRN and PCRNs meet to debrief challenges, share educational updates, support each other, and provide input for proposed palliative care improvements. All PCRN class graduates are entered into a database and are invited to the meeting. Although 800–900 names are on the roster, typically 10–20 nurses attend these bimonthly meetings. These meetings provide an opportunity for nurses to reflect on their shared experiences when caring for patients with serious illness. They ask for feedback and advice related to patient situations that they found challenging and they celebrate each other's successes and innovations when a situation went especially well.

3. *Weekly unit rounds*: Weekly palliative care rounds, conducted by the palliative care APRN with the palliative care social worker, were originated during the development of IMPACT-ICU and continued because of the benefit to clinical nurses who valued the accessibility, real-time coaching, and deep listening offered by the pair. A template (see example in Appendix 1) focuses the conversation and subtly educates the bedside nursing staff about the components of a palliative care assessment, beginning with the nurse's own compassion fatigue or distress and continuing to the patient's symptoms, family support, and communication challenges.

The procedure for implementing unit rounds might be reproduced in other environments. The palliative care APRN, in conjunction with the charge nurse, reviews the unit census and identifies patients and nurses who might benefit from a bedside check-in for coaching or support. The APRN and social worker approach the bedside nurse, make sure the time is convenient for them, begin by checking in on how the nurse is doing, and then progress through the template depending on the needs of the patient. The entire conversation is designed to be quick, 5–10 minutes per nurse.

The palliative care rounds template and procedure were modified depending on the needs of the unit. For example, some units adopted walking rounds with quick conversations about 3–6 patients, while others preferred a seated discussion in a conference room, focused on one patient who had been served by multiple nurses. Sometimes the unit was too busy for anyone to stop and discuss patients; on those days, the APRN and social worker would provide a treat (a cookie or a cup of coffee) and plan to come back another day. As nurses or other members of the interprofessional team became accustomed to the process, they began to proactively request a consultation or ask to "run something by you. . . ."

As an unexpected benefit, palliative care rounds provide the opportunity to identify recurring clinical issues and opportunities for quality improvement. For example, lack of consistency in the comfort care order sets used by ICU and acute care units was recognized as a problem that created conflict and delays during transitions of care. In response, a universal comfort care order set was developed and implemented for the entire medical center. In another example of palliative care rounds influencing practice, the PCRNs created a checklist to standardize the transition to comfort care and ensure a pre-transition huddle so that all members of the interprofessional team have an opportunity to address concerns (see Appendix 2). The ICU NPs continued this work by ensuring that the huddle preceding the comfort care transition was documented in the EMR.

The PCRN activities and professional development provide a model for bedside nurses to work closely with the interprofessional palliative care team to meet the needs of patients with serious illness and their families during hospitalization. The close working relationships between the PCRNs and the palliative care team are invaluable to ongoing patient and family care.

[a] Milic MM, Puntillo K, Turner K, et al. Communicating with patients' families and physicians about prognosis and goals of care. Am J Crit Care. 2015;24(4):e56–e64. doi:10.4037/ajcc2015855.

[b] Anderson WG, Puntillo K, Cimino J, et al. Palliative care professional development for critical care nurses: A multicenter program. Am J Crit Care. 2017;26(5):361–371. doi:10.4037/ajcc2017336.

Social Worker

Palliative social workers provide expert psychosocial assessment and intervention to patients and families affected by serious illness. The core principles of clinical social work—"start where the client is," embrace a "person in environment" approach, and focus on the strengths (as opposed to the deficits) of patients/families—are naturally aligned with the values of palliative care.[37] Palliative social workers use their empathic listening and psychosocial assessment and intervention skills in work with patients/families. They explore the patient/family's history, beliefs, values, relationships, communication styles, and coping mechanisms, and collaborate on plans of care as they evolve.[2] With expertise in conflict management and problem resolution, palliative social workers can be particularly skilled in the context of complex team and/or family dynamics.[37] In the hospital setting in particular, palliative social workers may be able to provide continuity of care that is not possible in settings where unit- or team-based social workers are precluded from following patients/families as they transition through the hospital system. The role is multidimensional and dynamic, and palliative social workers are encouraged to practice to the fullest extent of their training.[38] Increasingly, palliative social workers are offered opportunities to be involved in systems-level change through leadership, education, advocacy, administration, and research.[26]

The Larger Team

The interprofessional team in the hospital setting may also include many additional professionals with qualifications, skills, and experience to meet the needs of patients/families, including (but not limited to): pharmacists, physician assistants/associates, medical interpreters, mental health professionals, child life specialists, nursing assistants, nutritionists, respiratory therapists, physical and occupational therapists, speech and language pathologists, complementary and expressive arts therapists, community health workers, paramedics, emergency medical technicians, psychologists, psychiatric-mental health advanced practice registered nurses, case managers, traditional medicine practitioners, and volunteers.[2] In the hospital setting, palliative care teams also engage with primary and other specialty team members to assist with management and coordination of care. Additionally, hospital-based palliative care teams typically have relationships with home hospice organizations with which they work closely to coordinate transitions of care. It is important to recognize the unique expertise and contributions that each team member brings to the care they provide. Palliative care clinicians in the hospital can learn invaluable information from engaging with all team members with curiosity and respect.

Trainees

In an educational environment such as a teaching hospital, trainees across professions and levels of education become members of the consult team, especially where palliative care fellowships are offered. Core palliative team members have the opportunity to educate and mentor trainees, though their learning needs may interface and can at times compete with the care needs of patients/families. On teams with rotating clinicians, full-time team member(s) are ideally designated to serve as cornerstones of continuity to ensure that trainees receive education and attention.

Team Interactions

Palliative care team members have interactions with each other throughout the day, extending beyond the team workspace to their care on the floors, in joint visits and family care conferences, and through a constant stream of electronic communication. Within these clinical day-to-day interactions, the healing scope and distinctive contributions of each team member are highlighted (see Box 12.2).

Box 12.2 Patient/Family Narrative

Mr. B is a 75-year-old male who has been diagnosed with stage 4 chronic obstructive pulmonary disease (COPD). He is a widow; his wife died just 8 months ago of cancer. Mr. B has 1 child, a 42-year-old son, John, daughter-in-law Maggie, and 2 young grandchildren, ages 10 and 7. Mr. B used to work on a farm but had to stop about 10 years ago because of progressive shortness of breath and deconditioning. John is a pastor at a local church and Maggie is an elementary school teacher. Mr. B now spends most of his time with his grandchildren, whom he describes as the "light of my life."

Mr. B is admitted to the hospital with shortness of breath. This is his third admission in 3 months. He came through the Emergency Department at the insistence of his son and daughter-in-law as they noticed he had not gotten out of bed for several days except to use the bathroom due to feeling short of breath, weak, and fatigued. A palliative care consultation is received from the primary medical team, requesting assistance with symptom management and discussion of next steps in care. After reviewing the consultation, the palliative care nurse practitioner and social worker decide to do a joint visit to meet Mr. B. A discussion with the primary physician and bedside nurses prior to meeting Mr. B reveals that he has declined to take the morphine that has been prescribed for his shortness of breath. Upon arrival at the bedside, the clinicians ask Mr. B for permission to visit, and once granted, bring in chairs to be sure they are sitting at eye level with him. Using a conversational approach to their assessment, they ask Mr. B about life at home, which reveals more details about his shortness of breath and confusion about his medication regimen. They learn about his grief over the death of his wife and his fear about not seeing his grandchildren grow up. Mr. B shares that he does not want to "abandon" or "disappoint" his family, but he also wants to focus on "enjoying time with them" rather than "coming back and forth to the hospital all the time."

To address his shortness of breath, the nurse practitioner and social worker approach Mr. B with curiosity and learn about the symbolic meaning he ascribes to morphine. Mr. B shares that he saw his buddies take morphine in Vietnam and more recently watched his wife receive the medication for pain. The nurse practitioner and social worker give Mr. B the time and space to share the narrative of his experience in combat and his wife's illness; they bear witness to his experience and offer empathy. The clinicians jointly provide gentle education about the use of opioids to treat shortness of breath. They focus on how improved symptom control could also help Mr. B achieve his goal of being more active with his grandchildren. The nurse practitioner informs Mr. B that he follows a "start low, go slow" approach and offers reassurance that the palliative care team will continue to closely monitor and support him. Both clinicians remind Mr. B that he is always the "captain" of his medical care. The palliative social worker speaks with Mr. B about additional interventions to help with his shortness of breath. She returns later that day on her own and, in collaboration with Mr. B, uses a passive muscle relaxation and imagery intervention. Mr. B selects the experience of being at the beach—where he and his wife loved to go on vacation—and is guided through the sounds, colors, textures, sights, and smells of that place, which Mr. B shares he finds calming and comforting. The experience is recorded so Mr. B can continue to use the intervention post-hospitalization.

To address next steps in care, with Mr. B's permission, the nurse practitioner schedules a family meeting with Mr. B's son and daughter-in-law. Mr. B requests that his extended family—siblings and nieces/nephews be included as well. Given the relationship that the palliative social worker has begun to foster with Mr. B and the potential for spiritual concerns to arise given that John is a pastor, both the palliative social worker and chaplain decide to attend the meeting, along with the palliative care nurse practitioner and primary team resident physician. The nurse practitioner ensures that a pre-conference huddle is scheduled so all clinicians can be "on the same page" prior to the family meeting. The primary team resident physician facilitates the brief pre-conference huddle with the palliative care team. The clinicians agree that the plan for the family meeting will be to provide Mr. B and his family with an update on Mr. B's condition and offer them space to share questions and concerns. Given Mr. B's worsening condition, they will introduce the idea of a transition to a comfort-oriented plan of care. The palliative care nurse practitioner, social worker, chaplain, and primary team physician discuss the potential challenges with this situation to ensure they all feel prepared and supported going into the family meeting.

In conversations leading up to the family meeting, the palliative care team learns the following information from John and Maggie, which is discussed in the pre-conference meeting. Given the recent death of his mother, John is overwhelmed with the idea of his father dying. John also has extended family who believe that "God works miracles" and Mr. B will one day be cured of his COPD through prayer. John feels the emotional and moral weight of his family's belief system as well as his own religious struggle and sense of suffering with whether this desired miracle could occur.

Mr. B and John attend the meeting in person, with the rest of the family participating via videoconference. The meeting commences with introductions of Mr. B, the family, and all healthcare team members. The primary team resident physician then carefully and compassionately offers a summary of the patient's circumstances and challenges. Silence follows. The palliative social worker picks up on the nonverbal cues from John and the family of the importance to revisit the patient's wife's recent death and their immense grief. Many tears and remembrances of her follow, and grief support is provided. Mr. B invites the meeting back to the topic of his healthcare and requests the team's plan of care recommendation. With gentle clarity, the team recommends a shift toward a comfort-oriented care plan. As expected, family members speak to their hope of a miracle. The chaplain then shares that the entire team joins them in that hope as well. When the family appear surprised, John declares how much he believes the team cares for his father and shares this hope. He shares, however, that he believes the miracle has been that his father lived this long. Mr. B concurs. After carefully weighing what he has experienced, seen, and heard from his family and the healthcare team, Mr. B tearfully shares that it is now time for him to focus on his shortness of breath at home and "go to heaven with my wife when my time comes." Mr. B, John, and Maggie agree that Mr. B will transition to John and Maggie's home with hospice services.

As the healthcare team exits the conference, extended family members leave the videoconference call, and Mr. B requests to return to his hospital room to rest, the palliative care team members linger with John. They acknowledge again his grief around his mother's death and his emotions related to his father's illness. John begins to cry. Without rushing him, they process the family meeting and how it felt for John to hear Mr. B speak about his hopes and goals at this point in his life. As their conversation ends, the palliative care team provides John with reassurance that they will make all necessary arrangements to ensure a smooth transition to his home with hospice services.

As the palliative care team gathers for their rounds the next day, the nurse practitioner requests extra time for those who could stay after to process Mr. B's family meeting. The nurse practitioner, social worker, and chaplain all share relevant background information and a summary of the family meeting. The nurse practitioner also vulnerably expresses his emotional struggles as his own father had died at the same age and of the same illness. The nurse practitioner, social worker, and chaplain provide and receive support from each other, as well as the palliative care team members not involved in Mr. B's care. Along with processing the clinical details of this situation and focusing on their shared plan of care, these clinicians did something unique to palliative care teams. These interprofessional members recognized that the privilege of caring for patients with serious illness and their families can result in both a heightened sense of their own vulnerability, as well as an immense sense of shared meaning and team strengthening.

Challenges of Interprofessional Teams in the Hospital Setting

Equity and Equality

As palliative care teams operate within larger healthcare institutions and systems, a power differential often exists between professions within these systems, where hierarchical and paternalistic models have historically afforded the most power to physicians. Other professions such as social workers and chaplains may find themselves to be "guests in host settings," practicing within organizations whose mission and decision-making models have been defined by higher-status physicians in ways that can stymie the bio-psycho-social-spiritual approach to care and lateral approach to management favored by palliative care teams.[40] This reality has significant implications for palliative care team dynamics and functioning. For example, in most palliative care teams, physicians and advanced practice nurses can bill for services in a way that helps contribute to the financial stability of the team, whereas social workers and chaplains are typically salaried clinicians who do not bill.[40] Palliative care program administrators and leaders, many of whom are physicians and are used to working within the fee-for-service model, must learn to advocate to the hospital or parent organization leadership for the financial support and resources for all members of the team.

Another important consideration for palliative care teams is time expectations. What are the work-hour expectations for each team member? What are the on-call, time-off service, and continuing education allotments? Are all core team members offered designated administrative days to pursue projects or research? In teaching institutions, are all team members invited to apply for academic appointments? If they are eligible to apply, are all team members supported to take advantage of this opportunity? What, in turn, are the implications of these policies for each profession's perceived value and worth on the team? While there are no straightforward solutions, each institution and team is encouraged to acknowledge and grapple with these questions to promote team cohesion, effectiveness, equity, and wellness.

Professional Identity

With the lack of universal interprofessional education opportunities for all healthcare clinicians, individuals are often not exposed to the expertise of other professions with which they are expected to work collaboratively.[20,21] This can lead to misconceptions about roles and responsibilities, as well as mismatched expectations, which can result in conflict, frustration, and demoralization among team members. For example, how often are clinical social workers seen as primarily discharge planners, chaplains called only for their prayers before discontinuation of a ventilator in the ICU, and nurse practitioners misperceived as "mid-level" as opposed to independent clinicians? Knowledge of each other's training, approach to care, and scope of practice can foster respect for each other's skills, knowledge, and expertise and is crucial for strong team functioning.

Role Overlap

The transdisciplinary[§] model of palliative care posits that interdependence among team members is expected as a result of skills that overlap and roles that are shared.[41] As Opie observed, "clinically, members are involved in role release rather than role retention as

---

[§] The process this framework is pointing to is more accurately described as *transprofessional*, since it illustrates the collaboration and synergy between professions rather than disciplines. However, in this chapter and throughout the book, the term *transdisciplinary* is used since it is currently the word most commonly used in the literature to signify this form of team collaboration. When we refer to interprofessional, it is within this framework of working at the transdisciplinary collaborative level. It is referring to an advanced level of professional synergy.

they seek to develop a common knowledge base."[42(p40)] This may mirror the nature of the patient or family's experience, where needs are not partialized, but rather woven together and presented as an evolving narrative to responsive professionals.

Based on the National Consensus Project for Quality Palliative Care, palliative care team members are expected to develop generalist palliative care knowledge/skills in all domains of care and serve as specialists in the domains related to their own profession (see Chapter 3).[2] In practice this means that all team members, regardless of professional background, can complete spiritual, psychosocial, and pain/symptom screenings. The outcome of this screen can then prompt a timely referral to the specialist palliative care clinician for further assessment and intervention. For example, a nurse may complete a spiritual screening which reveals that a patient is experiencing spiritual/existential distress. After generalist-level responses to this information are offered, such as empathic listening and supportive presence, the nurse can involve the chaplain for more in-depth spiritual assessment and intervention.[30] Similarly, social workers and chaplains, as physical symptom generalists, screen for physical pain/symptoms, complete further assessment/intervention within their scope of practice (e.g., nonpharmacologic interventions) and refer to their physician, nurse practitioner, and/or pharmacy colleagues for potential pharmacologic intervention.

When professional boundaries and responsibilities are challenged, however, patient care can be hampered.[43] The psychosocial nature of many palliative care consults, together with the strong interest in psychosocial interventions which draw many medical practitioners to this field, create a situation that is ripe for role ambiguity and team conflict,[44] which can negatively affect patient/family care.[45] For example, more than one team member may have the skills to address a given concern, such as facilitating a family meeting or clarifying patient/family goals, values, and preferences. The team's critical task in these situations is to recognize the unique skill sets and expertise that each clinician brings to the table, and to strike a balance between role flexibility and exclusivity so that patient/family needs are met in the most effective and timely way possible.[41,42] When the dynamics of mutuality, respect, and interdependence infuse team relationships, blurred boundaries are expected, rather than perceived as a threat to individual expertise.[41] The Center to Advance Palliative Care (CAPC) suggests completing an assessment of team roles[46] to identify existing ambiguity and having the team work together to clarify/intervene where there may be areas of confusion or concern.

Opportunities and Strengths of Interprofessional Collaboration

Synergy

Palliative care team members combine their experience, skills, and knowledge to produce enhanced results,[23] which generates what Krout[47(p36)] terms "synerdisciplinary" care. With their own education and expertise, each team member approaches patient and family encounters through their own lens and recognizes different cues from the patient/family and nuances of the interaction. With the shared goal to improve quality of life, palliative care team members confer about their observations, which can lead to care that far surpasses what any one person can offer on their own and better addresses the scope of patient/family needs. When a profession's perspective is absent from a team, those nuances are lost.[23]

Quality of Care

Integration of palliative care into health systems has led to significant improvements in the quality of patient care with a simultaneous reduction in costs.[48-50] Specialized palliative care teams that work effectively and cooperatively improve patient and caregiver outcomes, which includes enhanced symptom management, quality of life, and patient satisfaction; increased hospice utilization; reductions in family distress; and more successful interactions with patients/families.[18,48,51] In particular, inpatient palliative care consultation services have been associated with improved communication between patients and clinicians; enhanced patient perception of emotional support; higher patient satisfaction; and decreased pain, dyspnea, and nausea.[46] Increased patient satisfaction with care can be attributed to the interprofessional palliative care team's ability to address the patient/family's desire for information and guide them through healthcare decision-making.[48]

Protection against Burnout

The team approach to palliative care can serve as a protective mechanism that softens and diffuses the stresses, responsibilities, and emotions that are inherent to work in healthcare in general and palliative care specifically. In a study of palliative care clinicians who had been working in the field for over 5 years, Webster and Kristjanson[52] found that the interprofessional team was identified as a strong source of support and helped participants to balance the sadness and satisfaction of their work over time. Interprofessional palliative care team members in the hospital can also provide companionship based on mutual experience. The respect and support exchanged by team members can enhance job satisfaction and the sense that one is making a meaningful contribution. On a broader level, palliative care teams often support referral teams with moral distress and resiliency, even when the original consult is for a specific clinical recommendation. Palliative care team members individually, or the team as a whole, may also participate in hospital-wide well-being and/or ethics committees, Schwartz Center Rounds,[53] and other such activities that are focused on clinical and moral sustainability for healthcare professionals.

Best Practices for Hospital-Based Interprofessional Palliative Care Teams

Effective palliative care team functioning is multifaceted and takes investment and continuous commitment to ensure its success. Palliative care by definition is not one-size-fits-all. Therefore, "best practices" for one patient/family or team may not work well for another, though the National Consensus Project does emphasize best practices for effective care delivery that are imperative for every palliative care practitioner to embrace.[2] While it is important to adhere to these guidelines, the true best practice for interprofessional palliative care teams in the hospital is to be continually attuned to patient/family and team needs and adjust accordingly.

Communication

Knowledge of one's own and others' roles and openness to embrace the team concept are key elements of collaborative practice.[20] However, arguably the most important component to an effective interprofessional team is impeccable formal and informal communication both within the team and with others with whom team members interact, especially referral practitioners.[23] Effective communication involves authenticity, active listening, and thoughtful speaking, which foster trust and respect for each team member and profession.

Balancing Professional and Team Identity

Palliative care teams balance individual professional identity with team identity. Ideal individual attributes of team members include self-awareness, especially of one's own strengths and weaknesses; the ability to set aside one's own beliefs to provide person-centered care; and a spirit of inquiry, curiosity, and humility, all of which contribute to a positive team and patient experience. To foster a culture of psychological safety, team members strive to be fully present, to display empathy, and to converse respectfully so that the interprofessional team is comfortable in taking risks, challenging each other, and exploring creative solutions.[54] Palliative care by nature involves complex approaches to complex issues. As such, the most effective teams invite diversity of experience and opinion, increase connections with each other, reduce power differentials, distribute control, and embrace uncertainty.[17]

Roles and Relationships

It can be a formidable task to clarify roles within the palliative care team, but to engage in such a process carries great potential for professional growth and optimal patient/family care. Toward this end, 2 questions might be asked by all team members during the assessment and intervention process with patients/families. First, what skills or training does each clinician bring to the team that can be optimized in the care of this patient? Each team member possesses specialized education and skills, distinctive qualities, as well as specific communication and relationship styles that may create a natural connection with patients/families who often bring a unique set of cultural, historical, or generational norms to care encounters. Over time, team members come to acknowledge and respect both these tangible and intangible qualities that enhance each clinician's ability to provide care. When faced with a situation in which a patient/family may share more information with one member of the team or express a preference to see a particular clinician instead of another, the team "starts where the client is" and, within reason, adjusts the provision of care to best meet the needs of the patient/family despite potential feelings of slight.

The second, related question that all team members need to ask is: Whose needs are being met by this plan of care? While a number of needs often coexist—systemic, programmatic, educational, and/or personal—patient/family needs always take precedence. If such precedence is given, appropriate use of team members' unique skill sets will naturally follow. This kind of differential care planning is possible within teams where expertise, mutual respect, and patient needs drive decisions.

Team Leadership and Composition

Although palliative care teams ideally embrace a lateral structure, effective leadership of the team remains vital to team functioning. Leadership of a palliative care team may look different for each program and may evolve in various ways. For example, teams that have historically been led by physicians or nurses will function differently than those teams where leadership rotates based on the established care plan and primary needs of the patient/family. Effective leadership with a lateral structure depends on the ability to build a culture of safety, share vulnerability, and establish purpose with a common goal.[55]

Staffing
Team composition of hospital-based palliative care services across the United States varies greatly, based mostly on hospital size and time since the program's inception.[19,56] Though staffing has grown overall, the National Palliative Care Registry data show that only 42% of hospital-based programs that participated in the study reported a full, core interprofessional team (i.e., chaplain, nurse practitioner or registered nurse, physician, social worker)[19,56] as recommended by the National Consensus Project for Quality Palliative Care.[2] Further, of the 347 adult palliative care programs that shared data about their hospital-based program composition, only 54.4% include a chaplain and 67.7% include a social worker in the core team.[19,57] None of the chaplains and few of the social workers in these programs

hold full-time equivalent positions with palliative care.[19,56] These data demonstrate that, despite the overall growth of palliative care teams, there is much work to be done to actualize the goal of truly interprofessional care.

It is complex to calculate staffing needs for specialist palliative care services, and little published evidence exists to suggest best practice. Most of the current data indicate the number of physicians who are needed per population but do not take into consideration the interdependence of other team members.[25] Staffing needs are often multifactorial and depend on patient demographics, geographical location, access to primary palliative care, competency levels of clinicians, and models of care.[25] CAPC has resources to assist institutions with such considerations as they contemplate and form their palliative care teams.[57]

Leadership Model

In medium and large hospital palliative care departments, the distinction between clinical leadership skills and program leadership skills is important. Some assume that a skillful physician will be equally skillful as an administrative/program leader, but the 2 skill sets are very different. The Dyad Leadership Model provides for a good balance of responsibilities and strengths, where there is a medical leader and a separate administrative leader who co-manage the palliative care program (personal communication with Katy Hyman, MDiv, BCC, email communication, July 23, 2020, and September 14, 2020). It can strengthen the program, patient care, and decision-making processes to have 2 people make decisions, sometimes together, sometimes separately, in their own domains. For example, program directors design marketing materials, set schedules, oversee budgets, serve as a liaison to hospital administration, and handle human resources issues like yearly assessments. The medical director may establish criteria for referrals, initiate new clinical efforts and protocols (e.g., outpatient clinic, palliative sedation), and serve as a liaison to the hospital medical staff structure. Jointly, the program director and the medical director may establish an on-call structure and strategize about how palliative care fits within the overall hospital structure. Since some responsibilities overlap, these 2 leaders must work well together, or leadership tension can destroy the program.

Interprofessional Collaboration in Practice

Team Rounds

The importance of interprofessional team clinical rounds cannot be overstated. In many settings, hospital-based palliative care teams will meet each weekday to review a daily census, discuss pertinent patient/family care needs, and explore plans of care. These meetings offer a chance for information sharing,[58] but also afford the space for collaboration and the opportunity to care for one another.[59] This meeting also becomes, with time, a means for team members who represent various professions to know one another's scope of professional practice through the assessments provided, interventions described, and language used.[60]

Brennan and colleagues[59] undertook a quality-improvement initiative to enhance their team's communication and efficiency within clinical rounds. The study revealed team members' perceptions that rounds were physician- and nurse-centric and satisfaction with rounds was low; the quality-improvement process included a conscious effort to alter how rounds were operationalized to encourage equal participation, with significantly improved satisfaction after the changes were implemented.[59] The important takeaway is to engage a similar process for customized and iterative adaptations to be made within each team's culture and unique environments.

Joint Visits

An important decision commonly faced by inpatient palliative care consult teams is to determine which team member or members should perform the initial consultation and subsequent visits with a given patient/family. In the hospital environment, palliative care team members are often able to engage in joint visits in which 2 or more core team members visit the patient simultaneously (the term "NOMA" or "No One Meets Alone" describes these joint visits). This model can maximize the team's ability to adopt a multifaceted approach to patient care; enhance efficiency and continuity of care as information is received by multiple team members in real time; provide valuable opportunities for team learning and debriefing; and minimize the time and energy required of patients/families. This "group approach" is, however, sometimes either unrealistic or unhelpful to patients/families. Each member of the team often needs to see patients/families individually to offer intervention in their specialized domains which would not be appropriate to do in a group setting. Further, some patients/families who are seen by one team member are relieved at not being overwhelmed by a "sea of white coats," especially in the hospital, where chairs are often limited and rooms are small. If multiple professionals are involved from one team, some patients/families may become confused about whom to contact for follow-up information and assistance. As always, palliative care clinicians strive to provide individualized person-centered care that is responsive to these preferences.

Interprofessional Approach to Pain and Symptom Management

Physical symptoms can reflect a complex interaction of physical, social, emotional, spiritual, existential, and practical concerns, aptly described as "total pain."[61] The concept of total pain has important implications for the palliative care team. It suggests that to achieve optimal symptom management, team members with different expertise need to work together to understand and address the multiple factors that impact both the symptom itself and the person who experiences it.[62] Continuous multidimensional assessment and inclusion of pharmacologic and nonpharmacologic interventions for pain and symptoms are paramount.[62]

Facilitating Patient and Family Communication

Assistance with decision-making processes is one of the most common reasons for palliative care consultation in the hospital environment,[63] and the ability to facilitate such conversations is among the core competencies for palliative care teams.[2] Negotiations about who attends and leads such meetings are imperative and should be based on patient/family need, team member expertise, relationship with patient/family, and availability. Although it is important to consider the number of people present at such meetings so as not to overwhelm patients/families (including trainee considerations), the presence of primary, specialty, and palliative care teams together can be beneficial, as this gives all clinicians the opportunity to hear the same information exchange to/from clinicians and patient/family.

Team Wellness

Although palliative care professionals often find intrinsic rewards in their work, it is important to consider the intensity that clinicians experience when they routinely bear witness to serious illness and profound grief/loss.[2] An estimated one-third of all palliative care team members feel burned out from both clinical work and systemic challenges (e.g., pathological altruism, racism, trauma), which can lead to team conflict, substandard patient care, and even the decision to leave the field altogether.[64] When team wellness is prioritized, it can help mitigate these challenges.[65] To create a healthy team requires investment from all members to plan and implement strategies that promote individual and systemic wellness during times of both stability and crisis.[65] For example, a debrief after a difficult patient/family encounter or a weekly pause to reflect on patients who have died can be built into routine team processes.[65] Additional team-based strategies may include the designation of a quiet space that staff can use to regroup or rejuvenate, implementation of a buddy system for routine check-ins, development of a "code lavender" response for when a team member needs urgent support, a few minutes dedicated to "team self-care" during team rounds, and cultivation of opportunities for social connection outside of patient care. Teams can create healthy boundaries around work expectations to foster wellness, such as a pause to consultations for lunch, no responses to emails during nights/weekends/time off, or even a cap to consults when demand exceeds staff availability. With regard to team expansion, teams can advocate for new staff based on data-driven need and desirable outcomes, so team members are not stretched beyond their limits before new staff is recruited. CAPC recommends that team members participate in a team assessment to determine function and wellness and to design customized interventions based on the unique needs of each team.[66]

Conclusion

The expectations for the interprofessional team in the hospital setting are to work interdependently and to represent their individual professions as well as the collective team. This requires commitment to the team approach to care, as well as education about how to work effectively on an interprofessional team. While the challenges of working on a palliative care team must be acknowledged, the strengths and opportunities available through this work can have synergistic results and the potential to lead to improved quality of life and enhanced practitioner and team well-being.

Discussion Questions

1. A social worker and physician work together on a hospital-based inpatient palliative care consultation team. The team receives a consultation to assist with complex communication and decision-making with a 75-year-old patient with end-stage liver disease. The palliative social worker and physician review the consult order and chart briefly and notice that the patient has significant symptoms, a long history of substance use disorder, and is estranged from his family. Given this history and current needs, they decide to do a joint initial visit with the patient. What are some points to consider, discuss, and agree upon together before they enter the room? How are their roles different? How might they overlap?

2. With what you have learned in this chapter, engage in a dialogue with your team members to compare and contrast the core tenets, perspective, and contributions for each profession on your inpatient palliative care team. Where does overlap exist? What are areas of potential conflict? How might this knowledge change views of and interactions with colleagues?

Additional Resources

American Academy of Hospice and Palliative Medicine (AAHPM):
   http://aahpm.org
Center to Advance Palliative Care (CAPC):
   http://www.capc.org
City of Hope Pain and Palliative Care Resource Center:
   https://prc.coh.org
Palliative Care Network of Wisconsin Fast Facts:
   https://www.mypcnow.org/fast-facts/
Hospice and Palliative Nurses Association (HPNA):
   https://advancingexpertcare.org/
National Association of Social Workers (NASW) Standards for Palliative and
   End of Life Care:
   https://www.socialworkers.org/LinkClick.aspx?fileticket=xBMd58Vw
   Ehk%3D&portalid=0

National Hospice and Palliative Care Organization (NHPCO):
www.nhpco.org
National Palliative Care Research Center:
http://www.npcrc.org
Social Work in Hospice and Palliative Care Network (SWHPN):
http://www.swhpn.org
Social Work Network in Palliative and End-of-Life Care Listserv:
https://peach.ease.lsoft.com/scripts/wa-peach.exe?SUBED1=SW-PALL-
EOL&A=1
Transforming Chaplaincy:
https://www.transformchaplaincy.org/

References

1. World Health Organization (WHO). WHO definition of palliative care. 2020. Accessed June 12, 2020. https://www.who.int/cancer/palliative/definition/en/.
2. Ferrell BR, Twaddle ML, Melnick A, Meier DE. National Consensus Project clinical practice guidelines for quality palliative care guidelines, 4th edition. *J Palliat Med.* 2018;21(12):1684–1689. doi:10.1089/*J Palliat Med*.2018.0431.
3. National Quality Forum. A national framework and preferred practices for palliative and hospice care quality. 2006. Accessed June 12, 2020. https://www.qualityforum.org/Publicati ons/2006/12/A_National_Framework_and_Preferred_Practices_for_Palliative_and_Hospi ce_Care_Quality.aspx.
4. Center to Advance Palliative Care (CAPC). What is palliative care? GetPalliativeCare. 2020. Accessed June 10, 2020. https://getpalliativecare.org/whatis.
5. Meier DE, Beresford L. The palliative care team. *J Palliat Med.* 2008 Jun;11(5): 677–681. doi:10.1089/J Palliat Med.2008.9907.
6. Stark D. Teamwork in palliative care: an integrative approach. In: Altilio T, Otis-Green, S, eds. *Oxford Textbook of Palliative Social Work*. Oxford University Press; 2011:415–424.
7. Connor SR. Development of hospice and palliative care in the United States. *Omega (Westport)*, 2007; 56(1):89–99. doi:10.2190/om.56.1.h.
8. Lutz S. The history of hospice and palliative care. *Curr Probl Cancer*, 2011; 35(6):304–309. doi:10.1016/j.currproblcancer.2011.10.004.
9. Kübler-Ross E. *On Death and Dying*. Collier Books/Macmillan; 1970.
10. Phillips, D. Balfour Mount. Palliative Care McGill. Accessed October 2, 2021. https://www. mcgill.ca/palliativecare/portraits-0/balfour-mount.
11. LeGrand SB, Walsh D, Nelson KA, Davis MP. A syllabus for fellowship education in palliative medicine. *Am J Hosp Palliat Care.* 2003 Jul–Aug;20(4):279–289. doi: 10.1177/ 104990910302000410.
12. Ferrell B, Wittenberg E, Neiman T. A historical perspective of palliative care communication. In: Wittenberg E, Ferrell BR, Goldsmith J, et al., eds. *Textbook of Palliative Care Communication*. Oxford University Press; 2016:10–13.
13. Center to Advance Palliative Care (CAPC) and National Palliative Care Research Center. America's care of serious illness: a state-by-state report card on access to palliative care

in our nation's hospitals. September 2019. Accessed August 10, 2020. https://reportcard. capc.org/.

14. Hughes MT, Smith TJ. The growth of palliative care in the United States. *Annu Rev Public Health*. 2014;35:459–475. doi:10.1146/annurev-publhealth-032013-182406.

15. Quill TE, Abernethy AP. Generalist plus specialist palliative care-creating a more sustainable model. *N Engl J Med*. 2013;368:1173–1175. doi: 10.1056/NEJMp1215620.

16. Cintron A, Meier DE. The palliative care consult team. In: Bruera E, Higginson I, von Gunten C, Ripamonti C, eds. *Textbook of Palliative Medicine*. Hodder Arnold Publications/Oxford University Press; 2006:259–265.

17. O'Donnell AE, Schaefer KG, Stevenson LW, et al. Social worker-aided palliative care intervention in high-risk patients with heart failure (SWAP-HF). *JAMA Cardiol*. 2018 Jun;3(6):516–521. doi:10.1001/jamacardio.2018.0589.

18. Ciemins EL, Brant J, Kersten D, Mullette E, Dickerson D. Why the interdisciplinary team approach works: insights from complexity science. *J Palliat Med*. 2016;19(7): 767–770. doi: 10.1089/*J Palliat Med*.2015.0398.

19. Rogers M, Heitner R. Latest trends and insights from the National Palliative Care Registry™ [webinar]. August 13, 2019. Accessed May 20, 2021. https://www.capc.org/events/recorded-webinars/latest-trends-and-insights-from-the-national-palliative-care-registry/.

20. Gellis ZD, Kim E, Hadley D, et al. Evaluation of interprofessional health care team communication simulation in geriatric palliative care. *Gerontol Geriatr Educ*. 2019 Jan–Mar; 40(1): 30–42. doi:10.1080/02701960.2018.1505617.

21. Institute of Medicine (IOM). *Measuring the Impact of Interprofessional Education on Collaborative Practice and Patient Outcomes*. National Academies Press; 2015 Dec 15. doi:10.17226/21726.

22. World Health Organization (WHO). Framework for action on interprofessional education and collaborative practice. 2010. Accessed June 12, 2020. http://www.nap.edu/catalog/10027/crossingthequalitychasm-a-new-health-system.

23. Youngwerth J, Twaddle M. Cultures of interdisciplinary teams: how to foster good dynamics. *J Palliat Med*. 2011 May;14(5):650–654. doi:10.1089/J Palliat Med.2010.0395.

24. Donesky D, Anderson WG, Joseph RD, Sumser B, Reid TT. TeamTalk: interprofessional team development and communication skills training. *J Palliat Med*. 2020 Jan;23(1):40–47. doi:10.1089/jpm.2019.0046. Epub 2019 Aug 5. PMID: 31381469.

25. Henderson JD, Boyle A, Herx L, et al. Staffing a specialist palliative care service, a team-based approach: expert consensus white paper. *J Palliat Med*. 2019 Nov;22(1):1318–1323. doi:10.1089/J Palliat Med.2019.0314.

26. Dahlin C, Coyne P, Goldberg J, Vaughan L. Palliative care leadership. *J Palliat Care*. 2019; 34(1): 21–28. https://doi.org/10.1177/0825859718791427.

27. Meier DE, Beresford L. Advanced practice nurses in palliative care: a pivotal role and perspective. *J Palliat Med*. 2006 Jun;9(3):624–627. doi:10.1089/jpm.2006.9.624.

28. George T. Role of the advanced practice nurse in palliative care. *Int J Palliat Nurs*. 2016;22(3):137–140. doi:10.12968/ijpn.2016.22.3.137.

29. van Dusseldorp L, Groot M, Adriaansen M, van Vught A, Vissers K, Peters J. What does the nurse practitioner mean to you? A patient-oriented qualitative study in oncological/palliative care. *J Clin Nurs*. 2019 Feb;28(3-4):589–602. doi:10.1111/jocn.14653.

30. Donesky D, Sprague E, Joseph D. A new perspective on spiritual care: collaborative chaplaincy and nursing practice. *ANS Adv Nurs Sci*. 2020;43(2):147–158. doi:10.1097/ANS.0000000000000298.

31. Damen A, Labuschagne D, Fosler L, O'Mahony S, Levine S, Fitchett G. What do chaplains do: the views of palliative care physicians, nurses, and social workers. *Am J Hosp Palliat Care*. 2019;36(5):396–401. doi:10.1177/1049909118807123.

32. Lucas AM. Introduction to the discipline for pastoral care giving. *J Health Care Chaplain.* 2001;10(2):1–33. doi:10.1300/j080v10n02_01.

33. Jeuland J, Fitchett G, Schulman-Green D, Kapo J. Chaplains working in palliative care: who they are and what they do. *J Palliat Med.* 2017;20(5):502–508. doi:10.1089/J Palliat Med.2016.0308.

34. American Academy of Hospice and Palliative Medicine (AAHPM). Palliative doctors. Accessed September 9, 2020. https://palliativedoctors.org/palliative/doctor.

35. Landzaat LH, Barnett MD, Buckholz GT. Development of entrustable professional activities for hospice and palliative medicine fellowship training in the United States. *J Pain Symptom Manage.* 2017;54(4):609–616.e1. https://doi.org/10.1016/j.jpainsym man.2017.07.003.

36. Schroeder K, Lorenz K. Nursing and the future of palliative care. *Asia Pac J Oncol Nurs.* 2018 Jan–Mar;5(1)4–8. doi:10.4103/apjon.apjon_43_17.

37. Mulkerin M. Palliative care consultation. In: Altilio T, Otis-Green, S, eds. *Oxford Textbook of Palliative Social Work.* Oxford University Press; 2011:43–52.

38. Sumser B, Remke S, Leimena M, Altilio T, Otis-Green S. The serendipitous survey: a look at primary and specialist palliative social work practice, preparation, and competence. *J Palliat Med.* 2015 Oct;18(10):881–883. doi:10.1089/jpm.2015.0022.

39. Dane BO, Simon BL. Resident guests: social workers in host settings. *Soc Work.* 1991; 36(3):208–213.

40. Goldberg JG, Scharlin M. Financial considerations for the palliative social worker. In: Altilio T, Otis-Green, S, eds. *Oxford Textbook of Palliative Social Work.* Oxford University Press; 2011:709–718.

41. Bronstein LR. A model for interdisciplinary collaboration. *Soc Work.* 2003 Jul; 48(3):297–306. https://doi.org/10.1093/sw/48.3.297.

42. Opie A. *Thinking Teams, Thinking Clients.* Columbia University Press; 2000.

43. Klarare A, Hagelin CL, Fürst CJ, Fossum B. Team interactions in specialized palliative care teams: a qualitative study. *J Palliat Med.* 2013 Sep;16(9):1062–1069. doi:10.1089/J Palliat Med.2012.0622.

44. O'Connor M, Fisher C. Exploring the dynamics of interdisciplinary palliative care teams in providing psychosocial care: "everybody thinks that everybody can do it and they can't." *J Palliat Med.* 2011 Feb;12(2):191–196. doi:10.1089/J Palliat Med.2010.0229.

45. Christ GH, Blacker, S. Improving interdisciplinary communication skills with families. *J Palliat Med.* 2005 Aug 29; 8(4): 855–856. https://doi.org/10.1089/J Palliat Med.2005.8.855.

46. Center to Advance Palliative Care (CAPC). Interdisciplinary team roles. Quick tips #4: Role clarity for a highly effective interdisciplinary team. 2018. Updated January 23, 2020. Accessed July 25, 2020. https://www.capc.org/toolkits/building-and-supporting-effective-palliative-care-teams/.

47. Krout RE. A synerdisciplinary music therapy treatment team approach for hospice and palliative care. *Aus J Mus Ther.* 2004 July;15:33–45. https://www.austmta.org.au/system/files/4_krout_a_synerdisciplinary_music_ther.pdf.

48. Gade G, Venohr I, Conner D, et al. Impact of an inpatient palliative care team: a randomized controlled trial. *J Palliat Med.* 2008 Mar;11(2):180–190. doi:10.1089/J Palliat Med.2007.0055.

49. Kamal AH, Gradison M, Maguire JM, Taylor D, Abernethy AP. Quality measures for palliative care in patients with cancer: a systematic review. *J Oncol Pract.* 2014 Jul;10(4): 281–287. doi:10.1200/JOP.2013.001212.

50. Meier DE. Increased access to palliative care and hospice services: opportunities to improve value in health care. *Milbank Q.* 2011 Sep;89(3)343–380. https://doi.org/10.1111/j.1468-0009.2011.00632.x.

51. Smith TJ, Temin S, Alesi ER, et al. American Society of Clinical Oncology provisional clinical opinion: the integration of palliative care into standard oncology care. *J Clin Oncol.* 2012;30:880–887.

52. Webster J, Kristjanson LJ. Long-term palliative care workers: more than a story of endurance. *J Palliat Med.* 2004 Jul;5(6):865–875. https://doi.org/10.1089/10966210260499050.

53. Schwartz Rounds and Membership. The Schwartz Center for Compassionate Healthcare. Accessed May 11, 2021. https://www.theschwartzcenter.org/programs/schwartz-rounds/.

54. Duhigg C. What Google learned from its quest to build the perfect team. *New York Times Magazine.* 2016 Feb 25. https://www.nytimes.com/2016/02/28/magazine/what-google-learned-from-its-quest-to-build-the-perfect-team.html.

55. Coyle, D. *The Culture Code: The Secrets of Highly Successful Groups.* Bantam; 2018.

56. Rogers M, Meier DE, Heitner R, et al. The National Palliative Care Registry: a decade of supporting growth and sustainability of palliative care programs. *J Palliat Med.* 2019 Sep;22(9):1026–1031. doi:10.1089/jpm.2019.0262.

57. Center to Advance Palliative Care (CAPC). Building and supporting effective palliative care teams. 2020. Accessed July 12, 2020. https://www.capc.org/toolkits/building-and-supporting-effective-palliative-care-teams/.

58. Verhaegh KJ, Seller-Boersma A, Simons R, et al. An exploratory study of healthcare professionals' perceptions of interprofessional communication and collaboration. *J Interprof Care.* 2017;31(3):397–400. doi:10.1080/13561820.2017.1289158.

59. Brennan CW, Kelly B, Skarf LM, Tellem R, Dunn KM, Poswolsky S. Improving palliative care team meetings: structure, inclusion, and "team care." *Am J Hosp Palliat Care.* 2016;33(6):585–593. doi:10.1177/1049909115577049.

60. Gadamer HG. *Truth and Method.* 2nd rev. ed. Weinsheimer J, Marshall DG, trans. Continuum; 2004.

61. Saunders C. Care of patients suffering from terminal illness at St. Joseph's Hospice, Hackney, London. *Nurs Mirror.* 1964 Feb;14:vii–x.

62. Cagle J, Altilio T. The social work role in pain and symptom management. In: Altilio T, Otis-Green S, eds. *Oxford Textbook of Palliative Social Work.* Oxford University Press; 2011:271–286.

63. Bischoff K, O'Riordan DL, Marks AK, Sudore R, Pantilat S. Care planning for inpatients referred for palliative care consultation. *JAMA Int Med.* 2018 Jan;178(1):48–54. doi:10.1001/jamainternmed.2017.6313.

64. Kamal AH, Gradison M, Maguire JM, Taylor D, Abernethy AP. Quality measures for palliative care in patients with cancer: a systematic review. *J Oncol Pract.* 2014 Jul;10(4): 281–287. doi:10.1200/JOP.2013.001212.

65. Center to Advance Palliative Care (CAPC). Strategies for maximizing the health/wellness of palliative care teams. 2019. Accessed September 22, 2020. https://www.capc.org/documents/98/.

66. Shanafelt TD, Noseworthy JH. Executive leadership and physician well-being: nine organizational strategies to promote engagement and reduce burnout. *Mayo Clin Proc.* 2017;92(1):129–146. doi:10.1016/j.mayocp.2016.10.004.

Appendix 1

Primary Palliative Care Assessment: Rounding Record

Date _____ Unit/Bed _____ Bedside RN _____ Completed by _____

"Have you taken the PC Training or ICU Communication Workshop?"   ☐ Yes   ☐ No

If yes, how did the trainings affect your practice? Are there other classes or workshops you would like?

Patient Name: MRN: Age: Sex:	Hospital Admission Date: _____/_____/_____ ICU Admission Date: _____/_____/_____
	Palliative Care consult active for this patient? ☐ No ☐ Yes – CNS only ☐ Yes – full team

Primary Service: ☐ Critical Care   Primary Attending _____

Surgical Services: ☐ Transplant_____   ☐ OHNS ☐ General Surgery ☐ Neurosurgery ☐ Vascular

☐ Orthopedic   ☐ Surgical Oncology   ☐ Urology   ☐ Cardiothoracic   ☐ Adv Lung

☐ Thoracic   ☐ Other _____

Medical Services: ☐ General Medicine   ☐ Neurology   ☐ Cardiology   ☐ Malignant Hematology

☐ Other _____

STEP 1: "Does your patient have a serious illness?" ☐ YES   ☐ NO

Check the disease category for patient's primary serious illness:

☐ Chronic disease exacerbation _____   ☐ Cancer _____

☐ Acute event _____   ☐ Advanced neurological disease

☐ End stage organ disease _____

☐ Sepsis   ☐ Poor surgical outcome   ☐ Multi-organ failure   ☐ Other _____

Current medical care: ☐ intubated ☐ trach ☐ pressors ☐ CVVH ☐ ECMO ☐ IABP ☐ LVAD

☐ other _____

"Have you had a chance to build rapport with the patient or family?" ☐ YES   ☐ NO

"Is social worker following the patient?" _____ Name _____

"Are the chaplains following the patient?" _____ Other key staff involved with patient? _____

Code Status _____ **Advance Directive** ☐ Yes ☐ No   **POLST** ☐ Yes ☐ No

DPOA _____

Recommendations/Plan:

STEP 2: Screen for and Develop Plan to Address Palliative Care Needs – bedside RN assessment

1. **"Does your patient have uncontrolled or difficult to manage symptoms?"** Check all that apply

   ☐ Pain ☐ Restless ☐ Anxious ☐ Tired ☐ Thirsty ☐ Hungry ☐ Nauseated ☐ Scared

   ☐ Shortness of breath/dyspnea ☐ Delirium/confusion ☐ Sad/depressed

   ☐ bloating/abdominal fullness ☐ Other _____

   Plan of care _____

   _____

2. **"Is the patient/ family emotionally distressed or struggling to cope?"** ☐ Yes ☐ No ☐ Family not present
   ☐ No family/SO ☐ Family non-English-speaking ☐ Patient sedated/delirious/altered

   Plan of care _____

   _____

3. **"Do you sense there are any spiritual, religious, or cultural needs?"**

   ☐ Yes ☐ No ☐ Not sure

   Plan of care _____

   _____

4. **"Do you have concerns about the quality of patient/family-clinician communication about prognosis and goals of care?"**

   ☐ Yes ☐ No

5. **"Does the patient/family seem to understand the medical situation and be aware of options?"** ☐ Yes ☐ No

   Plan for addressing identified needs:

STEP 3: "Are there important upcoming decisions?" ☐ Yes ☐ No

☐ Trach ☐ ECMO ☐ PEG ☐ surgery ☐ LVAD ☐ Dialysis ☐ Weaning ☐ Withdrawal of support ☐ Disposition
☐ Not a transplant candidate ☐ Awaiting transplant

Challenges:

STEP 4: (If applicable)

1. "Have you, as the bedside RN, discussed the patient's prognosis and goals of care with the patient/family?"
   ☐ Yes ☐ No Comment:

2. "Do you know the patient's past course of illness?"
   ☐ Yes ☐ No Comment:

3. "Have you, as the bedside RN, discussed the patient's prognosis and goals of care with the physicians?"
   ☐ Yes ☐ No

4. "Has there been a family meeting for this patient?"
   ☐ No ☐ Not sure ☐ Yes → "Did you attend?" ☐ Yes ☐ No; "Did you participate?" ☐ No ☐ Yes

5. "What factors have challenged your involvement in the above discussions for this patient?"
   ☐ Lack of skill/training ☐ Family not available ☐ MD not available ☐ Unfamiliar with pt
   ☐ Lack of time ☐ Difficulty with family ☐ Difficulty with MD ☐ Not invited to meeting
   ☐ No coverage ☐ Language barrier ☐ Worried about patient's or family's reactions
   ☐ Pt sedated/unable to communicate

Plan for addressing above challenges?

Appendix 2

Transition to Comfort Care: ICU Huddle Checklist

• All comfort care orders are written by ICU including discontinue all other active orders that may conflict with comfort care.

REQUIRED to be present (provider who will be writing the comfort care orders must be present)	OTHER participants as able
ICU Attending/Fellow	Chaplain
ICU Resident/NP	Pharmacist (for complex pain management)
Primary Team Attending/Resident	Social Worker
Bedside RN & Charge RN	Palliative Care if consulting
Respiratory Therapist	Clinical Nurse Specialist
Topics for Discussion	**Notes**
What do the patient/family know about what to expect?	
Is this patient someone who might benefit from IP Hospice evaluation? Call XXX-XXXX for evaluation.	
What special requests/goals do patient/family have?	
What is the plan for family physical/virtual presence?	
Cultural/religious preferences (before/after death?)	
What else does the family need?	
What is the plan for analgesia and sedation? How tolerant to opioids and benzos is this patient? If complex (e.g., pt with status epilepticus on multiple gtts, make sure to include Pharm input)	Infusion: starting rate = _____, × 4 = _____ Bolus: current effective dose = _____, × 4 = _____
What is the plan for vent and O2 support weaning? Does our plan align with family expectations?	
What is the sequence for withdrawal of other life-sustaining therapies (vasopressors, inotropes, IVFs, TF, AICD, CRRT, ECMO, etc.)?	
Anticipated trajectory? Transfer to acute care?	
Anticipated/potential challenges? If any, what is plan to address them?	
Are all staff comfortable with the plan?	
Primary Team: Has Donor Network West been notified? Autopsy discussed? Medical Examiner case?	
ICU team: Who will complete the comfort care huddle note in EMR? (use.CCHUDDLE dot phrase)	
Name (Initials/MRN): Unit/Bed:	Nurse: Date:

13

Critical Care, Emergency Department, and Crisis Scenarios

Lawrence Chyall and Cathy Dundas

Key Points

- All critical care clinicians (nurse, physician, social worker, chaplain, pharmacist, therapists) have a role in the provision of primary palliative care.
- Palliative care is delivered in a team. Powerful established teams and interprofessional collaboration are inherent to the work in the ICU and ED.
- Supporting each other to practice at the top of our scope creates a synergy that complements each other.

To someone entering the intensive care unit (ICU), the sights and sounds, including alarms, movement, communication, and procedures, may seem chaotic. However, for someone entrenched in this environment, it is a smooth choreographed dance of superlative teamwork, respect, and communication, which paves the way for supportive, dignified care and, at times, transitions to end of life. Teams strive to provide holistic, evidence-based answers to empower patients, families, and team members in order to offer physical healing, enhance communication, and bolster spiritual and emotional coping skills.[1] To bear witness to the outcomes of this graceful care allows one to reflect on the complexities of delivering high-quality interprofessional care and communication and to develop the skills to promote this kind of seamless interprofessional teamwork.

The ICU, emergency department (ED), and other hospital settings where patients have or are at risk of organ failure, rapid decline, and death (collectively termed "critical care" in this chapter) share 2 important features with palliative care—they are dependent on an interprofessional team for optimal functioning,[1] and they constantly face life-and-death situations. Both of these features can enhance collaboration between the critical care providers and the palliative care team, and they can also contribute to inadvertent misunderstandings and assumptions. For example,

---

Box 13.1. Physician Perspective

Michelle M. Milic, MD

From the earliest days of medical school training, we are taught to put the patient first. Compassionate and holistic care focused on a patient's values may shift as the disease progresses and care goals change. As providers, we need to be flexible with our approach and explore the deeper meaning of disease, hope, and well-being. The intense experiences of caring for the critically ill are the foundations of interprofessional care. For example, during my Pulmonary and Critical Care fellowship at Boston Medical Center, working without a consultative specialty palliative care service, I quickly recognized and learned to rely on the contributions of each of the diverse members of the ICU team. Impassioned bedside nurses, calming social workers, centering spiritual care providers, pharmacists, and others were present on daily rounds and at family meetings, providing a unique perspective and working together to support patients, families, and other team members. Addressing symptom relief concurrently with spiritual and psychological support, this well-integrated team provided the elements of what is now termed *primary palliative care*. This interprofessional collaboration, with mutual respect and teamwork, has a profound effect on how teams care for not only patients and families, but also each other. Team dynamics and the complexities of care and communication may lead to distress and burnout of all team members. These experiences provide a wealth of opportunities for individual and interprofessional team learning, acknowledging individuals' strengths, and role-modeling respect and collaboration. Caring for vulnerable, critically ill, and often underserved populations underscores that all patients must be treated with dignity and respect, receive the same level of high-quality care, and have their care aligned with their personal values.

---

before you read further, take a moment to stop and think about whom you expect to take the lead on a chapter focused on critical care. Are you surprised that a physician is not a coauthor for this chapter? Do you notice a bias about your approach to this chapter, given that fact? In contrast to critical care teams where physicians often assume a leadership role given the nature of the work and the need for rapid decisions, palliative care teams often strive to embrace the unique perspective of every team member with a flattened hierarchy in the leadership structure (see Box 13.1).

A given culture shares a common language, mutual understanding, purpose, knowledge, and belief structure,[2] not only in society, but also in many work or other team environments.[3] Common assumptions, behavioral norms, values, and procedures are foundational to a culture. Each of the professions, in both the critical care and the palliative care teams, practices within a profession-specific culture[4] as well as a shared culture

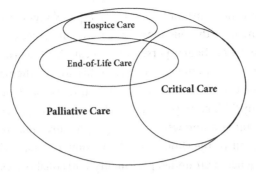

Figure 13.1. By definition, all patients in a critical care unit are seriously ill and therefore appropriate for palliative care services. Ideally, the palliative care and critical care interprofessional teams work together to optimize the care of the patients in the critical care unit.

Source: Aslakson RA, Cox CE, Baggs JG, Curtis JR. Palliative and end-of-life care: Prioritizing compassion within the ICU and beyond. *Crit Care Med*. 2021 Oct 1;49(10):1626–1637. doi:10.1097/CCM.0000000000005208. PMID: 34325446. Reprinted with permission from publisher.

of their critical care[5,6] or palliative care discipline[7,8]* (see Figure 13.1), leading to unique and intersecting shared mental models.[9] The purpose of this chapter is to explore best practices for interprofessional primary and specialty palliative care within fast-paced settings with frequent crisis scenarios, using a cultural lens and focused on the synergy of multiple interacting interprofessional teams.

Intensive Care Unit (ICU)

Patients admitted to the ICU have at least one form of organ failure (for example, respiratory, cardiac, or renal failure), hemodynamic instability, or respiratory insufficiency. These are the most critically ill and vulnerable patients in the hospital. Critically ill patients experience a myriad of symptoms including pain, thirst, dyspnea, and anxiety, to name a few.[10-12] They often undergo uncomfortable procedures, delirium, disorientation of day and night cycles, limited ability to communicate when intubated on a ventilator, and they describe a sense of isolation.[13] Complex physiologic changes demand detailed intricate care from the primary ICU team of physicians, nurses, respiratory therapists, pharmacists, and others, as well as multiple consulting services. The culture of the ICU varies from unit to unit, with some commonalities including a need for particular clinical training

---

* Although often used interchangeably, "discipline" refers to a branch of knowledge, while "profession" refers to an occupation that requires special education and/or prolonged training and a formal qualification. In this book, we have attempted to standardize the use of the term "profession" when referring to occupations such as chaplaincy, medicine, nursing, and social work, but occasionally the term "discipline" is used, especially when focused on the theory and knowledge development of the professions.

and expertise and the constant concern for rapid patient decline.[14] Minute-to-minute management of the outcomes and frequent reassessment and treatment adjustments attract a particular personality to care for the critically ill. One qualitative study contributed to the sparse data in this area by thematically coding self-described personality and work-related traits of intensivists. Common themes were collated to embody 9 different personas, including, among others, "the Fixer" who is a multi-tasker, functioning well under high pressure, and working well to support the team, as well as "the Diplomat" who is compassionate with a high degree of emotional intelligence, a grounded personality, and collaborates with others.[15] The intensive care unit features fast-paced, emergency interventions, complex communication with patients, families, and other providers, and rapid assessment and treatment.

More than 500,000 patients in the United States die following admission to the ICU every year. In America, approximately 20% of deaths occur in or around the time of an ICU stay,[16] and in addition to the high mortality rate there is also high morbidity within the ICU population. Hua and colleagues performed a retrospective cohort study of 53,124 ICU admissions and found that approximately 14% of them met one or more triggers for palliative care consultation. Extrapolating this percentage out to the national ICU census, an estimated 1.1 million patients may require palliative care consults.[17] These critically ill patients have a high symptom burden which is often uncontrolled. Fifty percent of patients who have an ICU length of stay (LOS) of at least 3 days requiring any form of life-sustaining treatment will die, and less than one-third will return to their baseline in 6 months.[18] For those who survive, there is advanced chronic illness or chronic critical illness after discharge.[19] In a robust study of more than 1300 critically ill patients, those receiving a tracheostomy for long-term ventilator support, or a percutaneous feeding tube, or both, had a 1-year mortality of 62%, 60%, and 64%, respectively.[20] Importantly, we are recognizing the longer-term outcomes of advanced clinical care and life support, including neurologic, psychiatric, and cognitive complications. For example, ICU delirium is associated with increased mortality 0–30 days after discharge.[21] Additionally, up to 10% of ICU survivors may develop post-traumatic stress disorder (PTSD) in response to their ICU stay.[22] Chronic complications, disability, and loss of functional status may lead to impaired quality of life and emphasize the need for supportive symptom management in conjunction with or instead of aggressive treatments based on shared decision-making between patient and provider.

Nurses, physicians, therapists, pharmacists, and other team members employed in the ICU setting manage complex symptoms and must work to align with patients and families to clarify treatment risks, benefits, and goals based on patient values. Additionally, ICU staff are keenly aware that treatment in the ICU carries a heavy symptom burden and seek to minimize the suffering for both the patient and their family. Many intensivists and ICU nurses recognize that advanced interventions may not be congruent with a patient or family's values and therefore seek to understand the patient and family's perspective so that appropriate treatments can be offered. Conversely, families may request advanced therapies that will not provide meaningful benefit to the patient.[23]

Prognostication can be challenging, with a high rate of morbidity and mortality and the potential for rapid clinical decline related to multisystem organ failure, compounded by clinical uncertainty, rapid turnover of patients, and frequent staffing changes. By the nature of the trajectory of certain illnesses, the clinical course may feel like it accelerates. End of life may approach rapidly, producing increased risk of patient and family distress. Not only is the ICU a stressful place for patients, but families report anxiety, PTSD, and complicated grief following an ICU admission.[24] Working in a high-risk environment can also lead to provider moral distress, burnout, and PTSD.[25-27] Palliative care has been shown to reduce ICU length of stay, increase family satisfaction, and decrease conflict over goals of care.[28-31] Although there are benefits of improved symptom assessment and patient comfort, incorporating palliative care in the ICU has no effect on mortality.[32]

Given the complexities of care, symptoms, and need for support, virtually all ICU patients have some palliative care need, and all ICU staff are primary palliative care clinicians.[33] Although not necessarily recognized as such, the ICU team works within the domains of quality palliative care, including identification and management of active symptoms, complex communication with patients, families, and multiple team members, as well as patient and family psychosocial, emotional, and spiritual support.[34] Although the literature supports the benefits of palliative care in the ICU,[35] providing complex care that addresses both palliative and disease-directed treatment in those with critical illness can be challenging. Barriers may include ICU culture such as "we aren't ready for palliative care yet," variable education, experience, and interest in the focus on symptom management or complex goals of care discussions, and competing demands for time with other critically ill patients. The uncertainty of prognostication, which may be challenging and inaccurate, complicates the process of supporting patients and families to set expectations for recovery, survival, or chronic critical illness.[36-37]

A study performed at 3 diverse medical centers consisting of patient and family focus groups described 4 pillars to high-quality ICU palliative care, including: (1) clinical care centered on the patient and focused on comfort, dignity, and the specific individual; (2) timely, complete, and clear communication addressing the patient's illness, prognosis, and treatment options; (3) patient-focused shared medical decision-making that incorporates patient values; and (4) care for the family, including visitation and support.[38] Despite the clear benefits of incorporating palliative care in the ICU,[35] multiple barriers to the integration of these systems include unrealistic expectations of the patient and family, insufficient training of physicians in communication skills, misperceptions about palliative care, and failure of system or culture change to improve primary palliative care or to integrate specialist palliative care.[1,39]

Interprofessional care is increasingly recognized as a pillar of high-quality care in the ICU.[40] The type of palliative care interventions that are typically required in the ICU include communication interventions, ethics consultations, educational interventions, specialty palliative care team involvement, advance care planning (ACP),[41,42] and end-of-life anticipatory guidance and care. However, given the complexities of ICU patient care, the model for optimal collaboration between palliative care and the ICU team is not well defined.[43,44] A more supportive and integrated system of care and collaboration must be developed to incorporate palliative care into the ICU ecosystem. This will involve systematic education and skills training focused on communication and interprofessional support for clinician teams.[45] Improving communication and functionality in an ICU can improve the work culture and create a sense of camaraderie, trust, and support, which in turn builds the essential trust necessary for teamwork.

Factors Unique to Palliative Care in the ICU

Palliative care in the ICU is influenced by numerous factors unique to this setting. The availability of advanced technologies for resuscitation and aggressive treatment can contribute to the sense that patients or families are "giving up" if they choose a less aggressive approach to care. The availability of advanced technologies can also cloud the prognosis—the perception that something else might be able to keep this person alive can interfere with the clarity of difficult conversations.[46] The high-technology interventions that may keep people alive can lead to confusion for family members who are attempting to select the best treatment pathway.

Intensivists, critical care nurses, and other ICU team members are highly trained with expectations and requirements for ongoing skill development. They tend to take pride in their abilities to rapidly and precisely identify and solve problems. Optimally, ICU team members embrace the skills of symptom management, conversing with patients and families about the type of care that aligns with their personal values, and attention to future quality of life if the current treatment plan is successful. These collectively are primary palliative care skills.[33]

Primary versus Specialty Palliative Care in ICU

There are not enough palliative care providers or team members available to provide consultative palliative care to all ICU patients who have palliative care needs[17]; therefore, the interprofessional ICU team can be trained to provide a foundational level of palliative care, or "primary palliative care," for all ICU patients as part of their usual care. Ideally, the ICU clinicians recognize their primary palliative care role, screen for informational and emotional needs of patient and family, and assess for distressing symptoms. Bedside clinicians can take additional continuing education courses in palliative care to enhance their knowledge and skills (see Chapter 10). When appropriate, ICU teams can embrace the palliative care consultation as an opportunity to learn from the specialist about best practices, and incorporate this learning into their own practice. In addition to the tangible "results" of a palliative care consultation such as a change in code status, primary providers may appreciate and learn from the subtler tasks, such as facilitating nuanced communication within a complex family system to enhance family support, building rapport and trust, and supporting the potential for a shift in the patient's goals of care over time. Ultimately, the ICU and palliative care teams can participate in ongoing respectful dialogue about their respective contributions, strengths, and limitations related to optimizing patient care.[47]

Resources are available to assist ICU team members in learning best practices for primary palliative care. IMPACT-ICU[48,49] and ELNEC-critical care[50,51] are 2 educational resources specifically designed for ICU nurses who want to integrate primary palliative care in their practice. During IMPACT-ICU, nurses practice effective communication skills in 3 palliative care scenarios—talking to a family member of a critically ill patient, talking to a physician, and communicating to support the patient, family, and team during a family meeting. ELNEC-critical care translates the literature, using the National Consensus Project (NCP) Guidelines as a framework, for application to nursing practice in the critical care setting. The "Improving Palliative Care in the ICU" (IPAL-ICU) initiative has taken the lead in exploring and publishing recommendations for integrating palliative care in the ICU.[52] VitalTalk communications training has been adapted for ICU clinicians.[53]

The *logistic and business factors* related to ICU care can impact the perception of the value of palliative care. Morbidity, mortality, and cost are carefully measured and reported throughout the United States. This includes medical, surgical, neurosurgical, and cardiovascular ICUs, where metrics of morbidity and mortality, use of extracorporeal membrane oxygenation (ECMO), transplant outcomes, and cost are all scrutinized. Although the cost of surgical and trauma ICU care is front-loaded, with the highest daily costs at the start of ICU admission and declining quickly after the first few days of care,[54] pressure exists to minimize ICU length of stay. Often a major turning point in care, which is frequently a decisive moment for the initiation and continuation of goals of care discussions for ICU patients, relates to the need for placement of a tracheostomy and/or permanent feeding tube. Given that limitations in procedures, plans for longer-term life-sustaining therapies, or a transition to comfort care should ideally be made before these invasive treatments are selected, the timing of these decisions may introduce a time pressure to the work of the ICU and palliative care teams. One approach is to initiate early and recurrent discussions with the patient or surrogate decision-maker in order to prepare for the possible trajectory of care. Another approach to therapeutic interventions is to consider a time-limited trial of invasive therapies or life support and to assess for clear, predefined metrics in the patient's clinical response and physiological improvement. This may strengthen trust and shared decision-making, allowing families time to process the complexities of rapidly changing care, putting the patient's goals and values at center stage in the decision-making process, and allowing time for patients to meet clearly identified metrics of improvement over the course of days while providing support to families during this time of uncertainty. The time-limited trial has been shown in one study of 3 academic West Coast hospitals to reduce non-beneficial treatments, median ICU LOS from 8.7 to 7.4 days, and median hospital LOS from 14.2 to 10.7 days ($p = 0.01$). Importantly, the initiation of the first scheduled family meeting was greatly reduced from 5.5 days to 1.0 day ($p = <0.001$).[55] This occurred without having an impact on hospital mortality or patient and family satisfaction, which was already high in these settings. It appears that one of the most important interventions as evidenced in this study is communication; formal family meetings occurred more frequently and earlier in the clinical course, and these were more likely to address topics necessary for effective shared decision making.

The *physiological focus* of ICU culture can sometimes be a barrier to providing palliative care which strives to understand the patient in the context of their full human experience. Although ICU care strives for a curative approach to organ dysfunction, there is always room for a palliative intervention for symptom management and patient and family support. In some instances, as curative options decrease and palliative interventions increase, the treatment approaches intersect, and palliation becomes the dominant therapy for the patient.

Patients are admitted to the ICU in response to actual or risk of failure of one or more organ systems. Intensivists, ICU nurses, and critical care respiratory care professionals are experts in human physiology and in treating organ failure. By necessity, interprofessional conversation in the ICU has a physiological focus. Patients may initially be conceptualized as a group of organ systems in need of treatment, rather than integral people embedded in a familial and cultural context. This viewpoint can be taken up by family members as they begin to see their loved one in ways similar to clinicians, inquiring about specific organs and systems ("How was his blood pressure overnight?"). While this organ systems approach may be necessary to provide optimal, detailed ICU treatment, it can be in conflict with seeing a patient holistically. Ultimately, this may complicate conversations focused on goals of treatment and values-based decisions, as one may ask, "what would he/she *think of this situation?*" The desire for particular physiological outcomes may not be realistic in the setting of the patient's underlying medical issues and critical illness. While focusing on the specifics of organ failure, details of physiologic metrics, and blood work, clinicians may keep away from a holistic understanding of the general state of health and prognosis of the patient. Furthermore, there can be discordance in the messaging that ICU clinicians relay and what the family members hear, internalize, and interpret. A study by Zier and colleagues asked family members of ICU patients to review certain phrases stated by clinicians about a theoretical ICU patient ranging from a good outcome ("90% chance of survival") to a high risk of death ("5% chance of survival"), and interpret their likelihood of survival. The families' understanding was very similar to the clinicians when the likelihood of survival was good, but tended to be overly optimistic about the possibility of recovery when the likelihood of survival was poor.[56]

Although these were hypothetical patients, the families indicated that they needed to hold on to hope, and they believed that patient characteristics unknown to the clinicians would improve the patients' chances of survival. This study points out a common discordance between the focus and values of some families and ICU teams. The families are focused on any amount of hope and possibility related to unknown factors, while the ICU team are focused on data illustrating measured risk of survival and death.

Bedside critical care nurses experience moral distress and may not always feel as empowered to enter into challenging conversations with families about the patient's values and what the future may hold as they do in discussing medical/physiological information. Facilitated practice of communication skills in a safe environment, followed by a reflection session and self-care practices, has been shown to lead to improvements in self-reported confidence, as well as increased use of communication techniques with patients, families, and other providers. Engaging nurses and empowering them to elicit patient and family informational and emotional needs resulted in a focus group of nurses identifying a change in the culture of communication and teamwork in the ICU.[48]

A high-functioning ICU team experiences a symbiotic ebb and flow with a healthy palliative care team, so that both teams attune to where suffering exists within a patient and family, the ICU team continuously monitoring the patient, the palliative care team offering iterative opportunities to clarify goals and values, and ongoing back-and-forth collaboration between the teams as the patient's hospitalization unfolds. It is imperative that the palliative care team has a clear understanding of the possible medical or surgical interventions, the ICU team's baseline discussions with patient and family, as well as the fundamental details on expected clinical course and prognosis. This knowledge aids in continuity of information sharing and allows all team members to focus care and recommendations based on the patient's values.

Models of Palliative Care Embedded in ICU

Multiple models exist for how palliative care is embedded within an ICU service (Figure 13.2). No one model is best,[8] but depends upon the resources available, the type of ICU services provided, the expertise of the various team members, and the personalities of those involved. Palliative care by definition is dependent on the intersecting perspectives of multiple team members; ideally, the perspectives of nursing, social work, medicine, and spiritual care join in addressing the needs of the patient with critical illness. Realistically, all palliative care team members are not able to interact with every patient, especially in an ICU setting, and therefore, the specialty palliative care team members train and work with the ICU team to bolster their primary palliative care skills of holistic assessment and palliative care interventions for the patients in their care.

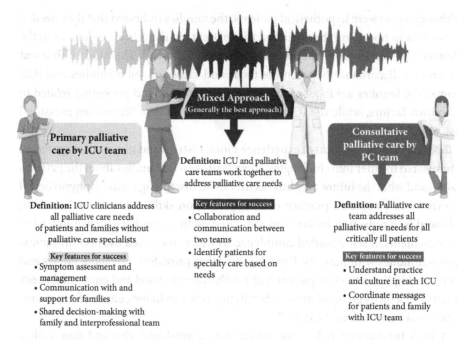

Primary palliative care by ICU team

Definition: ICU clinicians address all palliative care needs of patients and families without palliative care specialists

Key features for success
- Symptom assessment and management
- Communication with and support for families
- Shared decision-making with family and interprofessional team

Mixed Approach
(Generally the best approach)

Definition: ICU and palliative care teams work together to address palliative care needs

Key features for success
- Collaboration and communication between two teams
- Identify patients for specialty care based on needs

Consultative palliative care by PC team

Definition: Palliative care team addresses all palliative care needs for all critically ill patients

Key features for success
- Understand practice and culture in each ICU
- Coordinate messages for patients and family with ICU team

Figure 13.2. Models for integrating palliative care into the ICU.
Source: Curtis JR, Higginson IJ, White DB. Integrating palliative care into the ICU: A lasting and developing legacy. *Intensive Care Med*. 2022;48:939–942. https://doi.org/10.1007/s00134-022-06729-7. Reprinted with permission from Springer Nature.

Given that the ICU team already includes interprofessional members, sometimes the best model for providing specialty palliative care in the ICU involves an embedded palliative care team member whose primary assignment is ICU care. Depending on the needs of the ICU, this may be a nurse practitioner, nurse, social worker, or chaplain who joins the daily ICU rounds, interviews the patients/ families, and provides guidance on goals of care. Ideally, this palliative care team member serves as a bridge for the primary team and the specialty palliative care team, by attending daily palliative care team huddles and providing continuity for patients who are transferred from the ICU to the hospital floors. Efforts can be made to integrate the palliative care and the critical care teams and promote their highest level of functioning.[57] Memorializing and end-of-life rituals such as fingerprint charms, handprints, saving a swatch of hair, or a moment of silence after a code, can contribute to the integration of palliative care within the ICU team.

Sometimes, a palliative care physician serves as a consultant and specialty palliative care contact within the ICU. This is a common model in an academic hospital setting with a palliative care fellowship, where fellows, residents, and medical students are readily available. Given the strong physician influence already inherent in an ICU, this model may lose some of the benefit of the interprofessional palliative care team perspective, but serves well in training physician learners on their profession-specific educational objectives. A physician consultant can also serve to build confidence and trust early in the process of establishing a palliative care service. When the palliative care physician is integrated within a strong palliative care team, he/she can review the ICU cases and collaborate with his/her interprofessional colleagues to address unmet palliative needs, either individually or as a coordinated expert team.

Given the expertise of the critical care team, another model of palliative care is the use of a nurse, social worker, or chaplain as a mentor for primary palliative care within the ICU. Some palliative care teams, especially in teaching hospitals with palliative care fellows, may depend on the bedside nurses to contribute the nursing perspective. In this model, the palliative care team member collaborates with the charge nurse to identify patients with unmet palliative care needs, and rounds with the nurses and patients/families to assess the situation, to model problem-solving from a palliative care perspective, and to evaluate resolution of the concern. In a multisite study, 1110 charts were reviewed, and with appropriate nurse training and coaching, the ICU bedside nurses identified unmet palliative needs in 80% of the patients. These included an even distribution of symptom management, family distress/unmet support needs, and communication concerns. This coaching strategy can be used concurrently with other models of ICU palliative care[58] (see Appendix 1 in Chapter 12 for a sample of a rounding form).

Unique Profession-Specific Contributions of Palliative Care Team Members in the Critical Care Setting

Although the focus is predominantly physiological in the ICU because of the complexity of the diagnoses that lead to ICU admission, the psycho-social, spiritual, and cultural aspects of care are as important in ICU as they are elsewhere along the trajectory of illness.[1] Critical illness can often uncover interpersonal and familial challenges that have been dormant for years. Seriously ill patients admitted to the ICU experience severe spiritual and existential distress. Importantly, the cultural and spiritual aspects of care are complex, and by working together, the interprofessional palliative care team addresses ethnic, cultural, and spiritual aspects of health and illness to provide culturally respectful care of patients and families and aid in a shared decision-making model.[59-61]

Unfortunately, the chaplain is the member of the palliative care team who may be most likely to be missing from the ICU team. National guidelines from the American College of Critical Care Medicine Task Force suggest integration of spiritual care in ICU care.[62,63] Findings point to serious limitations in routinely providing care consistent with these guidelines. In most large spiritual care programs, chaplains respond to every code blue in the ICU, are scheduled 24/7 to respond to urgent and critical incidents, and at least one staff chaplain is assigned to the ICU(s) on an ongoing basis. It appears that in some institutions, chaplains may play their largest role in the medical ICU, when death or transition to comfort care is already expected.[64] In smaller spiritual care departments in community hospitals, just one chaplain may cover the entire hospital. Even in these smaller institutions, the chaplain spends a lot of time in the ICU for codes and end of life. Regrettably, some small, regional, or community hospitals rely solely or mainly on minimally trained volunteers from the community who may be ill-prepared for the professional trauma related to working in acute settings, instead of qualified board-certified professional healthcare chaplains on staff.

Illness in every culture has some association with spirituality or the existential dimension. Spiritual care is important for most people, but most clinicians are uncomfortable and untrained in talking about the subject.[65] Some hospital administrators do not accept the value of specialty spiritual care within healthcare,[66] some teams do not recognize the unique value that chaplains bring to the palliative care team beyond the psychosocial care provided by social workers and the holistic approach of nurses, and very few chaplains have specialty training in palliative care. Ernecoff and colleagues reported that spiritual care providers representing 13 ICUs across the country were present in only 2 of the 249 goals-of-care meetings examined, despite evidence that religion or spirituality was fairly or very important to 77% of the surrogate decision-makers.[67] Care provided by chaplains at end of life has been associated with increased satisfaction with care and decision-making by the families of patients who died in the ICU.[68] There is evidence that overall, chaplain-provided spiritual care in the ICU is underutilized and the spiritual care that is being provided by chaplains is underreported.[69,70]

When chaplains are integrated into the ICU team, the chaplain is able to proactively support gravely ill patients and their family surrogates in making difficult treatment decisions and assist them in coming to terms with the patient's condition.[71-74] Provision of spiritual support by the medical team during end-of-life discussions was associated with reduced aggressiveness of end-of-life care.[75] Experienced chaplains may play a role in assisting patients and families in decision-making, possibly by aligning their values and wishes with treatment plans and avoiding non-beneficial aggressive measures.[76] Early intervention by chaplains who are well integrated into their ICU team may assist patients and their loved ones in coming to terms with grave illness and making difficult treatment decisions.[77]

Choi and colleagues found that both ICU physicians and nurses welcomed the collaboration of chaplains when patients are dying or when talking about religious or spiritual topics. Nurses also appreciate the chaplain's presence during difficult conversations with families.[78] In a retrospective cross-sectional study of chaplain presence in one tertiary medical center's ICUs with over 4169 ICU admissions, 6% of patients were seen by chaplains and 80% of those who died were seen by a chaplain. Chaplains communicated with nurses after 57% of encounters and with physicians after 6% of encounters.[79] In addition to caring for patients and their families, chaplains are also trained to care for staff psychosocial and emotional needs. For these reasons, a well-trained specialty palliative care chaplain is vital in the care of critically ill patients, and may be an ideal choice to serve as primary palliative care mentor for an ICU team (see Chapter 3 on the roles and contributions of various team members).

The role of the palliative care social worker can easily morph into the case-management function of other social workers on the team. In an ICU staffed with intensivists, advanced practice providers, and bedside nurses to address the medical needs, a social worker serves as a strong palliative point of contact for patient and family. The palliative care social worker can meet with the patient or family on day one in the ICU to begin developing rapport, and then continue to follow up with goals of care conversations and support. Often the first day is focused on the traumatic event that prompted the ICU admission; subsequent early days consist of additional data gathering and values assessment, in preparation for discussing next steps in care. This requires the skills of active listening, expression of empathy, and skilled communication practices to address strong emotions, build trust and rapport, assist in identifying the medical power of attorney or surrogate decision-maker, and gather the collateral information that can be vital to the ongoing process of shared decision-making. Sometimes an intensivist can do this well and with compassion, and other times the intensivist focuses on the acute issues causing the critical illness, provides medical information, and depends on palliative care team members to provide emotional support to patients and families.

An interprofessional family meeting can be overwhelming for family members, especially when multiple specialties and "white coats" enter a conference room and are seated across from the family. However, the addition of supportive bedside nurses, social workers, or chaplains can aid the family in feeling more represented. The "4 Cs" of nursing support—convening a meeting, checking in with family, showing emotional support by caring, and continuing the conversation[80]—give a foundation for nursing support through communication skills with families. This active role allows for the bedside nurse to bring unanswered family questions or unmet emotional needs to the awareness of the other team members. Depending on the situation, other team members may also contribute to the palliative care of the critically ill patient. Ethics consultations may be helpful to parse out futility, which is a lack of physiologic benefit to the patient, or requests for inappropriate or non-beneficial care.[23]

Characteristics of a High-Functioning Team

Several characteristics, including humility, strong communication, trust, equity, compassion, self-reflection, grace, vulnerability, and openness to engage are especially important for the combined critical care and palliative care teams serving patients with life-threatening illness. Humility is an important ingredient for a high-functioning team. The need for simple humility spans the spectrum of expectations, prognosis, and what the future holds. No matter how experienced the provider is, prognostic uncertainty exists. Variations occur even with the best prognostic calculators in an age where patients and families experience prognostic uncertainty from multiple providers' estimates and internet searches. The biggest risk factor for severe traumatic brain injury (TBI) and nontraumatic intracranial hemorrhage (ICH) is having a doctor who thinks the patient will not survive.[81] A family's prayer for a miracle may coincide with a patient who is an outlier who defies all odds and survives despite a poor prognosis. Humility is attractive to patients and helps the team engage with them on the worst day of their life, during the worst grief they have ever experienced, and the most frightened they have ever been.

Humility spreads farther than prognosis; it needs to be represented with whole-person care, with culture, spirituality, and humanity. Cultural humility[82,83] is an important consideration when caring for patients with serious illness and their families. The cultural divide can be deepened with attempts to use telephone or video interpreters, especially in cultures that value eye contact and touch. When only 1 or 2 family members are invited to the hospital and the family would normally be filling up the waiting room, it may seem cold, heartless, and disconnected to not be inclusive and supportive of family needs for connection and support. This has never been more pronounced than during the COVID pandemic.[84] COVID-19, combined with the racial unrest of 2020, led to increased distrust and suspicion among some ethnic groups related to healthcare processes and visitation policies.[85,86]

The National Institutes of Health and the Institute of Medicine promote identifying healthcare disparities and addressing healthcare equity as top priorities of care and research. Healthcare disparities in critical care are well documented and multifactorial, and may include individual, community, and institutional factors.[87] In addition to quality and safety of care, the published literature highlights data on the racial and ethnic disparities in healthcare—the disparities in both palliative and critical care may intersect, creating a synergistic negative effect. Often, racial disparities become more pronounced at end of life, when some racial groups are perceived to be less likely to discontinue ventilation or pursue palliation, and racial minorities receive less palliative care, have more aggressive end-of-life care including CPR, and have fewer life-sustaining measures withdrawn.[88,89] Differences in communication content and styles include discussions of advance directives, use of life-sustaining therapies, and family-clinician communication. In one study, non-Whites engaged in fewer discussions of patients' wishes, and these conversations and decisions were less likely to be documented.[90]

Shrank and colleagues explored communication preferences in 2 ethnicities with varying socioeconomic status and found that non-Hispanic Whites were more exclusive when selecting family members to participate in family meetings and less interested in spiritual input. They were provided more information on medical conditions, treatment options, and discussions of quality of life. African American families preferred highlighting spirituality and prayer and were more inclusive in selecting family to participate in discussions.[91] One conclusion of this qualitative study was that exploration of communication preferences and fostering trust should be encouraged for clinicians serving various ethnic groups. The findings raise questions of implicit (unconscious) bias and the need for reflection to address the racial, ethnic, and cultural disparities in healthcare and communication.[92]

Addressing cultural humility and equity in healthcare will require multilevel changes in access, management, education, and communication. In addition, we need outcomes research as we move toward the goal of eliminating disparities.[93] In the COVID era, PTSD was found in 30%–60% of families with a loved one in critical care. In one study, this was significantly higher in the Hispanic population, and the families reported fewer "acts of compassion," described as "exceptional communication, developing more personal relationships, extra touches for patients (e.g., allowing a patient a Coca-Cola for breakfast), or addressing isolation head-on from clinicians."[94]

In palliative care conversations, the heightened state of panic and distress, combined with the potential for technical glitches, leads to difficulty in understanding. At the best of times, the interpreted conversations can be difficult due to cultural history, health literacy, and dialects. Some families may not have access to smartphones or video. Medical interpreters provide literal language interpretation of the words during a medical encounter, but the cultural nuance and context might be missing and may lead to misunderstanding.[95] Medical interpreters also struggle with translating words such as "palliative care," interpreting in the presence of family members who understand both languages, expressing sensitivity while remaining professional, and the interpreter's own emotions in a difficult conversation.[96] Using an English-speaking family member as a spokesperson may lead to unfortunate and devastating consequences, such as protecting family members from difficult news with subsequent distress when the news is finally relayed.[97] Pham and colleagues found that 55% of the ICU family meetings using professional interpreters had alterations in the content. These could be "additions, omissions, substitutions, or editorializations." Seventy-five percent were thought to have a potentially clinically significant consequence on the conversation and 93% of those likely to have a negative impact, which may include inadequate explanation of medical conditions or treatment recommendations, decrease in ability to provide emotional support to family, or editorializing by the interpreter.[98]

Self-reflection and openness to feedback are critically important characteristics for interprofessional teamwork on both the ICU and the palliative care teams. How do we normalize the practice of looking at the situation from the family's perspective? How can we center the patient and their family so that we understand the situation in a way that is reflective of *their* values as well as our own? Some clinicians may be reluctant to change their perspective. Not everyone has the training or the desire to provide primary palliative care, but in the ICU, advanced symptom management, participating in difficult conversations, exploring patients' and families' values, and ongoing adjustments to the care plan based on the patient's trajectory of illness are part of critical care practice. Palliative care requires humility, grace, vulnerability, understanding, and openness to engage, have the conversation, get to know a patient and their loved ones, inquire about values and preferences, and ultimately walk with them with compassion on their journey.

Critical Illness beyond the ICU

In addition to the ICU, critically ill patients are cared for in many other locations including pre-hospital emergency response, the ED, mass casualty, military conflict, the maternity ward, and in locations where people live without housing (see Box 13.2).

Box 13.2. Street Medicine Palliative Care Project

Tanya Majumder, Melanie Bien

People experiencing homelessness (PEH) often present in end stages of the disease process and die at earlier ages than the general population. PEH have unique palliative care needs, including family configurations, shelter/street at end of life, complex pain, comorbid mental illness, mistrust of medical systems, and management of active substance use. In many homeless care systems, team members are siloed in their work with chronically ill PEH, each trying to fill system gaps on their own without support or a guiding framework, causing profound distress, frustration, loneliness, and less effective overall care.

To address the needs of our team and patients, we developed a framework to guide palliative care for PEH: (1) engagement/outreach; (2) clinical care coordination; (3) trauma-informed patient-centered care (active listening to both verbal and nonverbal cues, meeting people where they are, and tending to patients' trusted relationships); (4) inquiry (what is important); and (5) grief support/closure (debrief and support for both care team and family members).

We hold monthly multidisciplinary team meetings to collectively identify and cultivate skills needed for successful palliative care with PEH. These meetings provide a safe space for our diverse team to lead, develop, and practice skills (listening, mindfulness, boundaries, and teamwork) and to discuss cases within an interprofessional framework. Our goals in these meetings are to decrease the isolation with this challenging work, ensure that we are addressing our own counter-transference, and to work collaboratively to provide the highest standard of care.

Case: Mr. A was a 74-year-old person who was unhoused for decades, living in a driveway. He had limited contacts with systems, so outreach, engagement, and trust building were crucial. Outreach was able to connect him to care, where he was diagnosed with end-stage renal disease. His rapport with one of the nurses on the team helped him connect with a physician and a social worker for a meaningful goals-of-care conversation. This conversation was instrumental in guiding his inpatient care when he decompensated and was admitted to the ICU. His care was focused on his values, and he died with care focused on comfort.

Emergency Department

"I demand the end-of-life act for my sister!" she screamed. A panicked nurse called the palliative care team looking for assistance to address this delicate topic. An immediate response from the palliative care social worker led to a calmed advocate who explained her sister was in pain (anyone could see her writhing in pain from a mere glance) and was dying, and therefore she demanded the End-of-Life Option Act, or Death with Dignity Act. Gentle empathy, active listening, validation, and redirection while developing rapport and gaining trust allowed this situation to ease its way into understanding that the palliative care team could immediately and effectively treat her sister in the moment with expertise and compassion. The palliative care physician arranged for an admission to address the intractable symptoms, and the palliative care pharmacist recommended a pain regimen taking into account her new renal failure. The patient's hospital care plan was focused on comfort for the patient and family and allowed for a natural death within days, with her family at her side. This dance of the interprofessional palliative care team can be spontaneous or a rhythm that develops over time. As the palliative care team learns each other's language, they develop a shared language, mannerisms, and cues, and the ability for a highly focused, compassionate holding of the patient and family develops. These skills are put to the test and often thrive in the ED setting, where emotions, fear, and pain are frequent human experiences (see Box 13.3).

Palliative care, particularly symptom management, has historically been a significant part of the care provided in the ED.[99] Patients come to the ED seeking treatment of trauma, acute illness, and exacerbation of chronic conditions, including managing the pain, dyspnea, and anxiety associated with many chronic diseases. ED providers help patients with chronic disease exacerbation decide if hospital admission is consistent with their preferences and goals. When admission and curative treatment are not wanted, ED providers arrange for safe disposition to skilled nursing or hospice.

The palliative care work possible in the ED is exponential.[100] It can be offered by enhancing the skills of the existing staff to recognize the needs of patients and families and provide the symptom management, communication, and complex decision-making necessary to care for those patients, or by a full complement of a palliative care team ready to serve the ED's primary team. Frontline team members, including bedside ED nurses who are fulfilled by the intensity of ED clinical practice and have a passion for and understanding of palliative care, become palliative care allies. Screening for palliative care needs for patients in the ED and referral for specialty palliative care is not yet standardized, but early evidence suggests its benefits.[101] Providers who learn the unique offerings of a palliative care team begin consulting and partnering to improve patient care in a plethora of situations. Discharge from the ED straight to hospice becomes a reality. Focused admissions for comfort care or general in-patient hospice (GIP) are accomplished with patients' values at the forefront as a plan of care is developed.

Box 13.3. Palliative Emergency Medicine

Tara M. Coles and Masha Rand Rosenthal

Palliative emergency medicine (PEM) leverages interprofessional expertise to support the provision of patient- and family-centered, goal-concordant care in the ED. Early integration of palliative care in acute care environments serves the needs of a growing population of patients with chronic and complex conditions presenting with related medical crises, severe symptoms, and issues related to caregiver burden and distress. Research in this area suggests multiple benefits, such as improved patient and family satisfaction, improved hospital outcomes, and cost savings, among others.[a]

Since its recognition as a medical specialty in 1979, emergency medicine (EM) has evolved beyond its core mission of evaluating, resuscitating, and stabilizing the acutely ill or injured to include a central role in caring for patients presenting for "crisis care" at various stages of chronic, complex illness.[b,c] In 2006, the American Board of Emergency Medicine (ABEM) joined 9 other specialties in sponsoring Hospice and Palliative Medicine (HPM) for subspecialty training and certification. PEM developed in recognition of the role the ED plays in setting the care trajectories and addressing the complex physical, spiritual and psychological needs of patients and families in crisis.[a,b]

The interprofessional (IP) team model inherent to both EM and palliative care makes the ED an opportune environment to "screen and intervene" for unmet, often unrecognized, palliative care needs.[a,c] Engaging the spectrum of IP team members (emergency medical services, unit clerks, nurses, nursing assistants, advanced practice providers, pharmacists, physicians, social workers, chaplains) in the design and implementation of PEM protocols and processes allows best-practice guidelines to be tailored to the unique characteristics of each ED.

Several ED-specific screening tools for identifying patients with palliative care needs exist. Common criteria include presence of a serious illness (at any stage), along with secondary markers such as functional decline, uncontrolled symptoms, escalating need for caregiver support, or frequent ED visits. Alternatively, the surprise question ("not surprised if the patient died within 12 months") is a simple and rapid screening measure that may indicate the need for further palliative care interventions.[a,c]

Multiple models for integrating palliative care into ED care have emerged:

1. Training ED providers and staff in primary palliative care skills (e.g., communication skills, symptom management, familiarity with advance care documents) often driven by ED palliative care champions or in collaboration with inpatient palliative care;
2. Driving early referral to palliative care from the ED;

Box 13.3 Continued

3. Embedding palliative care providers within the ED (initiatives have used MD, NP, RN, or SW);
4. Creating a dedicated ED consult sub-team for real-time palliative care consults in the ED in hospitals with large inpatient PC services[a-c];
5. Partnering with community-based palliative care and hospice groups.

Engaging the spectrum of disciplines in integrating palliative care with EM, we can address patient and family suffering from the outset, decrease caregiver fatigue, and foster EM clinical team cohesion and resiliency, while simultaneously improving hospital resource utilization and quality of care.[a,c]

[a] Loffredo AJ, Chan GK, Wang DH, et al. United States best practice guidelines for primary palliative care in the emergency department. *Ann Emerg Med.* 2021 Nov;78(5)658–669.

[b] Lowery DS, Quest TE. Emergency medicine and palliative care. *Clin Geriatr Med.* 2015 May;31(2)295–303.

[c] George N, Bowman J, Aaronson E, Ouchi K. Past, present, and future of palliative care in emergency medicine in the USA. *Acute Med Surg.* 2020 Mar 18;7(1):e497.

[d] Wang, DH. Beyond code status: Palliative care begins in the emergency department. *Ann Energ Med.* 2017 Apr;69(4):437–443.

Family conferences with the palliative care team in the ED can become beacons of support amid chaos and fear. A space, literal or figurative, is created to hold and honor the embodied person on the gurney. The cause or mechanism of injury matters little to the dying person. Whether the illness is caused by a stroke, heart attack, trauma, or life-ending cerebral hemorrhage, it is in these moments when one realizes the fragility of life and what little control one has over the natural dying process. This can lead to internal grief and a search for meaning of life and suffering. The gentle touch, a soft word, the presence of holding a space for emotions to be felt, honored, and guided is a sacred encounter like no other. The mother losing her daughter, the elderly wife in fear of her long-time husband being permanently altered, the estranged brother trying to understand his sister's plight—it all comes together in the ED, where palliative care plays an important, unique, and necessary role. When the primary ED team jumps into action to save lives, as they are expertly trained to do, the palliative care team supports that process by getting to know not only the patient but the person in the bed. The palliative care chaplain is attuned to the spiritual suffering of the moment and serves as a creator of peace, while the palliative care social worker attends to the physiological and emotional chaos that is churning and becomes a producer of balance. The physician provides direction and treatment options, thereby creating the plan and next steps. Even amidst this chaos, peace, hope, calm, direction, and breath can be regained. The expert guidance of the palliative care interprofessional team helps move the fear and destruction of the ED visit into an experience more reasoned and understood.

Mass Casualty

A recent example of a mass casualty event (Box 13.4) is the COVID-19 pandemic,[102] a unique experience in the history of American healthcare and the world. This pandemic has created trauma from the triage process, devastating loss for many families, and caregiver and provider moral distress and burnout.[103,104] The social and political complexity of the global health crisis and confusion with evolving epidemiological knowledge inadvertently led to greater spread of the virus, with early transfers between institutions leading to outbreaks in skilled nursing facilities and in correctional facilities. Visitor limitations increased distress when patients were declining and family members were unaware of the natural progression of disease.[105] The family system is the focus of palliative care, and accompanying loved ones is a central tenet of support. Changing and inconsistent visitation policies contributed to moral distress for staff and caregivers. Overall, patients in facilities experienced adverse effects, including loneliness and isolation, which increased the rate of decline or contributed to delirium. For many, physical and mental health issues were exacerbated as necessary healthcare was delayed or refused due to fear of COVID-19.

Box 13.4. Expanding Palliative Care into the World of Mass Casualties

---

Michelle Neveu

Even though it has been more than a decade, hearing the term "mass casualty" takes me straight back to the trauma bay at a military hospital in Bagram, Afghanistan, in 2009. I can still see the crowded room and smell the combination of blood, sweat, gasoline, and gunpowder. As military medical personnel, we were well trained to handle these triage situations quickly and efficiently to save as many lives as possible with the resources we had available. Unfortunately, this also meant that those poor souls who sustained injuries deemed un-survivable were generally moved to a separate room, where we tried to manage their end-of-life symptoms before moving on to the next patient. As I reflect on my time since then as a registered nurse and now as a palliative care nurse practitioner, I am proud of the care that we were able to give to those who were saved, and also wonder if the end-of-life care that we provided could have been more robust and meaningful had we incorporated some palliative care concepts into our mass casualty training.[a] The training we received at the time included didactic courses, simulator training, and large-scale mass causality exercises, which focused on principles of triage and trauma care. Adding a few VitalTalk-style communication tools, including empathy statements and guidance on alleviating existential/spiritual distress, to the didactics training would then allow participants to integrate primary palliative care into the simulator training and exercises.

Box 13.4 Continued

I believe the most efficient way to improve care provided to mass casualty patients is to include primary palliative care training in our mass casualty curricula. Like most medical knowledge and skill, if taught early and practiced often, providing primary palliative care to our patients has the potential to become standard of care. During a mass casualty event, it is all hands on deck. If all members of the healthcare team understand the importance of connecting with the emotional and spiritual aspects of the human on the gurney while tending to their physical ailments, I believe we can provide the best whole-person care to our dying military members. Early palliative care interventions also have the potential to improve outcomes for those who survive, but may be left with lifelong physical and psychological disabilities.

While primary palliative care should be standard training for all healthcare providers who respond to mass casualty events (both military and civilian),[b] I also envision specialty palliative care teams playing a larger role in caring for those affected by mass casualties in the civilian setting. Whether it be an act of violence, a pandemic, or severe weather, the physical and psychological injuries that are sustained during these mass casualty events are complex. Suffering and distress resulting from mass casualty events can be minimized with careful preparation focused on 6S + C-E: supplies, staff, space, systems, sedation, separation, communication, and equity.[c] Specialty palliative care teams have the training and skills needed to attend to these difficult situations, and have the potential to improve short-term and long-term outcomes for both visible and invisible traumatic injuries. I am blessed to work for an organization that includes our palliative care team in our hospital's contingency response plan through automatic referrals to the palliative care team for severe trauma patients and those with diagnoses that meet specific criteria during large-scale illness or injury events. I hope that this practice will become standard for healthcare organizations around the world.

[a] Matzo M, Wilkinson A, Lynn J, Gatto M, Phillips S. Palliative care considerations in mass casualty events with scarce resources. *Biosecur Bioterror.* 2009 Jun;7(2):199–210. doi:10.1089/bsp.2009.0017. PMID: 19635004.

[b] Rosoff PM. Should palliative care be a necessity or a luxury during an overwhelming health catastrophe? *J Clin Ethics.* 2010 Winter;21(4):312–320. PMID: 21313865.

[c] Sullivan DR, Iyer AS, Enguidanos S, et al. Palliative care early in the care continuum among patients with serious respiratory illness: An Official ATS/AAHPM/HPNA/SWHPN Policy Statement. *Am J Respir Crit Care Med.* 2022;206(6):e44–e69. https://doi-org.ucsf.idm.oclc.org/10.1164/rccm.202207-1262ST

Conclusion

By the nature of their work, critical care clinicians are primary palliative care providers, bringing a set of skills to assess and manage distressing symptoms, provide patient and family support, and communicate effectively with patients, families, and other providers. Embracing a palliative care framework, including advanced symptom management and communication skills, will cause less moral distress and enhance outcomes. Coordination between critical care and palliative care teams will enhance the care that both teams provide, resulting in benefits for patients and their families. In the highest-functioning teams, no one jockeys for the primary role as a voice of authority; rather, it is a true team effort. This principle is demonstrated in the operating room, high-end restaurants, and complex religious rituals. High levels of trust, respect, humility, understanding, and flexibility are the "secret sauce" that makes interprofessional teamwork succeed, and nowhere is that truer than in critical care settings.

Case #1: What Can Go Wrong

A young woman was driving to meet her boyfriend when a fire truck struck her vehicle. Her mother, unaware of her dating status, believed the young woman was going to work. Her boyfriend came across the scene of the accident, saw her injuries, but did not accompany her to the hospital. In the busy trauma ED, multiple team members were present, including the neurosurgeon, intensivist, and ED physician. The palliative care social worker was briefed with a "one-liner" prior to meeting mom. This mother was overwhelmed with processing information regarding her daughter, a vibrant young woman, thriving this morning, starting college in mere weeks, now with devastating injuries. The mother hears the news from the neurosurgeon and intensivist that she has significant injuries and is likely brain dead. The intensivist provided a succinct and straightforward message to mother that the patient would be transferred to the ICU to complete the necessary brain death testing, and then left the palliative care social worker to support the mother. "How are you feeling? What did you hear before I arrived? What did you hear the intensivist say?"

During the subsequent days, the palliative care social worker supported the family to balance their hopes with expectations of devastating neurologic outcomes. The young woman was ultimately diagnosed with severe traumatic brain injury (TBI) and was given a poor prognosis for meaningful recovery. She was expected to require a tracheostomy for continued ventilator support, gastric feeding tube for nutrition, have no meaningful communication, and require complete care for all activities of daily living. She was presumed brain dead and now she is not.

Given their strong Catholic faith, the family viewed this as a miracle. The unit chaplain was contacted to help the team and family engage what a miracle means for this family and how the family's relationship to God, faith, and hope influences their decision-making. The patient's mother appreciated the suggestion of a Catholic priest visit for sacramental care. The next day, the young woman was twitching her eyes, and when her mother held her hand, the patient would reflexively weakly grasp her fingers. "She knows I'm here; I'm fighting for her, I won't stop. . . . She's my baby, nothing you say will change that."

This case allows us to reflect on the complexities of clinical care, prognostication, and communication. The message might have been, "This is traumatic and scary; we are worried about her and more tests are required to understand the extent of her injuries. We are concerned that her brain is damaged, and this could lead to brain death, despite all interventions and support." Instead, when the team said "brain dead" at the initial visit, hope was aroused when she ended up having some brainstem function. Then, when the young woman started blinking and closing her hands, the family interpreted this as a second miracle. The doctors were not consistent in the description of prognosis and quality of life to expect. All agreed that the young woman had sustained a traumatic global brain injury with limited expectation for meaningful recovery; however, as is often the case, there is no guarantee that she would not improve to some extent.

During several family conferences, we readdressed hope and reframed the mother's expectations. She visited the ICU daily, self-soothing, rocking and praying. Although the palliative care social worker doesn't typically pray with patients, led by spirit rather than by protocol, the palliative care social worker softly held the mother's hand and prayed that we would have some sort of peace and understanding and reassurance for the family. The palliative care social worker kept the language vague enough for her to keep her hope while not promising something the team could not deliver. Over their 3 or 4 days together, the mother was able to translate the information she was receiving into her own belief system and decided that she would continue to fight for her daughter until she hears from God that He is ready to take her. The mother did not want her daughter going to a long-term acute care (LTAC) center for the rest of her life. The patient was transferred to another hospital because of insurance requirements, and passed away a week later from respiratory complications.

Interprofessional Discussion about Case #1

- Interprofessional palliative care team: Who is this young woman? Who is the family? What are they hoping that we can achieve together? What are their fears? How best can the team work together to assess verbal and nonverbal prompts from family members? What communication skills can be used to clarify the medical information and the family member's understanding of the situation?
- Physician: What changes in messaging at the initial visit may have helped bridge the gap between the family and the medical teams? How do you

approach doing a values assessment? How might you approach a time limited trial? How might the approach differ if resources are limited (as in the COVID pandemic)?

- Nursing: What family dynamic may be affecting the mother's response to this accident? Disagreements occurred among nurses, some of whom saw this as futile care, and others could understand the desire for LTAC, given her age and acuity of the situation. Are the nurses experiencing moral distress?
- Social work: Is there more complex family dynamics at play here? What about when we knew that the young woman's response was part of the medical process? How do you support the boyfriend who resurfaces during the hospital stay?
- Chaplain: This mom has immense religious belief. Who is this young woman in the world? What is their role? Sometimes that alters expectations. What is the family's understanding of a miracle, and how does this influence decision-making and anticipatory loss? Are there signs of moral distress within the interprofessional team?

Case #2: Quality of Life Projections

A 30-year-old male immigrated from Central America with his mother, father, 2 sisters, and 2 brothers, all in their 30s. He worked as a construction worker, and one night after work was drinking and taking methamphetamine at a friend's house. The friend went to the garage to smoke a cigarette when he heard a gunshot. Upon returning to the house, he found the patient had shot himself in the head with a handgun. It was unclear if this was a suicide attempt or an accidental discharge since the patient was intoxicated and under the influence of multiple substances. The force of the gunshot caused a split and elevation of the cranium, which had the effect of relieving swelling, and preventing herniation and brain death. The neurocritical care doctor on duty told the family that he was at end of life, and transferred the patient to the ICU on comfort measures only so the family could see him. The family was praying for a miracle and viewed stopping life-sustaining treatment as abandoning the patient. Over multiple family meetings, it became clear that the individual's primary role in the family and world was as a son and brother and that he could continue to fulfill these roles on long-term life support. Once the treatment aligned the care plan with the family's values by performing a tracheotomy and preparing the patient for discharge to an LTAC, the family's stress was greatly reduced. Furthermore, giving up attachment to a specific outcome relieved the care team of their moral distress. Over the ensuing years the patient was liberated from the mechanical ventilator and eventually had his tracheotomy removed. He is interactive with other people for limited and intermittent periods of time and he is able to eat enough to live without enteral nutrition. His family visits regularly, and the patient remains a much-loved son and brother.

Interprofession Discussion about Case #2

- How does moral distress develop in a case such as this, and what are ways that the palliative care team can help address this?
- How does your professional and personal life experience contribute to your perspective on this case?
- How does the team use surrogate decision-makers to assess values and preferences, including quality of life, with varying treatment trajectories?

References

1. Donovan AL, Aldrich JM, Gross AK, et al.; University of California, San Francisco Critical Care Innovations Group. Interprofessional care and teamwork in the ICU. *Crit Care Med.* 2018 Jun;46(6):980–990. doi:10.1097/CCM.0000000000003067. PMID: 29521716.
2. Conerly TR, Holmes K, Tamang AL. *Introduction to Sociology.* 3rd ed. Rice University; 2021.
3. Kelly D. Understanding workplace culture. Int J Palliat Nurs. 2019 May 2;25(5):211. doi:10.12968/ijpn.2019.25.5.211. PMID: 31116657.
4. Dodek P, Cahill NE, Heyland DK. The relationship between organizational culture and implementation of clinical practice guidelines: a narrative review. JPEN J Parenter Enteral Nutr. 2010 Nov–Dec;34(6):669–674. doi:10.1177/0148607110361905. PMID: 21097767.
5. DeKeyser Ganz F, Engelberg R, Torres N, Curtis JR. Development of a model of interprofessional shared clinical decision making in the ICU. Crit Care Med. 2016;44(4):680–689. doi:10.1097/CCM.0000000000001467.
6. Baggs JG, Norton SA, Schmitt MH, Dombeck MT, Sellers CR, Quinn JR. Intensive care unit cultures and end-of-life decision making. J Crit Care. 2007. Jun;22(2):159–168 doi:10.1016/j.jcrc.2006.09.008. Epub 2007 Feb 8. PMID: 17548028; PMCID: PMC2214829.
7. Bruera E. The development of a palliative care culture. J Palliat Care. 2004. Winter;20(4):316–319. PMID: 15690835.
8. Curtis JR, Higginson IJ, White DB. Integrating palliative care into the ICU: a lasting and developing legacy. Intens Care Med. 2022 Mar;93(3):498–509. doi:10.1007/s00134-022-06729-7. Epub 2022 May 16. PMID: 35577992.
9. Floren LC, Donesky D, Whitaker E, Irby DM, Ten Cate O, O'Brien BC. Are we on the same page? Shared mental models to support clinical teamwork among health professions learners: a scoping review. *Acad Med.* 2018 Mar;93(3):498–509. doi:10.1097/ACM.0000000000002019. PMID: 29028635.
10. Devlin JW, Skrobik Y, Gélinas C, et al. Clinical practice guidelines for the prevention and management of pain, agitation/sedation, delirium, immobility, and sleep disruption in adult patients in the ICU. *Crit Care Med.* 2018;46(9):e825–e873. doi: 10.1097/CCM.0000000000003299. PMID: 30113379.
11. Leemhuis A, Shichishima Y, Puntillo K. Palliation of thirst in intensive care unit patients: translating research into practice. *Crit Care Nurs.* 2019;39(5):21–28. doi:10.4037/ccn2019544. PMID: 31575591.

12. Arroyo-Novoa CM, Figueroa-Ramos MI, Puntillo KA. Pain, anxiety, and the continuous use of opioids and benzodiazepines in trauma intensive care unit survivors: an exploratory study. *P R Health Sci J*. 2022. Sep;46(9):e825–e873. PMID: 36018737.

13. Zengin N, Ören B, Üstündag H. The relationship between stressors and intensive care unit experiences. *Nurs Crit Care*. 2020 Mar;25(2):109–116. doi:10.1111/nicc.12465. Epub 2019 Aug 13. PMID: 31407452.

14. Aslakson RA, Cox CE, Baggs JG, Curtis JR. Palliative and end-of-life care: prioritizing compassion within the ICU and beyond. *Crit Care Med*. 2021;49(10):1626–1637. doi:10.1097/CCM.0000000000005208. PMID: 34325446.

15. Dennis D, Knott C, Khanna R, van Heerden PV. Characteristics of the contemporary intensivist: a qualitative study. *J Emerg Med Crit Care*. 2022 Jul;8(1):6.

16. Angus DC, Barnato AE, Linde-Zwirble WT, et al.; Robert Wood Johnson Foundation ICU End-of-Life Peer Group. Use of intensive care at the end of life in the United States: an epidemiologic study. *Crit Care Med*. 2004 Mar;32(3):638–643. doi:10.1097/01.ccm.0000114816.62331.08. PMID: 15090940.

17. Hua MS, Li G, Blinderman CD, Wunsch H. Estimates of the need for palliative care consultation across United States intensive care units using a trigger-based model. *Am J Respir Crit Care Med*. 2014 Feb 15;189(4):428–436. doi:10.1164/rccm.201307-1229OC. PMID: 24261961; PMCID: PMC3977718.

18. Detsky ME, Harhay MO, Bayard DF, et al. Six-month morbidity and mortality among intensive care unit patients receiving life-sustaining therapy: a prospective cohort study. *Ann Am Thorac Soc*. 2017 Oct;14(10):1562–1570. doi:10.1513/AnnalsATS.201611-875OC. PMID: 28622004; PMCID: PMC5718567.

19. Morgan A. Long-term outcomes from critical care. *Surgery (Oxf)*. 2021 Jan;39(1):53–57. doi:10.1016/j.mpsur.2020.11.005. Epub 2020 Dec 17. PMID: 33519011; PMCID: PMC7836934.

20. Law AC, Stevens JP, Choi E, et al. Days out of Institution after tracheostomy and gastrostomy placement in critically ill older adults. *Ann Am Thorac Soc*. 2022 Mar;19(3):424–432. doi:10.1513/AnnalsATS.202106-649OC. PMID: 34388080; PMCID: PMC8937225.

21. Fiest KM, Soo A, Hee Lee C, et al. Long-term outcomes in ICU patients with delirium: a population-based cohort study. *Am J Respir Crit Care Med*. 2021 Aug 15;204(4):412–420. doi:10.1164/rccm.202002-0320OC. PMID: 33823122; PMCID: PMC8480248.

22. Marra A, Pandharipande PP, Patel MB. Intensive care unit delirium and intensive care unit-related posttraumatic stress disorder. *Surg Clin North Am*. 2017 Dec;97(6):1215–1235. doi:10.1016/j.suc.2017.07.008. Epub 2017 Oct 5. PMID: 29132506; PMCID: PMC5747308.

23. Bosslet GT, Pope TM, Rubenfeld GD, et al.; American Thoracic Society ad hoc Committee on Futile and Potentially Inappropriate Treatment; American Thoracic Society; American Association for Critical Care Nurses; American College of Chest Physicians; European Society for Intensive Care Medicine; Society of Critical Care. An official ATS/AACN/ACCP/ESICM/SCCM policy statement: Responding to requests for potentially inappropriate treatments in intensive care units. *Am J Respir Crit Care Med*. 2015 Jun 1;191(11):1318–1330. doi:10.1164/rccm.201505-0924ST. PMID: 25978438.

24. Anderson WG, Arnold RM, Angus DC, Bryce CL. Posttraumatic stress and complicated grief in family members of patients in the intensive care unit. *J Gen Intern Med*. 2008 Nov;23(11):1871–1876. doi:10.1007/s11606-008-0770-2. Epub 2008 Sep 9. PMID: 18780129; PMCID: PMC2585673.

25. Mason VM, Leslie G, Clark K, et al. Compassion fatigue, moral distress, and work engagement in surgical intensive care unit trauma nurses: a pilot study. *Dimens Crit Care Nurs*. 2014 Jul–Aug;33(4):215–225. doi:10.1097/DCC.0000000000000056. PMID: 24895952.

26. Hancock J, Witter T, Comber S, et al. Understanding burnout and moral distress to build resilience: a qualitative study of an interprofessional intensive care unit team. *Can J Anaesth*. 2020 Nov;67(11):1541–1548. English. doi:10.1007/s12630-020-01789-z. Epub 2020 Aug 26. PMID: 32844247.

27. Vincent H, Jones DJ, Engebretson J. Moral distress perspectives among interprofessional intensive care unit team members. *Nurs Ethics*. 2020 Sep;27(6):1450–1460. doi:10.1177/0969733020916747. Epub 2020 May 14. PMID: 32406313; PMCID: PMC8077224.

28. Campbell ML, Guzman JA. Impact of a proactive approach to improve end-of-life care in a medical ICU. *Chest*. 2003 Jan;123(1):266–271. doi:10.1378/chest.123.1.266. PMID: 12527629.

29. Azoulay E, Pochard F, Chevret S, et al. Impact of a family information leaflet on effectiveness of information provided to family members of intensive care unit patients: a multicenter, prospective, randomized, controlled trial. *Am J Respir Crit Care Med*. 2002 Feb 15;165(4):438–442. doi:10.1164/ajrccm.165.4.200108-006oc. PMID: 11850333.

30. Metaxa V, Anagnostou D, Vlachos S, et al. Palliative care interventions in intensive care unit patients. *Intensive Care Med*. 2021 Dec;47(12):1415–1425. doi:10.1007/s00134-021-06544-6. Epub 2021 Oct 15. Erratum in: Intensive Care Med. 2022. PMID: 34652465.

31. Lautrette A, Darmon M, Megarbane B, et al. A communication strategy and brochure for relatives of patients dying in the ICU. *N Engl J Med*. 2007 Feb 1;356(5):469–478. doi:10.1056/NEJMoa063446. Erratum in: *N Engl J Med*. 2007 Jul 12;357(2):203. PMID: 17267907.

32. Aslakson R, Cheng J, Vollenweider D, Galusca D, Smith TJ, Pronovost PJ. Evidence-based palliative care in the intensive care unit: a systematic review of interventions. *J Palliat Med*. 2014. Feb;17(2):219–235 doi:10.1089/jpm.2013.0409. PMID: 24517300; PMCID: PMC3924791.

33. Ito K, George N, Wilson J, Bowman J, Aaronson E, Ouchi K. Primary palliative care recommendations for critical care clinicians. *J Intensive Care*. 2022 Apr 15;10(1):20. doi:10.1186/s40560-022-00612-9. PMID: 35428371; PMCID: PMC9013119.

34. Ferrell BR, Twaddle ML, Melnick A, Meier DE. National Consensus Project clinical practice guidelines for quality palliative care guidelines, 4th edition. *J Palliat Med*. 2018 Dec;21(12):1684–1689. doi:10.1089/jpm.2018.0431. Epub 2018 Sep 4. PMID: 30179523.

35. Grabda M, Lim FA. Palliative care consult among older adult patients in intensive care units: an integrative review. *Crit Care Nurs Q*. 2021 Apr–Jun;44(2):248–262. doi:10.1097/CNQ.0000000000000358. PMID: 33595971.

36. Baggs JG. Prognostic information provided during family meetings in the intensive care unit. *Crit Care Med*. 2007. Feb;35(2):646–647. doi:10.1097/01.CCM.0000255163.16683.14. PMID: 17251713.

37. Nelson JE. Identifying and overcoming the barriers to high-quality palliative care in the intensive care unit. *Crit Care Med*. 2006 Nov;34(11 Suppl):S324-S331. doi:10.1097/01.CCM.0000237249.39179.B1. PMID: 17057594.

38. Nelson JE, Puntillo KA, Pronovost PJ, et al. In their own words: patients and families define high-quality palliative care in the intensive care unit. *Crit Care Med*. 2010 Mar;38(3):808–818. doi:10.1097/ccm.0b013e3181c5887c. PMID: 20198726; PMCID: PMC3267550.

39. Baker M, Luce J, Bosslet GT. Integration of palliative care services in the intensive care unit: a roadmap for overcoming barriers. *Clin Chest Med*. 2015;36(3):441–448. doi:10.1016/j.ccm.2015.05.010.

40. Curtis JR, Treece PD, Nielsen EL, et al. Integrating palliative and critical care: evaluation of a quality-improvement intervention. *Am J Respir Crit Care Med*. 2008;178(3):269–275. doi:10.1164/rccm.200802-272O

41. Curtis JR , Treece PD , Nielsen EL , et al. Randomized trial of communication facilitators to reduce family distress and intensity of end-of-life care. *Am J Respir Crit Care Med*. 2016;193(2):154–162. doi:10.1164/rccm.201505-0900OC.

42. Metaxa V, Anagnostou D, Vlachos S, et al. Palliative care interventions in intensive care unit patients [published correction appears in Intensive Care Med. 2022 Apr;48(4):516]. *Intensive Care Med*. 2021;47(12):1415–1425. doi:10.1007/s00134-021-06544-6

43. Rose L. Interprofessional collaboration in the ICU: how to define? *Nurs Crit Care*. 2011;16(1):5–10. doi:10.1111/j.1478-5153.2010.00398.x.

44. Reader TW, Flin R, Mearns K, Cuthbertson BH. Developing a team performance framework for the intensive care unit. *Crit Care Med*. 2009;37(5):1787–1793. doi:10.1097/CCM.0b013e31819f0451.

45. White DB, Angus DC, Shields A-M, et al. A randomized trial of a family-support intervention in intensive care units. *N Engl J Med*. 2018;378(25):2365–2375. doi:10.1056/NEJMoa1802637.

46. Akgün KM, Kapo JM, Siegel MD. Critical care at the end of life. *Semin Respir Crit Care Med*. 2015 Dec;36(6):921–933. doi:10.1055/s-0035-1565254. Epub 2015 Nov 24. PMID: 26600274.

47. Hua M, Fonseca LD, Morrison RS, Wunsch H, Fullilove R, White DB. What affects adoption of specialty palliative care in intensive care units: a qualitative study. *J Pain Symptom Manage.* 2021.Dec;62(6):1273–1282. doi:10.1016/j.jpainsymman.2021.06.015. Epub 2021 Jun 25. PMID: 34182102; PMCID: PMC8648909.

49. Boyle DA, Barbour S, Anderson W, et al. Palliative care communication in the ICU: Implications for an oncology-critical care nursing partnership. *Semin Oncol Nurs.* 2017 Dec;33(5):544–554. doi:10.1016/j.soncn.2017.10.003. Epub 2017 Oct 26. PMID: 29107532.

50. Grant M, Wiencek C, Virani R, et al. End-of-life care education in acute and critical care: the California ELNEC project. *AACN Adv Crit Care.* 2013 Apr–Jun;24(2):121–129. doi:10.1097/NCI.0b013e3182832a94. PMID: 23615009.

51. Ferrell BR, Dahlin C, Campbell ML, Paice JA, Malloy P, Virani R. End-of-life Nursing Education Consortium (ELNEC) Training Program: improving palliative care in critical care. *Crit Care Nurs Q.* 2007 Jul–Sep;30(3):206–212. doi:10.1097/01.CNQ.0000278920.37068.e9. PMID: 17579303.

52. Mosenthal AC, Weissman DE, Curtis JR, et al. Integrating palliative care in the surgical and trauma intensive care unit: a report from the Improving Palliative Care in the Intensive Care Unit (IPAL-ICU) Project Advisory Board and the Center to Advance Palliative Care. *Crit Care Med.* 2012;40(4):1199–1206. doi:10.1097/CCM.0b013e31823bc8e7

53. October TW, Wolfe AJ, Arnold RM. Putting prognosis first: impact of an intensive care unit team premeeting curriculum. *ATS Scholar.* 2021;2(3):386–396.

54. Dasta JF, McLaughlin TP, Mody SH, Piech CT. Daily cost of an intensive care unit day: the contribution of mechanical ventilation. *Crit Care Med.* 2005;33(6):1266–1271. doi:10.1097/01.ccm.0000164543.14619.00.

55. Chang DW, Neville TH, Parrish J, et al. Evaluation of time-limited trials among critically ill patients with advanced medical illnesses and reduction of nonbeneficial ICU treatments. *JAMA Internal Med.* 2021;181(6):786–794.

56. Zier LS, Sottile PD, Hong SY, Weissfield LA, White DB. Surrogate decision makers' interpretation of prognostic information: a mixed-methods study. *Ann Intern Med.* 2012;156(5):360–366. doi:10.7326/0003-4819-156-5-201203060-00008

57. Boyle D, Merrifield S, ICU &PC partnership: Three models in a large health system. Poster Presentation, CAPC, 2016.

58. Anderson WG, Puntillo K, Cimino J, et al. Palliative care professional development for critical care nurses: a multicenter program. *Am J Crit Care.* 2017;26(5):361–371. doi:10.4037/ajcc2017336.

59. Lichtenthal WG, Kissane DW. The management of family conflict in palliative care. *Prog Palliat Care.* 2008 Feb 1;16(1):39–45. doi:10.1179/096992608x296914. PMID: 24027358; PMCID: PMC3767457.

60. Gillilan R, Qawi S, Weymiller AJ, Puchalski C. Spiritual distress and spiritual care in advanced heart failure. *Heart Fail Rev.* 2017;22(5):581–591.

61. Roze des Ordons AL, Sinuff T, Stelfox HT, Kondejewski J, Sinclair S. Spiritual distress within inpatient settings: a scoping review of patients' and families' experiences. *J Pain Symptom Manage.* 2018;56(1):122–145.

62. Davidson JE, Powers K, Hedayat KM, et al. Clinical practice guidelines for support of the family in the patient-centered intensive care unit: American College of Critical Care Medicine Task Force 2004–2005. *Crit Care Med.* 2007;35(2):605–622.

63. Davidson JE, Aslakson RA, Long AC, et al. Guidelines for family-centered care in the neonatal, pediatric, and adult ICU. *Crit Care Med.* 2017;45(1):103–128.

64. Labuschagne D, Torke A, Grossoehme D, et al. Chaplaincy care in the MICU: examining the association between spiritual care and end-of-life outcomes. *Am J Hosp Palliat Med.* 2021;38(12):1409–1416.

65. Donesky D, Sprague E, Joseph D. A new perspective on spiritual care: collaborative chaplaincy and nursing practice. *ANS Adv Nurs Sci.* 2020 Apr–Jun;43(2):147–158. doi:10.1097/ANS.0000000000000298. PMID: 31922988.

66. Flannelly KJ, Weaver AJ, Handzo GF, Smith WJ. A national survey of health care administrators' views on the importance of various chaplain roles. *J Pastoral Care Counsel.* 2005;59(1-2):87–96. doi:10.1177/154230500505900109.

67. Ernecoff NC, Curlin FA, Buddadhumaruk P, White DB. Health care professionals' responses to religious or spiritual statements by surrogate decision makers during goals-of-care discussions. *JAMA Intern Med.* 2015;175(10):1662–1669.

68. Johnson JR, Engelberg RA, Nielsen EL, et al. The association of spiritual care providers' activities with family members' satisfaction with care after a death in the ICU. *Crit Care Med.* 2014;42(9):1991–2000.

69. Labuschagne D, Torke A, Grossoehme D, et al. Chaplaincy care in the MICU: describing the spiritual care provided to MICU patients and families at the end of life. *Am J Hosp Palliat Care.* 2020;37(12):1037–1044.

70. Ho JQ, Nguyen CD, Lopes R, Ezeji-Okoye SC, Kuschner WG. Spiritual care in the intensive care unit: a narrative review. *J Intensive Care Med.* 2018;33(5):279–287.

71. Jeuland J, Fitchett G, Schulman-Green D, Kapo J. Chaplains working in palliative care: who they are and what they do. *J Palliat Med.* 2017;20(5):502–508.

72. Bandini JI, Courtwright A, Zollfrank AA, Robinson EM, Cadge W. The role of religious beliefs in ethics committee consultations for conflict over life-sustaining treatment. *J Med Ethics.* 2017;43(6):353–358.

73. Wirpsa MJ, Johnson ER, Bieler J, et al. Interprofessional models for shared decision making: the role of the health care chaplain. *J Health Care Chaplain.* 2019;25(1):20–44.

74. Wirpsa MJ, Pugliese K, eds. *Chaplains as Partners in Medical Decision-Making: Case Studies in Healthcare Chaplaincy.* Jessica Kingsley; 2020.

75. Balboni TA, Balboni M, Enzinger AC, et al. Provision of spiritual support to patients with advanced cancer by religious communities and associations with medical care at the end of life. *JAMA Intern Med.* 2013;173(12):1109–1117.

76. Kirby M. Alma's story: "She's dying from a broken heart"—Mary telling the story of her sister Alma's death. In: Wirpsa MJ, Pugliese K, eds. *Chaplains as Partners in Medical Decision-Making: Case Studies in Healthcare Chaplaincy.* Jessica Kingsley; 2020:175–184.

77. Torke AM, Maiko S, Watson BN, et al. The chaplain family project: development, feasibility, and acceptability of an intervention to improve spiritual care of family surrogates. *J Health Care Chaplain.* 2019;25(4):147–170.

78. Choi PJ, Chow V, Curlin FA, Cox CE. Intensive care clinicians' views on the role of chaplains. *J Health Care Chaplain.* 2019;25(3):89–98. doi:10.1080/08854726.2018.1538438.

79. Choi PJ, Curlin FA, Cox CE. "The patient is dying, please call the chaplain": the activities of chaplains in one medical center's intensive care units. *J Pain Symptom Manage.* 2015Oct;50(4):501–516. doi:10.1016/j.jpainsymman.2015.05.003. Epub 2015 May 27. PMID: 26025278; PMCID: PMC4592806.

80. Krimshtein NS, Luhrs CA, Puntillo KA, et al. Training nurses for interdisciplinary communication with families in the intensive care unit: an intervention. *J Palliat Med.* 2013;19(3):347–363. doi:10.1007/s12028-013-9925-z.

81. Izzy S, Compton R, Carandang R, Hall W, Muehlschlegel S. Self-fulfilling prophecies through withdrawal of care: do they exist in traumatic brain injury, too? *Neurocrit Care.* 2013;19(3):347–363. doi:10.1007/s12028-013-9925-z.

82. Murray-García J, Tervalon M. The concept of cultural humility. *Health Affairs (Project Hope).* 2014;33(7):1303.

83. Tervalon M, Murray-García J. Cultural humility versus cultural competence: a critical distinction in defining physician training outcomes in multicultural education. *J Health Care Poor Underserved.* 1998;9(2):117–125.

84. Azoulay É, Curtis JR, Kentish-Barnes N. Ten reasons for focusing on the care we provide for family members of critically ill patients with COVID-19. *Intensive Care Med.* 2021. Feb;47(2):230–233. doi: 10.1007/s00134-020-06319-5. Epub 2020 Nov 24. PMID: 33231733; PMCID: PMC7685190.

85. Altman MR, Eagen-Torkko MK, Mohammed SA, Kantrowitz-Gordon I, Khosa RM, Gavin AR. The impact of COVID-19 visitor policy restrictions on birthing communities of colour. *J Adv Nurs.* 2021;77(12):4827–4835.

86. Roy S, Showstark M, Tolchin B, Kashyap N, et al. The potential impact of triage protocols on racial disparities in clinical outcomes among COVID-positive patients in a large academic healthcare system. *PloS One*. 2021;16(9):e0256763–e0256763.

87. Foreman, MG, Willsie SK. Health care disparities in critical illness. *Clin Chest Med*. 2006 Sep;27(3):473–486. doi:10.1016/j.ccm.2006.04.007.

88. Soto GJ, Martin GS, Gong MN. Healthcare disparities in critical illness. *Crit Care Med*. 2013 Dec;41(12):2784–2793. doi:10.1097/CCM.0b013e3182a84a43.

89. Degenholtz HB, Thomas SB, Miller MJ. Race and the intensive care unit: disparities and preferences for end-of-life care. *Crit Care Med*. 2003;31(5 Suppl):S373–S378.

90. Muni S, Engelberg RA, Treece PD, Dotolo D, Curtis JR. The influence of race/ethnicity and socioeconomic status on end-of-life care in the ICU. *Chest*. 2011 May;139(5):1025–1103.

91. Shrank WH, Kutner JS, Richardson T, Mularski RA, Fischer S, Kagawa-Singer M. Focus group findings about the influence of culture on communication preferences in end-of- life care. *J Gen Intern Med*. 2005;20(8):703–709.

92. Gonzalez CM, Deno ML, Kintzer E, Marantz PR, Lypson ML, McKee MD. Patient perspectives on racial and ethnic implicit bias in clinical encounters: implications for curriculum development. *Patient Educ Couns*. 2018 Sep;101(9):1669–1675. doi:10.1016/j.pec.2018.05.016. Epub 2018 May 20. PMID: 29843933; PMCID: PMC7065496.

93. Betancourt JR, Green AR, Carrillo JE, Ananeh-Firempong O 2nd. Defining cultural competence: a practical framework for addressing racial/ethnic disparities in health and health care. Public Health Rep. 2003;118(4):293–302. doi:10.1093/phr/118.4.293

94. Amass T, Van Scoy LJ, Hua M, et al. Stress-related disorders of family members of patients admitted to the intensive care unit with COVID-19. *JAMA Internal Med*. 2022 Jul-Aug;118(4):630.

95. Silva MD, Tsai S, Sobota RM, Abel BT, Reid MC, Adelman RD. Missed opportunities when communicating with limited English-proficient patients during end-of-life conversations: insights from Spanish-speaking and Chinese-speaking medical interpreters. *J Pain Symptom Manage*. 2020 Mar;59(3):694–701. doi:10.1016/j.jpainsymman.2019.10.019. Epub 2019 Oct 25. PMID: 31669199; PMCID: PMC7422717.

96. Kirby E, Broom A, Good P, Bowden V, Lwin Z. Experiences of interpreters in supporting the transition from oncology to palliative care: a qualitative study. *Asia Pac J Clin Oncol*. 2017 Oct;13(5):e497–e505. doi: 10.1111/ajco.12563. Epub 2016 Jul 20. PMID: 27435829.

97. Rosenberg E, Seller R, Leanza Y. Through interpreters' eyes: comparing roles of professional and family interpreters. *Patient Educ Couns*. 2008 Jan;70(1):87–93. doi:10.1016/j.pec.2007.09.015. Epub 2007 Nov 26. PMID: 18031970.

98. Pham K, Thornton JD, Engelberg RA, Jackson JC, Curtis JR. Alterations during medical interpretation of ICU family conferences that interfere with or enhance communication. *Chest*. 2008 Jul;134(1):112. doi: 10.1378/chest.07-2852. Epub 2008 Mar 17. PMID: 18347204; PMCID: PMC2693085.

99. Grudzen CR, Stone SC, Morrison RS. The palliative care model for emergency department patients with advanced illness. *J Palliat Med*. 2011 Aug;14(8):945–950. doi:10.1089/jpm.2011.0011. Epub 2011 Jul 18. PMID: 21767164; PMCID: PMC3180760.

100. Lamba S, DeSandre PL, Todd KH, et al.; Improving Palliative Care in Emergency Medicine Board. Integration of palliative care into emergency medicine: the Improving Palliative Care in Emergency Medicine (IPAL-EM) collaboration. *J Emerg Med*. 2014 Feb;46(2):264–270. doi:10.1016/j.jemermed.2013.08.087. Epub 2013 Nov 25. PMID: 24286714.

101. George N, Phillips E, Zaurova M, Song C, Lamba S, Grudzen C. Palliative care screening and assessment in the emergency department: a systematic review. *J Pain Symptom Manage*. 2016 Jan;51(1):108–119.e2. doi:10.1016/j.jpainsymman.2015.07.017. Epub 2015 Aug 31. PMID: 26335763.

102. Coccolini F, Sartelli M, Kluger Y, et al. COVID-19 the showdown for mass casualty preparedness and management: the Cassandra Syndrome. *World J Emerg Surg*. 2020 Apr 9;15(1):26. doi:10.1186/s13017-020-00304-5. PMID: 32272957; PMCID: PMC7145275

103. Godshall M. Coping with moral distress during COVID-19. *Nursing*. 2021 Feb 1;51(2):55–58. doi:10.1097/01.NURSE.0000731840.43661.99. PMID: 33953101.

104. Malliarou M, Nikolentzos A, Papadopoulos D, Bekiari T, Sarafis P. ICU nurse's moral distress as an occupational hazard threatening professional quality of life in the time of pandemic COVID 19. *Mater Sociomed*. 2021 Jun;33(2):88–93. doi:10.5455/msm.2021.33.88-93. PMID: 34483734; PMCID: PMC8385730.

105. Wendlandt B, Kime M, Carson S. The impact of family visitor restrictions on healthcare workers in the ICU during the COVID-19 pandemic. *Intensive Crit Care Nurs*. 2022 Feb;68:103–123. doi:10.1016/j.iccn.2021.103123. Epub 2021 Jul 28. PMID: 34456111; PMCID: PMC8315942.

14

Outpatient Palliative Care Clinics

Dulce M. Cruz-Oliver and Kafunyi Mwamba

Key Points

- Outpatient palliative care is an integral component to optimize health-care and requires support by health systems because relying solely on inpatient consultation is not sufficient. A combination of outpatient and inpatient interprofessional palliative care services provides the most comprehensive support for those living with serious illness.
- The composition of the outpatient palliative care interprofessional teams will vary depending not only on the settings, but also on the needs of the patient population and the resources and priorities of the health system.
- The independent and co-located outpatient palliative care clinics are the preferred models of delivery (as compared to embedded), given that they allow more freedom in scheduling, treatments or prescribing, and referrals.
- Early outpatient palliative care is the preferred approach because it allows for access to these services early enough to make a difference in a patient's quality of life.
- Current evidence demonstrating the benefits of palliative care is predominantly based in studies of patients with cancer. While patients with non-cancer illness share many of the same palliative care needs, more data are needed to prove effectiveness.
- More research on the effectiveness of the interprofessional team in outpatient palliative care is recommended, to determine the optimal approach to provide supportive care for patients with serious, life-threatening illness.
- Including outpatient palliative care in the training curriculum of interprofessional palliative team members will improve the workforce shortage.

According to the Worldwide Hospice and Palliative Care Alliance and the World Health Organization,[1] palliative care should be based not on prognosis or diagnosis, but on need, regardless of whether the person's care takes place at the primary or specialist levels of outpatient care. For the most part, palliative care teams in hospitals are now the rule, not the exception, because evidence shows their benefits in quality of service and cost savings.[2,3] However, once the patient is discharged from the hospital, or if they receive care mainly in the clinic setting, palliative care is still beneficial to the patient with serious illness. Patients who are nearing the end of life often have hospice available to them, as a mandated component of their insurance benefit (see Chapter 11), and patients with serious illness not enrolled in hospice may access palliative care either in the home (see Chapter 15) or clinic setting. Regardless of setting, high-quality palliative care is only possible when provided by an interprofessional team that includes a chaplain, social worker, physician, nurse, and other clinicians. Palliative care in the community setting and especially the outpatient clinic setting, needs further development as it is one of the most recent developments in the field.

A 2013 survey among 20 outpatient palliative care practices reported that most services were started by inpatient providers when they perceived poor quality of outpatient care.[4] The majority of referred patients had cancer diagnoses, followed by chronic obstructive pulmonary disease (COPD), neurologic disorders, and heart failure. The most common reasons for referral were pain management and determining goals of care. Eleven practices noticed staffing shortages, and 8 had wait times of a week or more for new patient appointments. Only 12 practices provided 24/7 coverage. Medical insurance and institutional support were the most common funding sources. The most commonly reported challenges included funding for staffing and being overwhelmed with referrals.[4] Although initiating outpatient palliative care at time of diagnosis for patients with advanced cancer allows for uniform access to this service early enough to make a difference, the standard of monthly visits from the time of diagnosis to death is not practical in most settings because there are insufficient resources to meet this demand.[5] This chapter describes the interprofessional team within the context of outpatient palliative care clinics, the impact of the interprofessional team on models of palliative care delivery and the populations they serve, and the challenges encountered in outpatient palliative care clinic implementation.

The Interprofessional Team in the Context of Outpatient Palliative Care Clinics

Patients with serious and life-limiting illness experience a multitude of care issues throughout their disease trajectory, ranging from physical symptoms, psychological distress, spiritual concerns, access to information, decision-making, and end-of-life care. These issues intersect with each other, fluctuate in intensity over the course of illness, and contribute to decreased quality of life and increased caregiver burden.[6] Historically, Dr. Cicely Saunders, who founded the modern hospice and palliative care movement, advocated that only an interprofessional team could relieve the "total pain" of patients with serious illness. Dr. Saunders described total pain as not only physical, but also psychological, social, emotional, and spiritual suffering.[7] In essence, to meet these needs, a team of professionals with specific skills is required to assess and care for patients and treat them as people, not as illnesses. Hui and colleagues[8] suggest that the team approach is the best way to provide optimal palliative care for outpatients with serious illness and their families.

Members of the Outpatient Palliative Care Team

The composition of healthcare professionals involved in outpatient palliative care depends on the settings, priorities, and the availability of resources.[9] Professionals on the team include physician, nurse, chaplain, social worker, and sometimes pharmacist, physiotherapist, and other healthcare professionals, who each contribute their unique expertise to support the patient's goals of care in a cohesive manner through coordinated communication, assessments, and interventions[8] (see Figure 14.1; see Chapter 3). Although not an exhaustive list, relatives, caregivers, volunteers, civil servants, and community members also contribute to the overall care of patients and need to be considered as members of outpatient palliative care

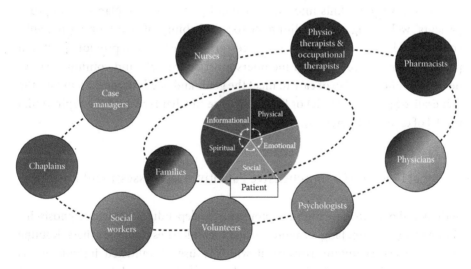

Figure 14.1. The palliative care team is interprofessional, with different members of the team providing different expertise, thus allowing a patient's needs to be addressed in a holistic (informational, physical, emotional, social, and spiritual) and timely fashion, augmenting the ability of family caregivers to support the patient. This implies that the professional employs their expertise in each unique team-based interaction (i.e., at clinic huddle and multiple or serial clinician visits) and each person's contribution as a professional is valuable because it brings an important knowledge base and skill set to the collaborative care of patients and their families.

Adapted with permission from Hui D, Hannon BL, Zimmermann C, Bruera E. Improving patient and caregiver outcomes in oncology: Team-based, timely, and targeted palliative care. *CA: Cancer J Clin.* 2018;68(5):356–376.

teams. This is particularly true in resource-poor settings, such as developing countries that have no access to palliative care. Likewise, in developed countries, most people die in the hospital, but some prefer being in their own homes. Care needs might be overwhelming to family members who have not been adequately prepared for this new role.[10] Consequently, family members need to be considered as team members of the outpatient palliative care team in addition to being part of the unit of care, and deserve social support for their contributions, especially at the end of life.

The composition of outpatient palliative care teams will continuously evolve, depending on the trajectory of the illness and on patient needs. All team members are not expected to participate at the same time in the clinic setting. For example, a patient visit may consist of a single or serial clinician evaluation, where different clinicians of the interprofessional team evaluate an aspect of patient care sequentially, or a multiple clinician evaluation, where 2 or more clinicians evaluate a patient at the same time. Patient outcomes depend on the skills of the diverse team members and their abilities to collaborate with each other.[11] A team huddle discussion of the patient's case may provide the opportunity for interprofessional input when an individual team member provides the direct patient care. The advantage of having different individuals bring their expertise and various skills into the outpatient palliative care plan is to improve patients' well-being and to diminish the probability of overlooking patients' concerns.[12] Having a team does not necessarily translate into providing optimal palliative care, however; team members must coordinate and communicate to develop a coherent plan of care to meet the goals and needs of the patient (see the Generalist-Specialist Model of Palliative Care in Chapter 3 and the aspirational model of care in Chapter 16).

What Does the Comprehensive Palliative Care Assessment Entail?

Seriously ill patients have high symptom burden depending on their diagnosis, including nausea, pain, fatigue, anorexia, and breathlessness, among others. Routine comprehensive symptom assessment with the use of validated instruments is indicated in the context of advanced disease.[13] A comprehensive assessment includes assessment of symptoms, quality of life, and spiritual and psychological concerns. Palliative care clinician specialists are prepared to screen for concerns in all domains of palliative care and to assess concerns within their own areas of practice. One commonly used instrument is the Edmonton Symptom Assessment Scale (ESAS)[14,15] which assesses symptoms—namely pain, dyspnea, anxiety, and fatigue—that are the most significant predictors of quality of life. The Canadian Problem Checklist (CPC) is another instrument that assesses spiritual and psychosocial concerns that are common and can be addressed by the palliative care approach.[16] In some cases, family caregivers also complete a screening tool to assess caregiver burden[17,18] or well-being.[19] The initial assessment concludes with treatment recommendations for the referring providers who are overseeing the patient's care. In other words, patients with serious illness such as cancer are referred to the interprofessional palliative care team from the primary or specialist treating team, such as oncologists. The interprofessional palliative care team provides an extra layer of support, with attention to pain and symptom management and adjustment to serious illness, and provides recommendations back to the referring team for ongoing relief of symptoms and improved quality of life while the patient is going through treatment.

A retrospective qualitative analysis of provider documentation demonstrated that standardized evaluations (psychosocial assessment, spiritual well-being, and caregiver support), symptoms (mood, pain, and mental status), treatment recommendations (counseling or new medication), and advance directive completion were the most common activities documented in an outpatient palliative care clinic.[20] Providers were more likely to evaluate general pain, hospice awareness, and discuss/recommend hospice in delayed (>12 weeks after diagnosis) palliative care ($p = 0.035$) compared to early (<12 weeks of diagnosis) palliative care, though it should be noted that palliative care involvement 12 weeks post-diagnosis is considered "early" in the cancer trajectory in most contexts.[20] Earlier outpatient palliative care referrals, ideally at the time of diagnosis, are recommended to allow for maximum benefit of services. In this context, the question remains why patients diagnosed with serious illness are not referred early enough to the interprofessional palliative team.

Models of Care Delivery

Palliative care is recognized as a leader in modeling team-based collaborative practice and communication.[21] A study in outpatient palliative cancer care demonstrated that the interprofessional team of palliative care specialists in stand-alone clinics remains the gold standard for ambulatory palliative care because the overlap of roles has the greatest impact on multiple patient and caregiver outcomes, such as fewer hospitalizations and emergency department (ED) visits, improved symptom management and quality of life, and overall survival.[6] Palliative care is a model that is beneficial throughout the disease trajectory and can be delivered alongside other disease-directed therapies. This is one reason why the outpatient palliative care clinic must be designed to meet the unique needs of stakeholders, including patients and families, referring providers, and institutions. Literature suggests convening focus groups before implementation and using stakeholder satisfaction surveys after implementation to ensure that the planned or offered services are meeting the needs of those served.[22] There is a need for sustained investment in specialist palliative care clinician training and for scaling of existing effective models of delivery, such as the independent, co-located, or embedded model, based on an institution's needs.[6]

Independent Model

In the independent model, besides having its own space and administrative support, the outpatient palliative care team creates its own referral process that independently evaluates patients and generates revenue in a sustainable manner.[22] In addition, the outpatient palliative care team (physicians, nurse practitioners, chaplains, and social workers) has full control of scheduling the patients and determining the length of the visits by taking into consideration the needs of the patients and their family caregivers.[23] For the most part, the team members meet in joint visits to perform comprehensive palliative care assessments and interventions. The visit concludes with the team providing recommendations to the referring team, which may include facilitating the transition from the clinic to other services such as home care or hospice.

Co-Located Model

In the co-located model, the palliative care clinic is at the same location as the oncologist or specialty clinic, and the time of appointments is coordinated close to oncology or specialty appointment time to decrease travel burden on seriously ill patients. This model follows the same principles of the independent model in terms of their interprofessional team approach and consultation role with referring specialists.[22]

Embedded Model

In the embedded model, the members of the outpatient palliative care team are incorporated into a multidisciplinary clinic. This means that they do not have full control of scheduling the patients. In addition, the space and administrative support are shared with other specialties in the clinic, which presents financial implications.[24] In the embedded model, although patients are initially referred based on the provider's discretion, trigger criteria may be established on the basis of advanced illness and an ESAS score greater than 5 on one or more symptoms. In a study on an embedded outpatient palliative care clinic for COPD and heart failure (HF) patients, the inpatient palliative care team, which included hospital case managers, pulmonary physicians, and nurses, referred patients with advanced COPD and HF to the outpatient palliative care clinic for goals of care and symptom burden management. As outcomes, the impact of the embedded clinic resulted in a reduction of office visits by 53%, a reduction of triage phone calls by 92%, and out of the 57 patients enrolled in the outpatient palliative care clinic, only 5 patients were readmitted to the hospital and 3 patients were seen in the ED.[25] Patients with access to the embedded model encountered palliative care as outpatients more often and earlier in the case of patients with advanced serious illness.[26] As indicated previously, referring at the time of diagnosis of life-limiting illness for early palliative care is preferred. Nonetheless, this depends on institutional resources and priorities.[27]

Outpatient Palliative Care Clinic Populations

Palliative care is essential for patients with serious chronic and advanced illnesses. Evidence suggests that interprofessional teams working in outpatient palliative care clinics are able to meet the needs of patients diagnosed with cancer and non-cancer serious illness.[28]

Patients with Cancer

Various randomized controlled trials (RCTs) demonstrate the benefits of early outpatient palliative care for patients with advanced cancer with regard to survival, quality of life, and mood; symptom intensity did not change in response to early outpatient palliative care.[29-31] Generally, early palliative care is defined as care offered within 3 months of advanced metastatic disease diagnosis.[32] One of the seminal studies, by Temel and colleagues,[31] compared patients with metastatic lung cancer referred at time of diagnosis to a palliative care clinic (following the co-located model with a team consisting of advanced-practice nurses and physicians) with those with standard oncologic care. Patients in the concurrent care group had fewer hospital admissions, less chemotherapy at end of life (EOL), better quality of life, were referred to hospice earlier, and lived 2.5 months longer than control patients.[31] With the development of immunomodulators and targeted therapies, the outpatient palliative care needs of patients with cancer are transitioning to a focus on managing novel side effects, coping with prognostic uncertainty, and embracing survivorship.[33]

Inpatient consultation alone does not provide the same level of benefits as a combination of outpatient and inpatient palliative care.[5] Avoiding terminal hospitalization is arguably more important for those with incurable malignancies, and meeting this goal may require relationship building and coordination of care that can only occur when concurrent outpatient palliative care is available in addition to inpatient palliative services.[5] Outpatient palliative care delivered by interprofessional stand-alone clinics[34] can play a particularly important role in facilitating EOL

Table 14.1 Proposed Oncology Referral Criteria for Outpatient Palliative Care[36]

Criteria		Category
Distress	Severe physical symptoms	Need-based criteria
	Severe emotional symptoms	
	Request for hastened death	
	Spiritual or existential crisis	
Care needs	Assistance with decision-making/care planning	
	Patient request	
Neurologic	Delirium	
	Brain or leptomeningeal metastasis	
	Spinal cord compression or cauda equine	
Within 3 months of diagnosis of advanced/incurable cancer of patients with median survival ≤1year		Time-based criteria
Diagnosis of advanced cancer with progressive disease despite second-line systemic therapy (incurable)		

discussions over time and helping patients refine their goals of care. However, the optimal timing and nature of these interventions need to be studied further.[35]

Patients who meet any one of the criteria listed in Table 14.1[36] are appropriate for referral.[37] Despite the strong evidence in favor of,[37] and the enthusiastic support for early specialist palliative care referral in clinical guidelines[38] concurrent with primary palliative care delivered by oncology teams, referral is often initiated on the basis of patient needs (need-based, or by physician discretion when patient presented with distress or neurological symptoms or other care needs), instead of where the patient is along the disease trajectory (timed-based, or by diagnosis trigger).[35] This discrepancy occurs partly because existing palliative care programs often do not have the necessary infrastructure to accommodate universal early referrals, and need-based referrals are more intuitive to referring oncologists.[35] However, discretionary referral alone, while more sustainable than seeing every patient from time of diagnosis, may be insufficient to identify all of those who might benefit from palliative care services.[5] The cutoffs for referrals may need to be individualized for each institution, depending on the tools used, the local availability of interprofessional specialist palliative care, and the level of primary palliative care delivery by the oncology team (see Figure 14.2).[35,37] The use of standardized referral criteria should complement, not replace, clinical judgement to facilitate appropriate referrals.[35]

Non-Cancer Patients

Current evidence demonstrating the benefits of palliative care is predominantly based on studies of patients with cancer. While patients with non-cancer illness share many of the same palliative needs as patients with cancer, like pain and

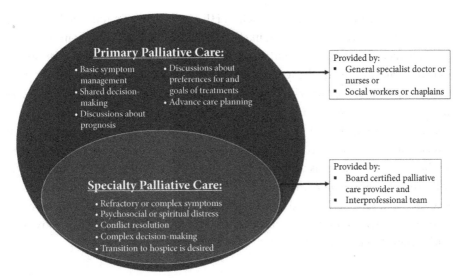

Figure 14.2. Primary versus specialty palliative care. Irrespective of population served by the outpatient palliative care clinic, basic palliative care needs can be provided by primary care or disease-specific specialists, and the complex palliative care needs by an interprofessional palliative care team of clinicians.

Adapted from Chuzi S, Pak ES, Desai AS, Schaefer KG, Warraich HJ. Role of palliative care in the outpatient management of the chronic heart failure patient. *Curr Heart Fail Rep.* 2019;16(6):220–228.

breathlessness, they also have worse functional impairment and higher levels of anxiety and depression.[40] While 3–4 months of continuity by an interprofessional team are needed to realize the full benefit of early outpatient palliative care, findings are mixed in terms of symptoms, quality of life, resource utilization, and cost effectiveness among patients with serious illness (both cancer and non-cancer).[41] Among the reasons for these findings are the diverse structure of interventions (single professional vs. interprofessional, or direct patient care vs. consultation only), lack of definition of usual care in the control arm, and other study design variability, such as the use of referral rather than screening for eligibility.[41] Rabow and colleagues[42] reported that palliative consultation services using the embedded model for patients with cancer, heart failure, and COPD improved dyspnea, anxiety, and spiritual well-being, but not pain or depression. Consultation included a comprehensive care team intervention approach composed of a social worker, nurse, chaplain, pharmacist, psychologist, art therapist, volunteer coordinator, and 3 physicians, collaboratively addressing physical, emotional, and spiritual needs. Consultation did not change ED visits, specialty clinic visits, or hospitalization, probably because consult recommendations were not followed by primary care physicians (PCPs) and referral was time-based (prognosis) rather than need-based.[42]

A recent population-based study by Quinn and colleagues[43] found that, similar to patients dying from cancer, palliative care in either the outpatient or inpatient setting was associated with 12%, 12%, and 41% reduction in the rate of ED visits, hospital admissions, and intensive care unit admissions, respectively, in patients dying from chronic organ failure, such as HF, cirrhosis, and stroke. Palliative care was also associated with increased likelihood of dying at home, where most people prefer to die, and a recognized indicator of high-quality EOL care.[43] The same group of investigators performed a systematic review and meta-analysis in non-cancer illness and palliative care interventions. They had similar results where palliative care interventions decreased ED visits, hospitalizations, and symptoms, though they did not improve quality of life—potentially due to high risk of bias in one included study, differences between specialist and non-specialist interventions, or the possibility that "usual care" is influenced by palliative care principles over time.[44] The following sections explore the evidence behind outpatient palliative care specific to patients with HF, COPD, and neurological disease. Outpatient palliative care can also serve patients requiring perinatal palliative care (see Box 14.1), liver (Box 14.2) and kidney disease (Box 14.3).

Box 14.1. Perinatal Palliative Care

Erin M. Denney-Koelsch

Perinatal palliative care (PPC) seeks to provide interdisciplinary supportive care to pregnant people and their families in the setting of life-limiting fetal conditions throughout the pregnancy, birth, and early infancy.[a] PPC is both unique and similar to other fields within palliative care. Compared to other types of palliative care, PPC seeks to care for 2 patients, part of the time during which one of them (the fetus) is within the other (the mother). The challenges are profound in this population in parental decision-making, ethical considerations, and sense of loss of a dreamed of future.

Our ability to detect fetal abnormalities through ultrasound or prenatal blood testing has dramatically increased in recent decades. About 2% of pregnancies are found to have life-limiting fetal conditions, usually in the mid-second trimester (between 18 and 20 weeks). This knowledge leaves parents with many weeks of knowing of the baby's tenuous condition prior to delivery. This time period can be extremely difficult, with profound feelings of grief, loss of the imagined pregnancy and future parent-child relationship, and challenging decisions to be made about mother and baby's care.[a] They are faced with decisions of termination versus continuation of the pregnancy, how to monitor the pregnancy for mother's and baby's health, mode and timing of delivery, and how much to intervene in the delivery room to resuscitate and stabilize the baby.[a]

Unlike a sudden and unexpected premature birth, miscarriage (fetal death at <20 weeks), or stillbirth (fetal death at >20 weeks), the window of time from diagnosis until birth offers a unique opportunity for interdisciplinary supportive care. Most clinicians who care for these families entered the field through pediatric palliative care or perinatal loss bereavement care. In both groups, the clinicians saw the value of earlier involvement, establishing a therapeutic

Box 14.1 Continued

relationship over time, and offering all the supports of an interdisciplinary team to help families through a heartbreaking situation.

Perinatal palliative care teams work with the teams of obstetrics, maternal-fetal-medicine, neonatology, genetics counseling, pediatric subspecialists (e.g., surgery, cardiology, neurology, etc.), and sometimes hospice.[a] Often, each of these teams has an interdisciplinary team of its own with, at a minimum, physicians, nurses, and social workers. Often, they also have child life specialists, chaplains, music or art therapy, and others. As a group, these teams seek to support mother's health, fetus and baby health, and the entire family unit, including the other parents and siblings.

The large number of people who may interact with these families necessitates having someone as a primary source of contact, usually a fetal care coordinator who may be part of the obstetrical or palliative care teams. The care coordinator uses the guiding principles of fostering perinatal parenting, seeing and treating the baby as a person, and using relationship-based care to create a "safe space" for the parents.[b] They provide a place to ask questions, share their hopes and fears, and to work on a unified birth plan that honors the family's wishes and values within medical feasibility.

Perinatal palliative care is a growing field with many centers currently establishing and building their programs; standards of care are just being defined. There is a growing body of literature and several books that provide significant detail on the interdisciplinary nature of this important and growing field.[a]

[a] Denney-Koelsch E, Côté-Arsenault D, eds. *Perinatal Palliative Care: A Clinical Guide.* Springer Nature; 2020.

[b] Côté-Arsenault D, Denney-Koelsch E, Elliott G. Creating a safe space: How perinatal palliative care coordinators navigate care and support for families. *Int J Palliat Nurs.* 2021 Oct 2;27(8):386–400.

Box 14.2. Outpatient Experience with Liver Disease

Leslie Montes Ferris and Amy W. Johnson

Patients with end-stage liver disease (ESLD) have unique and complex needs. Managing symptoms is paramount, along with addressing psychosocial stressors, mental health, and caregiver and family support to improve quality of life. Providing support with an interprofessional palliative care team helps to establish goals of care, advance directive planning, and stabilization of symptoms. A major focus of our interventions is to determine and articulate an acceptable quality of life for the patient and family.

Patients with ESLD suffer from pain, fatigue, muscle cramps, and depression, as well as numerous complications from the failing liver, including volume overload, episodes of confusion, bleeding, and repeat hospitalizations. Due to altered drug metabolism and the patient's frail state, symptom management is challenging and

Box 14.2 Continued

best addressed by both the palliative care and hepatology providers, and pharmacy specialists. Hepatic encephalopathy is one of the more difficult complications to address and affects compliance with medical recommendations, inability to drive or work, and increased reliance on a caregiver.

Patients with ESLD diagnosis often face a myriad of emotional, and psychosocial stressors. Some common themes that emerge with this population are the following:

- loss of self-identity and independence;
- ambivalence in adhering to treatment goals and medication management;
- excessive burden of care and caregiver burnout;
- anticipatory grief, life impact, and adjustment to serious illness;
- survivors' guilt for taking an organ from another person;
- history of substance use disorder, often associated with liver disease in blaming themselves for their diagnosis.

Given these challenges, our palliative care service is embedded within our hepatology clinic and covers patients ranging from those working toward getting listed for transplantation, those actively on the transplant list, those ineligible for transplant, and those with hepatocellular carcinoma. Our team consists of a physician, clinical social worker, and registered nurse. Patients are typically seen by the physician and clinical social worker, and phone support in between visits is provided by the registered nurse. In addition, the clinical social worker offers emotional support and counseling services to patients, caregivers, and families scheduled separately from these visits. This population must navigate the possibility of transplantation, and our team assists with support and plans no matter the outcome. We help navigate the prognostic uncertainty and manage symptoms as safely as we can, while addressing their mental health and acceptance of the *new normal*. Thus, interprofessional skills are imperative to the continuum of care in the hepatology service line.

The journey of ESLD is difficult for both the patient and family members. A palliative care team can join them on their journey to offer guidance as they navigate the complexities of their illness while enhancing their quality of life.

Heart Failure (HF)

The development and assessment of the impact of outpatient palliative care programs are still in their infancy.[45] However, 3 recent clinical trials demonstrated that structured palliative care interventions may improve quality of life, spiritual well-being,[46] depression,[46,47] fatigue,[47] and advance care planning documentation[48] in HF. However, only one study[47] used a collaborative team of social worker, registered nurse, palliative

Box 14.3. Kidney Disease

Christine Corbett and Daniel Lam

Outpatient kidney palliative care supports patients with kidney disease across the continuum, including those who forgo or withdraw from dialysis. For those who forgo dialysis and opt for integrated kidney and palliative care, this is called conservative kidney management. Patient complexity requires a comprehensive interprofessional team and collaboration across specialties whether programs are housed in the division of nephrology or palliative care.

At University Health, an urban safety net hospital in Kansas City, Missouri, referrals for kidney palliative care come from primary care, nephrologists, and palliative care providers. Patients declining vascular access or dialysis, or those who desire goals of care conversations, should be referred.

The role and skill set of each team member are invaluable and intersect with high-quality, person-centered patient care. Ideally, a medical director (nephrologist or palliativist), nurse practitioner, nurse, chaplain, social worker, and pharmacist specializing in pain management are available. The medical director has oversight over policy, program structure, and often provides direct patient care. The nurse practitioner also provides education and patient care.

At the initial visit, education regarding the program is discussed, including the patient-centered approach to care, appointment frequency, and so on. During subsequent visits, goals of care conversations are held with patient and family, and wishes are documented. Additionally, symptoms are discussed and addressed. Research indicates that patients with kidney disease may suffer more symptom burden than patients with cancer who are receiving chemotherapy.

Challenges of outpatient kidney palliative care include minimizing emergency room visits. Social workers, chaplains, and residents are available after hours for troubleshooting. There may be discrepancy between family and patient wishes, so ethics consultation may be required to mitigate.

Patients who initially opt for dialysis also have high palliative care needs. From an interprofessional team perspective, the structure of the dialysis team shares similarities to hospice and palliative care teams. Like hospice, the Medicare ESRD Program mandates an interdisciplinary team for dialysis care delivery. At minimum, the team must include a physician, a registered nurse, a masters-prepared social worker, and a registered dietician. This provides unique opportunities to promote interprofessional primary palliative care and to strengthen the impact and utilization of secondary palliative care for dialysis patients.

Northwest Kidney Centers (NKC) is a nonprofit dialysis provider in Washington State with an embedded kidney palliative care team model to improve palliative care access. Each team member of the kidney palliative care team serves as a palliative care champion and coordinates with their interprofessional

Box 14.3 Continued

counterparts in the dialysis facility. Outpatient palliative care teams caring for end-stage kidney disease patients may cultivate relationships to promote primary palliative care champions within the dialysis team.

The interprofessional team members of the kidney palliative care team at NKC share similar skills, but also have specific skills connected to their role with the aim to work in concert to meet the diverse palliative care needs of patients, including serious illness communication, symptom management, legacy work, and complex care coordination.

In summary, there are high palliative care needs across the advanced kidney disease population that will benefit from coordinated, high-quality interprofessional palliative care.

Sources: Davison SN, Tupala B, Wasylynuk BA, Siu V, Sinnarajah A, Triscott J. Recommendations for the care of patients receiving conservative kidney management: Focus on management of CKD and symptoms. *Clin J Am Soc Nephrol.* 2019;14(4):626–634.

Renal Physicians Association. *Shared Decision-Making in the Appropriate Initiation of and Withdrawal from Dialysis.* 2nd ed. 2010. https://cdn.ymaws.com/www.renalmd.org/resource/resmgr/Store/Shared_Decision_Making_Recom.pdf.

Weisbord SD, Fried LF, Arnold RM, Fine MJ, Levenson DJ, Peterson RA, Switzer GE. Prevalence, severity and importance of physical and emotional symptoms in chronic hemodialysis patients. *J Am Soc Nephrol.* 2005;16:2487–2494

Lam DY, Scherer JS, Brown M, Grubbs V, Schell JO. A conceptual framework of palliative care across the continuum of advanced kidney disease. *Clin J Am Soc Nephrol.* 2019;14(4):635–641.

physician, and cardiologist embedded with primary cardiologists; a chaplain was not included on the team. After social worker and nurse assessments, team discussion led to specific recommendations communicated to the primary cardiologist and enacted by the palliative nurse.[47] None of these trials showed differences in mortality or hospitalization rates between intervention and control arm. Nevertheless, the authors argue that these hard endpoints are overstressed, while the other patient-centered outcomes, such as symptoms and understanding of prognosis, are often not emphasized enough[45] and more emphasis is needed for integrating the interprofessional team approach. Calls for the integration of palliative care are growing in the care of HF patients, with the Joint Commission and Centers for Medicare and Medicaid Services mandating involvement of palliative specialists in managing patients considered for left ventricular assist device therapy.[45] Several key aspects of preparedness planning and detailed strategies[49] (see Table 14.2) for how the interprofessional team can engage with patients in these conversations have been described with a resultant increase in advance care planning.[50]

In caring for patients with heart failure, shared decision-making is challenging for a number of reasons, including the number of treatment options available, clinician uncertainty regarding prognosis, patients' poor prognostic awareness, the risk-benefit of therapy being offered, and lack of consensus regarding patient's goals and values.[45] Caregivers of patients with HF report impaired health status and high prevalence of depressive symptoms, which are related to patient disease burden. A secondary analysis

Table 14.2 A Team Approach to Goals and Values: Preparedness for LVAD[50] and Heart Transplant

CATEGORY *Team member who may provide discussion*	MEASURE TO BE CONSIDERED	SAMPLE STATEMENTS
Device failure *Entire team*	LVAD failure Transplant rejection	Can we take a moment to explore "what if scenarios?" If this didn't turn out the way you expected it, what would be most important to you? For example, if the LVAD stops working, death might result quickly. We can discuss changes in your care plan to maximize quality of life, preparing for changes in your health, and decisions about potential resuscitation.
Post-procedure QOL *Psychologist, social worker, and chaplain*	Artificial nutrition Hydration	How do you feel about needing a feeding tube long term if you are unable to eat or drink because of a complication, such as a stroke?
	Goals and expectations	What do you hope to achieve by getting a VAD/transplant? What are some things you look forward to doing after getting your VAD/transplant?
	Psychosocial assessment Social dynamics	What do you imagine recovering from surgery will look like? Tell me about support systems you have in place for yourself and caregiver. Are there other factors in your (your family's) life that might impact you during the recovery period?
	Spiritual, religious, existential preferences	What do you turn to when life is challenging like this—for example, God, prayer, journaling, nature, family, etc.? Are you able to turn to that now? How do these beliefs impact your view of life and death, your values, or attitudes toward a life-sustaining treatment such as a VAD?
Catastrophic complications *Physician and nurse*	Antibiotics long-term LVAD infection	Infections and treatment with antibiotics can impact QOL for some patients. Are there circumstances when you would want this treatment limited?
	Hemodialysis	If you have kidney failure you may require dialysis, and the center closest to you many not do this with a VAD. How do you feel about hemodialysis long term? What if you had to move to somewhere closer?
	Intracranial hemorrhage or stroke	If a stroke affected your QOL (discuss varying extent), how would you feel about continuing VAD therapy if you could not accomplish what was originally intended?
	Mechanical ventilation, long-term	If your lungs and breathing did not get better after you got your VAD/transplant and you needed to be on a breathing machine long term (including a tracheostomy), how do you feel about this?
	Review of postoperative morbidity and mortality	The surgeon has quoted a 20% mortality rate, which means there is a 1 in 5 chance you may not leave the hospital. What do you understand about your situation?
Progressive comorbid conditions *Social worker*	Postoperative plans for rehabilitation	What is your current plan for rehab after surgery? Have you thought about staying around the hospital or going back closer to home?

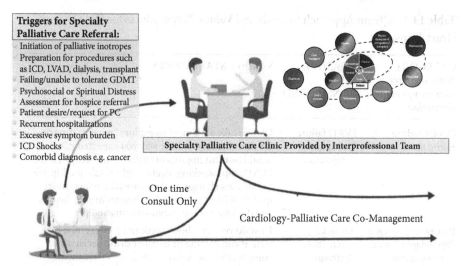

Cardiology/Heart Failure Clinic

Figure 14.3. When patients have one of the referral criteria that suggest advanced heart failure, evaluation by an interprofessional palliative care team is appropriate. Depending on patient needs, this may require a one-time consult or consistent co-management with the cardiology team to provide full support for the patient and their families.

PC = palliative care; ICD = implantable cardioverter-defibrillator; LVAD = left ventricular assist device; GDMT = guideline-directed medical treatment.

Adapted from Chuzi S, Pak ES, Desai AS, Schaefer KG, Warraich HJ. Role of Palliative Care in the Outpatient Management of the Chronic Heart Failure Patient. *Curr Heart Fail Rep.* 2019;16(6):220–228.

of a clinical trial showed that caregiver preparedness improved caregiver confidence, which contributed to their maintaining and dealing with HF signs and symptoms in the patient.[51] To meet the complex needs of HF patients and caregivers, it is imperative to have care coordination and collaboration among the 3 main medical specialties often involved, namely cardiology, palliative care, and primary care (see Figure 14.3). Moreover, the interprofessional palliative team (through serial clinic visits with an embedded or independent model) is crucial to provide optimal palliative care assisting in the shared decision-making and providing caregiver support.

Chronic Obstructive Pulmonary Disease (COPD)

Similar to national trends, few (2%–5%) patients living with COPD receive palliative care and it is considered, along with outpatient pulmonary rehabilitation, to be an underutilized service.[52] Of COPD patients who received palliative care in the outpatient setting using an embedded model with a single palliative specialist,[53] no patient had documented advance directives at the initial visit, but documentation increased to 61% for those who had follow-up appointments.[53] Most of these patients were Global Initiative for Chronic Obstructive Lung Disease (GOLD)[54] stage 3–4 and 72% were on oxygen at home. They were enrolled over 11 months and followed for 2 years.[53] Documented topics of discussion included symptoms (such as pain, breathlessness, and fatigue), psychological issues, and advance care planning.[53] These patients were most likely to experience physically distressing symptoms and the highest intensity of shortness of breath and anxiety.

The etiology of shortness of breath in COPD is thought to be both physiological and affective, with neurophysiological mechanisms causing distressing sensations, contributing to panic and anxiety; and anxiety and depression intensifying sensations of shortness of breath.[55] The sensation of breathlessness can result from stimulation of receptors in the lung and chest wall when central oxygen and carbon dioxide levels are out of balance. The respiratory muscles are unable to keep up with the neurological stimulus to breathe, or an imbalance exists between the distribution of inhaled oxygen and the capillaries involved in gas exchange. The sensation can be exacerbated by comorbidities and deconditioning. The lung and chest wall stretch receptors and the vagal receptors in the neck notify the brainstem respiratory centers that respond by increasing the ventilatory drive. A corollary discharge from the brainstem travels to the amygdala and limbic system adjacent to the "alarm" centers for other symptoms where fear and panic are unconsciously generated.[56]

Similar to "total pain," the concept of "total dyspnea" illustrates the holistic origin and potential treatment options for the distressing symptom of shortness of breath (see Figure 14.5). The concept of "total dyspnea" acknowledges the social, psychological, and spiritual influences on dyspnea and provides guidance for intervening holistically.[57] This approach allows the patient and practitioner to parse out the potential factors that may contribute and exacerbate dyspnea, including, for example, physical (air trapping with obstructive airways disease in COPD), social (feeling isolated and withdrawn from one's community or activities), spiritual (the significance of dyspnea in the existential realm or perhaps "self-inflicted disease

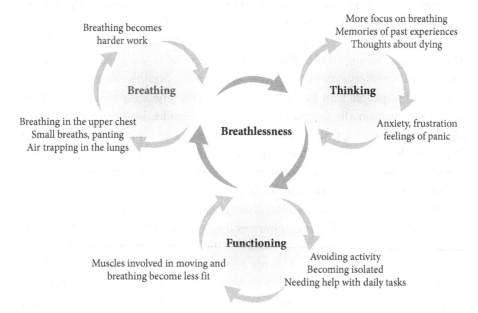

Figure 14.4. Schematic diagram to outline interventions for breathlessness.
Reproduced with permission of the Cambridge Breathlessness Intervention Service.

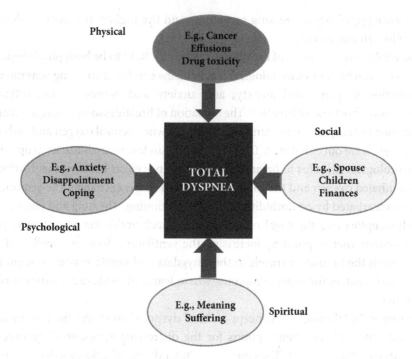

Figure 14.5. Total dyspnea.
Adapted from Kamal AH, Maguire JM, Wheeler JL, Currow DC, Abernethy AP. Dyspnea review for the palliative care professional: Assessment, burdens, and etiologies. *Journal of palliative medicine*. 2011;14(10):1167–1172.

with tobacco use"), and finally, the psychological (the anxiety and panic when breathing becomes labored). Each of these factors fuels the patient's perception of the dyspnea and contributes to the struggle to manage the symptoms effectively. An interprofessional team approach can help to support various aspects, triggers and determine the best individualized plan of care.

The Cambridge Breathlessness Intervention Service has developed the "Breathing-Thinking-Functioning (BTF) Model of Breathlessness" (see Figure 14.4) that can guide palliative interventions for people with chronic breathlessness.[58] Regardless of physiology, people who live with chronic breathlessness experience 3 primary factors that worsen the symptom: (1) breathing: ineffective breathing patterns; (2) thinking: cognitive patterns that worsen anxiety; and (3) functioning: reduced fitness and deconditioning. Although many patients have defects in all 3 areas, one is typically predominant, and focusing interventions to correct the predominant pattern can lead to improvement in breathlessness over time.[58]

While there have been no clinical trials on outcomes, observational data suggest that a nurse-led outpatient palliative care intervention with patient and family caregiver education[59] was associated with death outside of the hospital[60] and a positive impact in patients' self-management skills. Patients described how the professional relationship and availability of their palliative nurse made them feel safe, in control, and influenced their ability to self-manage their lives and prevent being hospitalized.[61] A review of treatments for dyspnea published between 1990 and 2019 revealed that the strongest evidence supported immediate-release opioids, oxygen to correct hypoxemia, a fan directed to the lower face, long-acting bronchodilators for COPD, and pulmonary rehabilitation.[62] Interventions that were classified as "likely to be effective" included sustained-release or subcutaneous opioids, short-acting bronchodilators for COPD, breathing management techniques, home-based exercise, breathlessness intervention programs, acupoints, and acupressure. The American Thoracic Society is the premier international professional organization of healthcare professionals and research scientists who focus on topics related to pulmonary care, critical care, and sleep.[63] They maintain a library of scientifically accurate educational materials for patients and families (see https://www.thoracic.org/patients/patient-resources/).

Pulmonary rehabilitation should be offered to all patients with moderate to severe COPD, whose dyspnea interferes with their daily activities despite optimal therapy.[64] Pulmonary rehabilitation is a holistic 8–12-week exercise-based intervention that incorporates patient education, stress reduction, and interprofessional treatment of any precipitating or exacerbating factors related to the patient's lung disease. Pulmonary rehabilitation and palliative care overlap in many of their characteristics, although pulmonary rehab typically incorporates more exercise training, and palliative care focuses more on advance care planning and spirituality (see Table 14.3).[65]

Dyspnea and functional capacity are important components for not only symptom management and quality of life, but also mortality.[66]

Neurological Diseases (Stroke, Dementia, and Parkinson's Disease)

Neurologists are often viewed as consulting physicians; however, patients living with chronic neurologic diseases such as multiple sclerosis, dementia, Parkinson's disease, or sequelae of stroke and traumatic brain injury often consider their

Table 14.3 Aspects of Care in Pulmonary Rehab versus Palliative Care

Aspects of Care	Pulmonary Rehab	Palliative Care
Holistic approach	++	+++
Interdisciplinary approach	++	+++
Patient centered	+++	+++
Based on patient preferences	+	+++
Family support	++	+++
Focus on disease modification	++	+
Principles applicable throughout disease	++	++
Focuses on symptom management and QOL	+++	+++
Focuses on maximizing functional status	+++	++
Promotes self-management strategies	+++	+
Psychological support	++	+++
Bereavement counseling	0	+++
Formal exercise training	+++	0
Promotes advance directives	++	+++
Spiritual dimension	0	+++

Source: Reticker AL, Nici L, ZuWallack R. Pulmonary rehabilitation and palliative care in COPD: Two sides of the same coin? 2012. https://doi.org/10.1177/1479972312441

neurologist as one of their primary physicians. Therefore, neurologists are positioned in both the outpatient and inpatient setting to address symptoms and improve quality of life for patients and caregivers, as well as facilitate EOL care. The neuro-palliative care subspecialty has emerged as a response to the multiple care needs of patients suffering from neurological diseases.[67] The patient's disease trajectory may be filled with prognostic uncertainty and multiple possible outcomes, such as death, persistent vegetative state, or improvement with wide-ranging disability, that require mastery in shared decision-making.[67-69] The role of the interprofessional palliative team is helpful in addressing the different aspects and complex needs of patients with neurological diseases.[43,70,71] One example of prognostic uncertainty and the key role of the interprofessional palliative team is the case of people living with Amyotrophic Lateral Sclerosis (see Box 14.4).

Box 14.4. Palliative Care for Amyotrophic Lateral Sclerosis

Elizabeth Lindenberger

Amyotrophic lateral sclerosis (ALS) is a neurodegenerative disease that causes progressive muscle weakness, functional disability, and death from respiratory failure. Although there is significant variability in survival time, the average life expectancy is 3–5 years. Patients with ALS may experience high levels of physical, spiritual, and existential distress, and the rates of caregiver stress are high. Palliative care is a critical component of ALS care, starting at the time of diagnosis and extending to the advanced stages and end of life.[a]

Interprofessional teamwork is the gold standard for ALS care and is associated with improved survival and quality of healthcare delivery. Interprofessional ALS centers exist nationwide, and many collaborate with the ALS Association. In these clinics, patients are seen by a variety of clinicians, including physicians, social workers, therapists, and others. While most of these clinics do not include specialty palliative care, increasingly, embedded palliative care models are developing, providing critical added support for patients and caregivers. Numerous models exist for interprofessional collaboration.[b] For example, a clinic might embed a palliative care clinician, (e.g., physician, nurse practitioner, or nurse), collaborate with a larger specialty palliative care outpatient team, or integrate a palliative care specialist periodically or specifically at more advanced stages. While selecting those with highest palliative care needs may be most resource efficient, there is also value to longitudinal palliative care involvement starting at the time of diagnosis. The best approach will depend on local resources and needs.

Patients with ALS experience an array of burdensome symptoms, including fatigue, muscle spasms, excessive secretions, dyspnea, weakness, speech and swallow impairment, and others. Palliative care may collaborate with all disciplines to help with symptoms. As an example, fatigue may be multifactorial, with possible causes including respiratory impairment, muscle weakness, or even depressed mood. Palliative care can also support patients with advance care planning, prognostic

Box 14.4 Continued

awareness, anticipatory guidance, and decision-making support. Longitudinal palliative care also offers important support to patients and caregivers in coping with the challenges of disease progression. Helping patients and caregivers adapt to disease progression is critical to promoting best possible quality of life. The availability of a specialist palliative care chaplain, while currently uncommon among ALS teams, is helpful in addressing existential concerns, as well as providing holistic palliative care and support for the patient and family.

Case Example: Palliative Care Embedded within the ALS Clinic

Ms. A is a 65-year-old woman with ALS, who has bilateral arm weakness, dyspnea on exertion, and mild dysphagia. She has lost 10 pounds over the past 6 months. Her husband cares for her at home. Ms. A reports finding mealtimes stressful, as her weak arms make self-feeding difficult, and she sometimes chokes on hard foods. At her most recent clinic visit, the ALS dietician offered suggestions for increasing caloric intake by adding high-protein, high-calorie smoothies. The speech-language pathologist (SLP) counseled her on altering food consistency to maximize swallowing safety (e.g., soft wet foods, such as adding gravy or extra sauces). The respiratory therapist measured her forced vital capacity (FVC) to be significantly decreased, at 50%, and the physician recommended initiation of noninvasive ventilation (NIV) at night. The palliative care clinician worked collaboratively with the team to explore her goals and assist with decisional support, particularly with regard to potential benefits of early feeding tube placement. During this discussion, Ms. A decided she wanted to pursue feeding tube placement to help reduce the stress of eating all her meals. She was encouraged to continue eating meals by mouth as tolerated and to use the feeding tube after meals to supplement nutrition. She became tearful during the visit and said, "it is so hard to talk about the future and what might happen." The palliative care clinician, along with the team social worker, acknowledged how difficult these conversations can be and offered a plan for continued support for addressing her concerns and needs over time. The social worker also met separately with the patient's husband to validate his perspective and offer support. The social worker referred Ms. A and her husband to ALS Association support groups.

In summary, palliative care is a critical component of comprehensive ALS care. Embedded palliative care offers patients and caregivers support with symptom management, advance care planning, anticipatory guidance, and coping. There are many potential models for incorporating specialty palliative care within ALS teams, and the most effective and pragmatic models may vary depending on local resources and needs.

[a] Everett E, Pedowitz E, Maiser S, et al. Top ten tips palliative care clinicians should know about amyotrophic lateral sclerosis. *J Palliat Med.* 2020;23:842–847.

[b] Phillips JN, Besbris J, Foster, L. Models of outpatient neuropalliative care for patients with amyotrophic lateral sclerosis. *Neurology.* 2020;95:782–788.

Persons living with Parkinson's disease have palliative care needs that begin at the time of diagnosis and continue throughout the course of the illness, including non-motor-symptom burden (such as pain, dementia, bulbar dysfunction affecting speech and swallowing, and GI symptoms such as constipation), caregiver distress, grief, and increased mortality. Primary palliative care refers to essential palliative care skills that may be practiced by a neurologist, including ongoing discussions about patient values and preferences, goals of care, assessment and management of a broad range of physical, emotional, social, and spiritual needs, attending to caregivers, and appropriate referrals to hospice.[72] A clinical trial that evaluated the effect of team-based outpatient palliative care embedded in neurology clinics in people with Parkinson's disease[73] compared to standard care demonstrated improved quality of life, non-motor-symptom burden, motor symptom severity, completion of advance directives, caregiver anxiety, and caregiver burden at 12 months. These benefits were greater for persons with higher palliative care needs.[74]

Patient and caregiver factors contribute to caregiver burden in persons living with neurological disease, such as Parkinson's disease and Alzheimer's disease, and they can be targets for future interventions to improve caregiver support.[75] Patients' comorbid conditions and dependence are associated with increased healthcare use and costs for caregivers.[64] Increases in caregiver depressive symptoms are associated with increases in multiple domains of caregivers' healthcare use and costs.[64] Primary care providers should integrate caregivers' needs in healthcare planning and delivery.[76] One way to detect a caregiver's palliative care needs is to screen for caregiver burden using the one question on overall burden from the ultra-short version and proxy rating Zarit Burden Interview: "Overall, how burdened do you feel caring for your relative?"[77] Activities aimed at teaching family caregivers, though highly important for dementia care, are not extensively practiced[78] and are one of the biggest contributions of outpatient palliative care.

Psychosocial and spiritual support may also be challenging for caregivers to provide as their loved one faces memory loss or decline in functioning. Advance care planning is a process that should ideally be visited many times throughout the course of this progressive illness as the patient's goals change.[79] Interprofessional palliative care team members can support this, as well as the ongoing and anticipatory grief of the caregivers and family.

As part of this robust area for research and aspirational clinical care for neurology patients, the Parkinson's Foundation has a Global Care Network with designated Centers of Excellence around the world. The Parkinson's Foundation is partnering with the University of Rochester Medical Center to make palliative care a standard of practice across all Centers of Excellence in the United States.[80]

Challenges of Outpatient Palliative Care Clinic Implementation

Starting and managing an outpatient palliative care clinic or embedded service can be complicated by barriers to access and by structural factors. A systematic review of studies examining barriers of access to outpatient palliative care identified a lack of knowledge about outpatient palliative care among health professionals, a lack of standardized referral criteria, and inequitable access to services as the primary barriers.[81] In addition, both healthcare professionals and patients associate palliative care with hospice care. Perhaps clarifying that palliative care is beneficial throughout the disease trajectory, and that it can be delivered alongside other treatments, may facilitate timely access and use of the outpatient palliative care team. Emphasizing the availability of concurrent palliative care while still receiving all disease-directed therapies may counter patients' perceptions that the healthcare team is giving up on them.

Despite the advantages of team-based approaches, an Australian survey showed that only one-third of clinics have a team-based approach.[82] The challenge remains to identify the team-based approach that works for a particular setting, and to measure its effectiveness in the provision of palliative care. Since palliative care is holistic in nature, the National Consensus Project (NCP) for Quality Palliative Care Guidelines[83] recommends, at minimum, the interprofessional team of physician, nurse, chaplain, and social worker, regardless of the settings. Additional challenges that compound the use of interprofessional team members in implementing outpatient palliative care include workforce shortages, healthcare structure and environment, and lack of high-quality research.

Barriers to Access

In 2010, the American Academy of Hospice and Plliative Medicine Workforce Task Force estimated an average 12,000-person shortage of palliative care physicians,[84] and the predicted number of palliative care physicians in 2030 will likely not be larger than it is today.[85,86] These findings result in a palliative-physician-to-serious-illness-person ratio of about 1:28,000 in 2030.[85] Estimates of additional team members' numbers in palliative care are lacking, though acknowledged shortages and gaps exist.[87,88] Because of scarce healthcare resources, it is impossible for all patients to receive palliative care from the time of diagnosis. Similar to cancer-targeted therapy, a more personalized approach to refer patients with higher current or anticipated supportive care needs may result in better outcomes. Provider specialists (i.e., physician, nurse, or social worker from disciplines of cardiology, oncology, neurology, and pulmonology) have an important role in providing primary palliative care, which includes basic symptom assessment and treatment, communication, decision-making, and referral to specialist palliative care.[37] Moreover, to meet the enormous challenge ahead to organize and disseminate sustainable goal-concordant care, there is a need for sustained investment in clinician training and the scaling of existing effective models of collaborative palliative care, as well as research to evaluate its effectiveness. For this reason, it is imperative that interprofessional palliative care training include a robust exposure to the outpatient setting with evidence-based approaches.

Structural Factors

Palliative clinics that operate in environments in which fee-for-service payment models predominate will need institutional support because clinics rarely generate enough revenue via billing to cover operational costs. However, in value-based payment environments, palliative clinics may contribute to care that improves revenue capture for pain management, depression screening, advance care planning documentation, and avoidance of ED visits. In both cases, clinic administrators should track data from the time of inception to help support value assessments.[89] To build an outpatient palliative care program in an institution, it is necessary to: (1) define the scope and benefits; (2) identify strategies to overcome common barriers to the integration of outpatient palliative care into serious illness care; (3) outline a business case; (4) describe successful models of outpatient palliative care; and (5) examine important factors in the design and operation of the clinic.[89]

Lack of High-Quality Research

High-quality studies are needed that evaluate the ability of outpatient palliative care to relieve suffering and how the integration of interprofessional palliative teams affects outcomes. Some research questions that still need to be addressed include the best timing, triggers, indications for, and optimal interaction among interprofessional palliative team members and benefits in patients with non-cancer illness.

Conclusion

The interprofessional team within outpatient palliative care clinics is of paramount importance to improve the quality of life for patients living with serious illness. Strong evidence for cancer patients and growing evidence for non-cancer patients supports the benefit of outpatient palliative care using an interprofessional team approach within an independent, co-located, or embedded model of care delivery. For this reason, palliative care training should include robust exposure to the outpatient setting to increase the interprofessional team workforce, and to expand research on the effectiveness of outpatient palliative care clinics.

Discussion Questions

1. Is there currently an outpatient palliative care clinic in your area? If so, what model is employed (independent, co-located, embedded)? Based on discussion in this chapter, identify primary benefits, challenges, and/or barriers facing the outpatient palliative care clinic(s) in your area. If no clinic exists what are the benefits, challenges, or barriers to implementing an outpatient clinic in your area?
2. What suggestions or strategies might be used to overcome challenges or barriers you identified in question 1?
3. Based on your population of interest or expertise, what are the unique considerations that should be accounted for in the provision of outpatient palliative care related to that population?

References

1. World Health Organization. Worldwide Hospice Palliative Care Alliance. Global Atlas of Palliative Care. Published 2020. Accessed September 26, 2022. file:///C:/Users/wallacecl/Downloads/WHPCA_Global_Atlas_DIGITAL_Compress.pdf.
2. Cruz-Oliver DM. Palliative care: an update. *Missouri Med*. 2017;114(2):110.
3. Khandelwal N, Benkeser D, Coe NB, Engelberg RA, Teno JM, Curtis JR. Patterns of cost for patients dying in the intensive care unit and implications for cost savings of palliative care interventions. *J Palliat Med*. 2016;19(11):1171–1178.
4. Smith AK, Thai JN, Bakitas MA, et al. The diverse landscape of palliative care clinics. *J Palliat Med*. 2013;16(6):661–668.
5. Blackhall LJ, Read P, Stukenborg G, et al. CARE track for advanced cancer: impact and timing of an outpatient palliative care clinic. *J Palliat Med*. 2016;19(1):57–63.
6. Hui D. Palliative cancer care in the outpatient setting: which model works best? *Curr Treat Options Oncol*. 2019;20(2):1–13.
7. Clark D. Total pain, disciplinary power and the body in the work of Cicely Saunders, 1958–1967. *Soc Sci Med*. 1999;49(6):727–736.
8. Hui D, Hannon BL, Zimmermann C, Bruera E. Improving patient and caregiver outcomes in oncology: team-based, timely, and targeted palliative care. *CA Cancer J Clin*. 2018;68(5):356–376.
9. Wiencek C, Coyne P. Palliative care delivery models. Paper presented at: Seminars in Oncology Nursing; 2014;30(4):227–233.
10. Caswell G, Hardy B, Ewing G, Kennedy S, Seymour J. Supporting family carers in home-based end-of-life care: using participatory action research to develop a training programme for support workers and volunteers. *BMJ Support Palliat Care*. 2019;9(1):e4.
11. Crawford GB, Price SD. Team working: palliative care as a model of interdisciplinary practice. *Med J Australia*. 2003;179(6):S32.
12. Rome RB, Luminais HH, Bourgeois DA, Blais CM. The role of palliative care at the end of life. *Ochsner J*. 2011;11(4):348–352.

13. Kelley AS, Morrison RS. Palliative care for the seriously ill. *N Engl J Med*. 2015;373(8):747–755.

14. Bruera E, Kuehn N, Miller MJ, Selmser P, Macmillan K. The Edmonton Symptom Assessment System (ESAS): a simple method for the assessment of palliative care patients. *J Palliat Care*. 1991;7(2):6–9.

15. Hui D, Bruera E. The Edmonton Symptom Assessment System 25 years later: past, present, and future developments. *J Pain Symptom Manage*. 2017;53(3):630–643.

16. Jammu A, Chasen M, van Heest R, et al. Effects of a cancer survivorship clinic: preliminary results. *Support Care Cancer*. 2020;28(5):2381–2388.

17. Macera CA, Eaker ED, Jannarone RJ, Davis DR, Stoskopf CH. A measure of perceived burden among caregivers. *Eval Health Prof*. 1993;16(2):204–211.

18. Preedy VR, Watson RR. *Handbook of Disease Burdens and Quality of Life Measures*. Vol. 4. Springer; 2010.

19. Tebb SS, Berg-Weger M, Rubio DM. The Caregiver Well-Being Scale: developing a short-form rapid assessment instrument. *Health Soc Work*. 2013;38(4):222–230.

20. Bagcivan G, Dionne-Odom JN, Frost J, et al. What happens during early outpatient palliative care consultations for persons with newly diagnosed advanced cancer? A qualitative analysis of provider documentation. *Palliat Med*. 2018;32(1):59–68.

21. Omilion-Hodges LM, Swords NM. Communication that heals: mindful communication practices from palliative care leaders. *Health Comm*. 2016;31(3):328–335.

22. Finlay E, Newport K, Sivendran S, Kilpatrick L, Owens M, Buss MK. Models of outpatient palliative care clinics for patients with cancer. *J Oncol Pract*. 2019;15(4):187–193.

23. Azhar A, Wong AN, Cerana AA, et al. Characteristics of unscheduled and scheduled outpatient palliative care clinic patients at a comprehensive cancer center. *J Pain Symptom Manage*. 2018;55(5):1327–1334.

24. Finlay E, Rabow MW, Buss MK. Filling the gap: creating an outpatient palliative care program in your institution. *ASCO*. 2018;38:111–121.

25. Fasolino T, Hollinger W. Embedded outpatient palliative care clinic for COPD & HF patients: structure, process and outcomes (S732). *J Pain Symptom Manage*. 2015;49(2):424.

26. Einstein DJ, DeSanto-Madeya S, Gregas M, Lynch J, McDermott DF, Buss MK. Improving end-of-life care: palliative care embedded in an oncology clinic specializing in targeted and immune-based therapies. *J Oncol Pract*. 2017;13(9):e729–e737.

27. Rabow MW, Dibble SL, Pantilat SZ, McPhee SJ. The comprehensive care team: a controlled trial of outpatient palliative medicine consultation. *Arch Internal Med*. 2004;164(1):83–91.

28. Rabow M, Kvale E, Barbour L, et al. Moving upstream: a review of the evidence of the impact of outpatient palliative care. *J Palliat Med*. 2013;16(12):1540–1549.

29. Bakitas M, Lyons KD, Hegel MT, et al. Effects of a palliative care intervention on clinical outcomes in patients with advanced cancer: the Project ENABLE II randomized controlled trial. *JAMA*. 2009;302(7):741–749.

30. Schwaederle M, Zhao M, Lee JJ, et al. Impact of precision medicine in diverse cancers: a meta-analysis of Phase II clinical trials. *J Clin Oncol*. 2015;33(32):3817–3825.

31. Temel JS, Greer JA, Muzikansky A, et al. Early palliative care for patients with metastatic non-small-cell lung cancer. *N Engl J Med*. 2010;363(8):733–742.

32. Bagcivan G, Dionne-Odom JN, Frost J, et al. What happens during early outpatient palliative care consultations for persons with newly diagnosed advanced cancer? A qualitative analysis of provider documentation. *Palliat Med*. 2018;32(1):59–68.

33. Temel JS, Petrillo LA, Greer JA. Patient-centered palliative care for patients with advanced lung cancer. *J Clin Oncol*. 2022;40(6):626–634.

34. Hui D. Palliative cancer care in the outpatient setting: which model works best? *Curr Treat Options Oncol*. 2019;20(2):17.

35. Hui D, Meng YC, Bruera S, et al. Referral criteria for outpatient palliative cancer care: a systematic review. *Oncologist*. 2016;21(7):895–901.

36. Hui D, Mori M, Watanabe SM, et al. Referral criteria for outpatient specialty palliative cancer care: an international consensus. *Lancet Oncol*. 2016;17(12):e552–e559.

37. Hui D, Hannon BL, Zimmermann C, Bruera E. Improving patient and caregiver outcomes in oncology: team-based, timely, and targeted palliative care. *CA Cancer J Clin.* 2018;68(5):356–376.

38. Ferrell BR, Temel JS, Temin S, et al. Integration of palliative care into standard oncology care: American Society of Clinical Oncology clinical practice guideline update. *J Clin Oncol.* 2017;35(1):96–112.

39. Chuzi S, Pak ES, Desai AS, Schaefer KG, Warraich HJ. Role of palliative care in the outpatient management of the chronic heart failure patient. *Curr Heart Fail Rep.* 2019;16(6):220–228.

40. Kieran Quinn: We need to raise awareness of the benefits of palliative care services for patients with terminal non cancer illness. TheBMJOpinion. Published 2020. Accessed July 15, 2020. https://blogs.bmj.com/bmj/2020/07/06/kieran-quinn-we-need-to-raise-awareness-of-the-benefits-of-palliative-care-services-for-patients-with-terminal-non-cancer-illness/.

41. Davis MP, Temel JS, Balboni T, Glare P. A review of the trials which examine early integration of outpatient and home palliative care for patients with serious illnesses. *Ann Palliat Med.* 2015;4(3):99–121.

42. Rabow MW, Dibble SL, Pantilat SZ, McPhee SJ. The comprehensive care team: a controlled trial of outpatient palliative medicine consultation. *Arch Intern Med.* 2004;164(1):83–91.

43. Quinn KL, Stukel T, Stall NM, et al. Association between palliative care and healthcare outcomes among adults with terminal non-cancer illness: population based matched cohort study. *BMJ.* 2020;370:m2257.

44. Quinn KL, Shurrab M, Gitau K, et al. Association of receipt of palliative care interventions with health care use, quality of life, and symptom burden among adults with chronic noncancer illness: a systematic review and meta-analysis. *JAMA.* 2020;324(14):1439–1450.

45. Chuzi S, Pak ES, Desai AS, Schaefer KG, Warraich HJ. Role of palliative care in the outpatient management of the chronic heart failure patient. *Curr Heart Fail Rep.* 2019;16(6):220–228.

46. Rogers JG, Patel CB, Mentz RJ, et al. Palliative care in heart failure: the PAL-HF randomized, controlled clinical trial. *J Am Coll Cardiol.* 2017;70(3):331–341.

47. Bekelman DB, Allen LA, McBryde CF, et al. Effect of a collaborative care intervention vs usual care on health status of patients with chronic heart failure: the CASA Randomized Clinical Trial. *JAMA Intern Med.* 2018;178(4):511–519.

48. O'Donnell AE, Schaefer KG, Stevenson LW, et al. Social Worker-Aided Palliative Care Intervention in High-risk Patients With Heart Failure (SWAP-HF): a pilot randomized clinical trial. *JAMA Cardiol.* 2018;3(6):516–519.

49. Swetz KM, Kamal AH, Matlock DD, et al. Preparedness planning before mechanical circulatory support: a "how-to" guide for palliative medicine clinicians. *J Pain Symptom Manage.* 2014;47(5):926–935; e926.

50. Woodburn JL, Staley LL, Wordingham SE, et al. Destination therapy: standardizing the role of palliative medicine and delineating the DT-LVAD journey. *J Pain Symptom Manage.* 2019;57(2):330–340; e334.

51. Vellone E, Biagioli V, Durante A, et al. The influence of caregiver preparedness on caregiver contributions to self-care in heart failure and the mediating role of caregiver confidence. *J Cardiovasc Nurs.* 2020;35(3):243–252.

52. Reticker AL, Nici L, ZuWallack R. Pulmonary rehabilitation and palliative care in COPD: two sides of the same coin? *Chron Respir Dis.* 2012;9(2):107–116.

53. Schroedl C, Yount S, Szmuilowicz E, Rosenberg SR, Kalhan R. Outpatient palliative care for chronic obstructive pulmonary disease: a case series. *J Palliat Med.* 2014;17(11):1256–1261.

54. Global Initiative for Chronic Obstructive Lung Disease. Global Strategy for the Diagnosis, Management, and Prevention of Chronic Obstructive Pulmonary Disease. *Am J Respir Crit Care Med.* 2013 Feb 15;187(4):347–365.

55. Chochinov HM, Johnston W, McClement SE, et al. Dignity and distress towards the end of life across four non-cancer populations. *PLoS ONE.* 2016;11(1):e0147607.

56. Booth S, Johnson MJ. Improving the quality of life of people with advanced respiratory disease and severe breathlessness. *Breathe.* 2019;15(3):198–215.

57. Kamal AH, Maguire JM, Wheeler JL, Currow DC, Abernethy AP. Dyspnea review for the palliative care professional: assessment, burdens, and etiologies. *J Palliat Med*. 2011;14(10):1167–1172.

58. Spathis A, Booth S, Moffat C, et al. The Breathing, Thinking, Functioning clinical model: a proposal to facilitate evidence-based breathlessness management in chronic respiratory disease. *NPJ Primary Care Resp Med*. 2017;27(1):1–6.

59. Broese JM, de Heij AH, Janssen DJ, et al. Effectiveness and implementation of palliative care interventions for patients with chronic obstructive pulmonary disease: a systematic review. *Palliat Med*. 2021;35(3):486–502.

60. Kraskovsky V, Schneider J, Mador MJ, Provost KA. Longer duration of palliative care in patients with COPD is associated with death outside the hospital. *J Palliat Care*. 2022 Apr;37(2):125–133.

61. Bove DG, Jellington MO, Lavesen M, Marsa K, Herling SF. Assigned nurses and a professional relationship: a qualitative study of COPD patients' perspective on a new palliative outpatient structure named CAPTAIN. *BMC Palliat Care*. 2019;18(1):24.

62. Campbell ML, Donesky D, Sarkozy A, Reinke LF. Treatment of dyspnea in advanced disease and at the end of life. *J Hosp Palliat Nurs*. 2021;23(5):406–420.

63. American Thoracic Society. Patient Resources. Accessed October 7, 2022. https://www.thora cic.org/patients/patient-resources/.

64. Spruit MA, Singh SJ, Garvey C, et al. An official American Thoracic Society/European Respiratory Society statement: key concepts and advances in pulmonary rehabilitation. *Am J Resp Crit Care Med*. 2013;188(8):e13–e64.

65. Reticker AL, Nici L, ZuWallack R. Pulmonary rehabilitation and palliative care in COPD: two sides of the same coin? *Chron Resp Dis*. 2012;9(2):107–116.

66. Celli BR, Cote CG, Marin JM, et al. The body-mass index, airflow obstruction, dyspnea, and exercise capacity index in chronic obstructive pulmonary disease. *N Engl J Med*. 2004;350(10):1005–1012.

67. Robinson MT, Barrett KM. Emerging subspecialties in neurology: neuropalliative care. *Neurology*. 2014;82(21):e180–182.

68. Frontera JA, Curtis JR, Nelson JE, et al. Integrating palliative care into the care of neurocritically ill patients: a report from the Improving Palliative Care in the ICU Project Advisory Board and the Center to Advance Palliative Care. *Crit Care Med*. 2015;43(9):1964–1977.

69. Mendlik MT, McFarlin J, Kluger BM, Vaughan CL, Phillips JN, Jones CA. Top ten tips palliative care clinicians should know about caring for patients with neurologic illnesses. *J Palliat Med*. 2019;22(2):193–198.

70. Kratzer A, Karrer L, Dietzel N, et al. [Symptom burden, health services utilization and places and causes of death in people with dementia at the end of life: the Bavarian Dementia Survey (BayDem)]. *Gesundheitswesen*. 2020;82(1):50–58.

71. Murray TM, Sachs GA, Stocking C, Shega JW. The symptom experience of community-dwelling persons with dementia: self and caregiver report and comparison with standardized symptom assessment measures. *Am J Geriatr Psychiatry*. 2012;20(4):298–305.

72. Lum HD, Kluger BM. Palliative care for Parkinson disease. *Clin Geriatr Med*. 2020;36(1):149–157.

73. Kluger BM, Katz M, Galifianakis N, et al. Does outpatient palliative care improve patient-centered outcomes in Parkinson's disease: rationale, design, and implementation of a pragmatic comparative effectiveness trial. *Contemp Clin Trials*. 2019;79:28–36.

74. Kluger BM, Miyasaki J, Katz M, et al. Comparison of integrated outpatient palliative care with standard care in patients with Parkinson disease and related disorders: a randomized clinical trial. *JAMA Neurol*. 2020;77(5):551–560.

75. Macchi ZA, Koljack CE, Miyasaki JM, et al. Patient and caregiver characteristics associated with caregiver burden in Parkinson's disease: a palliative care approach. *Ann Palliat Med*. 2020;9(Suppl 1):S24–S33.

76. Zhu CW, Scarmeas N, Ornstein K, et al. Health-care use and cost in dementia caregivers: longitudinal results from the Predictors Caregiver Study. *Alzheimers Dement*. 2015;11(4):444–454.

77. Kuhnel MB, Ramsenthaler C, Bausewein C, Fegg M, Hodiamont F. Validation of two short versions of the Zarit Burden Interview in the palliative care setting: a questionnaire to assess the burden of informal caregivers. *Support Care Cancer.* 2020;28(11):5185–5193.

78. Hallberg IR, Leino-Kilpi H, Meyer G, et al. Dementia care in eight European countries: developing a mapping system to explore systems. *J Nurs Scholarsh.* 2013;45(4):412–424.

79. Navia RO, Constantine LA. Palliative care for patients with advanced dementia. *Nursing.* 2022;52(3):19–26.

80. Dini M, Seshadri S, Norton S, et al. Implementing team-based outpatient palliative care in Parkinson's Foundation Centers of Excellence (COE): study design (P1-4.006). In: *AAN Enterprises*; 2022. https://www.mdsabstracts.org/abstract/implementing-team-based-outpatient-palliative-care-in-parkinsons-foundation-centers-of-excellence-coe-study-design/

81. Wentlandt K, Krzyzanowska MK, Swami N, Rodin GM, Le LW, Zimmermann C. Referral practices of oncologists to specialized palliative care. *J Clin Oncol.* 2012;30(35):4380–4386.

82. Wilcoxon H, Luxford K, Saunders C, et al. Multidisciplinary cancer care in Australia: a national audit highlights gaps in care and medico-legal risk for clinicians. *Asia-Pacific J Clin Oncol.* 2011;7(1):34–40.

83. National Consensus Project for Quality Palliative Care. *Clinical Practice Guidelines for Quality Palliative Care.* 4th ed. National Coalition for Hospice and Palliative Care; 2018.

84. Lupu D, American Academy of Hospice and Palliative Medicine Workforce Task Force. Estimate of current hospice and palliative medicine physician workforce shortage. *J Pain Symptom Manage.* 2010;40(6):899–911.

85. Kamal AH, Bull JH, Swetz KM, Wolf SP, Shanafelt TD, Myers ER. Future of the palliative care workforce: preview to an impending crisis. *Am J Med.* 2017;130(2):113–114.

86. Kamal AH, Bowman B, Ritchie CS. Identifying palliative care champions to promote high-quality care to those with serious illness. *J Am Geriatr Soc.* 2019;67(S2):S461–S467.

87. Thiel M, Mattison D, Goudie E, Licata S, Brewster J, Montagnini M. Social work training in palliative care: addressing the gap. *Am J Hosp Palliat Med.* 2021;38(8):893–898.

88. Parker J. Palliative care nursing curriculum could impact staff shortages. *Hospice News.* Published 2020. Accessed September 26, 2022. https://hospicenews.com/2020/06/09/palliative-care-nursing-curriculum-could-impact-staff-shortages/.

89. Finlay E, Newport K, Sivendran S, Kilpatrick L, Owens M, Buss MK. Models of outpatient palliative care clinics for patients with cancer. *J Oncol Pract.* 2019;15(4):187–193.

15

Home-Based Palliative Care

Niamh van Meines and Susan Enguídanos

Key Points

- Characteristics of home-based palliative care (HBPC) programs and services offered may be based on the individual payment structures arranged by insurance companies and medical groups.
- Lack of standardized payment systems for HBPC programs contribute to lack of universal access to HBPC.
- Interprofessional collaboration provides a structure that is aligned with the mission and vision of HBPC programs, through which successful achievement of patient outcomes may be achieved.

Introduction

Home-based palliative care (HBPC) emerged in response to the need for supportive care during serious illness for individuals who did not yet meet hospice criteria. Specifically, HBPC programs aim to provide interprofessional team-based care in the home, upstream from hospice and alongside disease-directed care. Although HBPC has been provided in the United States for more than 20 years, no standard payment or program structure exists for HBPC programs. In some contexts, the term *community-based palliative care* (CBPC) is used to describe an emerging field that seeks to integrate primary and specialty palliative and serious illness care with local healthcare systems.[1] In CBPC, care can be provided in specialty palliative care clinics, embedded in primary care or disease-focused specialty clinics, or provided at the place where the patient lives. In this sense, home-based palliative care is a subset of CBPC.

In this chapter, we present a brief history of HBPC and early research supporting these services, followed by an evidence-based model of HBPC care. We explore challenges to the growth of HBPC, including variation in HBPC funding, programs, and services, and the impact of telehealth on HBPC. The chapter concludes with a discussion of future directions for HBPC programs. Throughout the chapter, we focus on the collaborative relationships of the best HBPC interprofessional teams and their successes in achieving the goals of their programs. We examine profession-specific and synergistic contributions of the interprofessional team, where members of the HBPC team work collaboratively to achieve the patient's goals of care, as well as to meet the unique challenges of interprofessional palliative care practice in the home setting. See the HBPC case study in Box 15.1, which illustrates the value and role of HBPC in supporting a patient with serious illness who is living in the community and not ready for referral to hospice.

Box 15.1. Palliative Care Case Study

Bill Williams was a 54-year-old man who lived in rural California and was referred for HBPC due to his chronic obstructive pulmonary disease (COPD) and frequent exacerbations and hospitalizations requiring intensive care and ventilator support. He had comorbid conditions of congestive heart failure, hepatitis B, and a history of gastrointestinal bleed. He had significant difficulty following up with medical care and consistent medication use due to schizophrenia and substance use disorder involving methamphetamines and alcohol, and his COPD continued to progress due to persistent smoking. He resided intermittently in a homeless shelter and was a veteran. He received VA mental health services in the past; however, he had lost contact with his VA care team. He had not engaged with any spiritual care in recent years and had lost contact with his mother and sister who lived on the East Coast.

The HBPC team included oversight from a palliative care physician (MD) who attended the weekly interdisciplinary team meeting, monthly telehealth provider visits by a nurse practitioner (NP), and additional telehealth visits as needed for symptom management, weekly in-person or telehealth visits, and care coordination by a nurse case manager (RN), weekly in-person visits as needed by a social worker (SW), and weekly in-person visits from a community health worker (CHW) to check on Mr. Williams. HBPC services were provided at the homeless shelter where Mr. Williams spent most of his time. The SW was assigned as the primary contact as she had developed a trusting relationship with Mr. Williams and was most successful in partnering with him to implement his plan of care. His immediate care needs included applying for disability and Social Security benefits, enrollment on a Medicaid health plan, accessing Meals on Wheels, taking his medications as prescribed, and identifying other resources that were available to him. He had a positive relationship with the homeless shelter staff, and the HBPC team determined that his living arrangements were supportive and stable.

Goals of care included managing Mr. William's uncontrolled symptoms, assisting him with completing applications, and accompanying him to medical and social services appointments. The CHW provided transportation

Box 15.1 Continued

to appointments and accessed food and clothing to provide at each visit. The RN case manager established a medication management system and provided filled medi-sets to assist Mr. Williams with managing his medications. She further evaluated Mr. Williams's symptoms and offered support in risk-reduction behaviors specific to his substance use disorder. Changes to the plan of care were determined with the NP, who had a monthly telehealth visit with Mr. Williams to manage symptoms. Compliance with medication management improved with frequent check-ins with the RN, SW, and CHW who reported back to the RN regarding the expected presence or absence of medications in Mr. William's medi-set. Within a month, Mr. Williams received disability checks, had food and clothing, and his symptoms were improving. He abstained from substance use and avoided contacts who engaged in substance use. His mental health improved, and he endeavored to plan his future, which included advance care planning and completion of his advance directive. Thereafter, the palliative care team worked on re-establishing mental health services through the VA, and reconnecting with Mr. Williams's family to explore the potential for housing, care, and support. Successful interprofessional care to address Mr. William's complex medical and social issues was achieved through effective communication, coordination of care, identification of goals of care, planning and implementation of interventions among the MD, NP, SW, and CHW, which were discussed weekly in an interdisciplinary team meeting.

Unfortunately, Mr. Williams relapsed, had a myocardial infarction following methamphetamine use, and was re-hospitalized. His condition was grave, and he was placed on a ventilator, which was consistent with his advance directive. The SW visited him daily in the ICU, provided a supportive presence, contacted his family, and engaged the hospital chaplain to provide a spiritual presence. Together, the SW, chaplain, and family explored Mr. William's health condition and prognosis. They determined that removal of life support was the best choice given Mr. William's advance directive to remove life support if there was no hope of meaningful recovery. The SW was present at the time of compassionate extubation and remained with Mr. Williams until end of life. The RN case manager and SW provided support to family members, assisted in funeral arrangements, and remained in contact with the family to provide bereavement support. The HBPC team arranged an annual memorial led by the spiritual care counselor, where patients who received care from the HBPC team were remembered in a non-denominational memorial service.

History and Description of HBPC

Early U.S. HBPC programs were developed within managed-care organizations—healthcare companies or health plans focused on managed care as a model to reduce costs, institute preventive health strategies, and set treatment and financial guidelines, while maintaining a high quality of care.[2] HBPC was created in response to high rates of hospital deaths among patients with cancer, heart disease, and chronic obstructive pulmonary disease (COPD). Although home health services including skilled nursing, rehabilitation therapists, and home health aides are usually available for homebound patients after hospital discharge to assist the patient in regaining their strength and managing specific needs identified in their discharge plan,[3] HBPC provides a holistic approach and additional interprofessional support to the patient and family. In particular, a focus on palliative goals allows patients, families, and the interprofessional team to have meaningful discussions about practical treatment and care options specific to their serious illness. For patients in underserved rural areas, HBPC can be provided through telehealth technology, which is described in more detail below.

The first U.S. HBPC programs were modeled on hospice care, with similar features such as the interprofessional team and a 24-hour call center. Contrary to the hospice diagnostic and treatment criteria, HBPC eligibility was developed to increase access to supportive care by *not* requiring a 6-month life expectancy and allowing patients enrolled in HBPC to continue to access all eligible standard healthcare services.[4,5] HBPC focused on symptom management, quality of life, and aligning medical care with personal goals and values. While HBPC is not intended to substitute for hospice care, it provides an alternative for patients who may be eligible for hospice care but prefer to continue disease-directed treatments. Additionally, HBPC focuses on providing care upstream from hospice eligibility, in response to health needs of patients that emerge prior to the last 6 months of life. In this way, patients, family, and other caregivers have earlier access to supportive care during serious and advanced illness. Because HBPC is introduced earlier in a person's experience of the illness, the HBPC team members build meaningful and longer-term relationships with patients, families, and caregivers and focus on treatment options, decision-making, planning, and implementation of goals of care. In essence, HBPC redirects the patient and the interprofessional team to focus on the patient's "bucket list."[6]

Early HBPC programs used interprofessional teams, a physician, nurse, chaplain, and social worker, and research produced robust data to support the effectiveness of providing care in the home, both for patients and for health systems, through reduced healthcare costs.[4,5] These interprofessional team programs are considered the "gold standard" of HBPC, and this initial ideal is the model upon which credentialing agencies, such as the Joint Commission, have based their standards (see Table 15.1 for a comparison of the evidence-based model of HBPC to the diverse and unstructured nature of current HBPC services). In this evidence-based HBPC model, an interprofessional team provides an array of coordinated

Table 15.1 Comparison of "Gold Standard" HBPC versus Actual Practice

Description	Evidence-Based Home-Based Palliative Care Model	Current, Diverse Range of HBPC Services
Eligibility	• All advanced illness with an anticipated life expectancy of 1 year or less • Functional decline • Evidence of recent use of emergency room and hospitalizations	• Eligibility criteria determined by program and/or dictated by insurance reimbursement. Eligibility criteria based on prognosis may vary by program/payor.
Care decisions	• Can continue to pursue disease-directed treatment. • Team offers ongoing assistance with decision-making	• Patients may or may not continue to pursue disease-directed treatment depending on service policy and insurance. • Some teams rely on the primary care physician for care coordination.
Clinical interprofessional team	• Team includes physicians, nurses, social workers, chaplains, and home health aide or community health worker. • Team offers ongoing assistance with care coordination, decision-making, and disease management. • Team coordinates care for patients who may receive services from multiple community-based programs, specialists, and primary care providers.	• No regulatory requirement guiding the interprofessional team • Programs comprise various professions, and teams often differ significantly in composition from each other.
Goals of the HBPC service	• Pursuit of curative treatment and disease-directed therapies, along with pain and symptom management, and emotional and spiritual support. Management of illness and quality of life for as long as possible. Transfer to hospice when patient becomes eligible and consents.	• Goals may include prevention of hospitalization, management of defined chronic illnesses, management of seriously ill people where hospice enrollment is not yet appropriate or hospice care is declined for various reasons, and assistance with healthcare decision-making is needed.
Levels of care delivery	• There is no standard best practice for levels of care.	• Dependent on the structure and functions of the program, which may include home and/or telehealth visits, coordination with specialists and primary care providers, and community-based programs and services. HBPC may be provided in nursing facilities and assisted-living facilities.

Table 15.1 Continued

Description	Evidence-Based Home-Based Palliative Care Model	Current, Diverse Range of HBPC Services
Visit frequency	• Early HBPC trials established weekly visits, minimally.	• Visit frequency is defined by each discipline according to service structure and reimbursement requirements. • Palliative care programs are not bound by specific regulations; however, the program/provider must comply with requirements specific to medical necessity and documentation standards when billing for services under Medicare fee-for-service and/or various health plans.
Payment for services/ reimbursement	• There is no standard HBPC payment structure.	• Payment for palliative care services depends upon pay structure of the program. • Payment may come from Medicare Part B as standard payment per patient, per month, or some programs rely on donors, fundraising, and grants.

Sources: Brumley R, Enguidanos S, Cherin D. Effectiveness of a home-based palliative care program for end-of-life. *J Palliat Med*. 2003;6(5):715–724; Brumley R, Enguidanos S, Jamison P, et al. Increased satisfaction with care and lower costs: results of a randomized trial of in-home palliative care. *J Am Geriatr Soc*. 2007;55(7):993–1000; Cassel BJ, Kerr KM, McClish DK, et al. Effect of a home-based palliative care program on healthcare use and costs. *J Am Geriatr Soc*. 2016;64(11):2288–2295.

services to the patient, family, and caregivers. Similar to hospice care, HBPC services include profession-specific initial assessments, followed by pain and symptom relief, psychosocial and spiritual support, along with patient and caregiver education and training in disease and symptom management. HBPC also provides access to interprofessional team members, 24 hours a day, 7 days a week. The HBPC team holds regular case conferences to communicate patient, family, and caregiver needs and concerns and to coordinate care among team members. The interprofessional team coordinates with other healthcare providers involved with the patient, such as the primary care physicians and medical specialists, to ensure continuity of care and to communicate values and preferences as appropriate. The service aims to mediate early in the escalation of illness among high-risk populations through care management and coordination at home in collaboration with primary care teams.

Evidence of the Effectiveness of HBPC

HBPC has demonstrated improvement in patient satisfaction and in clinical outcomes. Studies examining HBPC and patient-level outcomes among patients with a wide range of comorbidities, including dementia, congestive heart failure (CHF), COPD, depression, and cancer, identify significant reductions in patient-reported pain, anxiety, depression, and fatigue.[7] Importantly, in a study of CHF, COPD, and cancer patients, those receiving HBPC were more likely to die at home than those who were not enrolled in HBPC,[5,8] a positive outcome in light of the fact that most individuals prefer to die at home.[9]

Along with improved patient-level outcomes, early trials demonstrated that receipt of HBPC resulted in lower rates of hospital death and reductions in costs of healthcare, ranging from 32% to 45% lower as compared to usual care without HBPC.[4,5] Other studies have found similar cost savings, largely driven by reductions in emergency room visits and hospitalizations.[10-13] In addition, growing evidence demonstrates that enrollment in HBPC reduces intensive care unit (ICU) days[13] and 30-day hospital readmissions[14,15] and increases enrollment and longer stays in hospice care.[10,11,16]

Early HBPC research focused on seriously ill patients with heart failure, cancer, and COPD with an estimated 1–2-year life expectancy.[5] Since these early studies, additional research has found evidence of HBPC cost effectiveness for patients with other diagnoses, including dementia.[10] In general, admission criteria may also include recent decline in functioning, increase in healthcare utilization such as emergency room visits and hospitalizations, and prognostication of limited life expectancy.[17]

The Interprofessional Team and Interprofessional Collaboration

The successful achievement of HBPC program goals hinges on the collection of people who are members of the HBPC interprofessional team and their complimentary, collaborative, and diverse skill sets. The look and feel of an HPBC program are defined by the contributions of each member of the interprofessional team, and the chemistry or synergy among them in achieving both patient and program goals. The collaborative interventions implemented to address the patient's goals of care and improve the quality of their lives are often specific to the profession providing the care. Who are the team members, what do they do, and why are there wide variations in the members of the HPBC team?

Care management is generally performed by nurses, chaplains, and social workers, with a focus on day-to-day management of pain and symptoms, discussions regarding treatment options, planning, support, and decision-making. The HBPC team facilitates goals-of-care conversations about the patient's and family's values, and aligns these values to guide the development of care plans and advance care planning. Members of the interprofessional team vary widely since the composition of the team is not dictated by a cohesive set of palliative care regulations. However, models of care that are increasingly prevalent based on requirements of health insurance plans include a provider (physician, physician assistant, or nurse practitioner), nurse, social worker, and chaplain. Additional members of the care team include community health workers, therapists, and artists, to name a few, and are dependent on goals of the HBPC program, funding, and other factors.

Factors that influence the composition of the HBPC team include the conceptual framework or design of the palliative care program from which the mission, vision, and goals are developed.[18] Often the team grows organically, beginning with people and professions with a desire to build a meaningful HBPC program focused on a set of ideals and goals, and a targeted patient population that would benefit from palliative care services. Similarly, initial development of palliative care services is dependent on the skills and expertise of the interprofessional team, many of whom occupy multiple roles, take on a host of additional responsibilities, and volunteer time and resources. Despite the desire to build the HBPC program based on a vision or mission, economic factors such as funding and reimbursement influences the successful creation of a functioning, self-sustaining palliative care program. Additional characteristics of HBPC programs are discussed in the following sections.

HBPC Agency Structure

HBPC is provided within a broad range of agency structures. HBPC services rarely function as free-standing organizations. Agency structure is dependent on factors such as physical location, populations served, reimbursement, and the cost of providing interprofessional team care. HBPC programs most commonly operate within or as a separate service line of home health agencies, hospice agencies, or hospitals.[19,20] Some health systems, medical groups, and physician practices also provide internal HBPC services to their patients and offer transitional care services following hospitalizations.[19] Within the umbrella of community-based palliative care (CBPC), both HBPC and clinic-based outpatient palliative care services may be offered (see Chapter 14).[20]

The implementation of the national measure, titled the Creating High-Quality Results and Outcomes Necessary to Improve Chronic Care Act (CHRONIC Act)[21] in 2017 resulted in the development of a wide range of HBPC services, including telehealth, care management, coordination of care, symptom management, care planning and decision-making, and 24-hour access to care and support, care that was not traditionally covered in the home. After approval of the CHRONIC Act, a rising number of health plans started to offer HBPC as a supplemental benefit, with the goal of expanding personal independence and improving quality of care for beneficiaries at home. This act further resulted in health plans recommending standards of practice aligned with the Clinical Practice Guidelines for Quality Palliative Care,[22] along with requirements for palliative care accreditation with the goal of setting standards and expectations for HBPC programs.[23]

Standards of Practice for HBPC Programs

As the numbers of HBPC programs increase, the development of standards of practice, the use of electronic medical records, and documentation of care and services have become more formalized. Standards of palliative care practice were developed by the National Consensus Project and are included in the Clinical Practice Guidelines for Quality Palliative Care [22] (see Chapter 1). The inclusion of HBPC coverage among some health insurance plans has led to the identification of quality indicators which are included in contracts between HBPC programs and health insurance plans, and requirements for the provision of services to health plan members. Quality indicators may include requirements for visit frequency, members of the palliative care team, and roles and responsibilities. Further, some health insurance plans and payers may require accreditation, policies and procedures, and standards of practice, along with outcome evaluation and development of program goals. Accreditation is achieved through Joint Commission Palliative Care Certification, Community Health Accreditation Partner: Palliative Care Certification (CHAP), and the Accreditation Commission for Health Care: Palliative Care Distinction (ACHC).[23]

Challenges to the Provision of HBPC Programs

Home-Based Palliative Care Payment Structures

Many challenges hamper efforts to expand access to HBPC. Despite strong early research attesting to the value of HBPC for both patients and the healthcare system, widespread replication of HBPC models has been slow. This lag can be traced to the absence of a system-wide funding stream to support HBPC. HBPC services are driven by the amount of funding provided by each payor. Comprehensive, team-based HBPC is not covered by the Medicare fee-for-service program. Because of this, for many years, HBPC was provided only by managed care organizations and the Veterans Association. Under these systems, per member per month payments cover all health services, which allows the health system to shift resources to provide care where needed most, including incorporating the HBPC model in the offerings.

The lack of Medicare funding has resulted in enormous variation in both the service and the number of disciplines of professional staff providing care.[24,25] Stakeholders among hospital systems, insurance programs, hospices, and in various and sundry clinical settings, as a result, have all participated in developing the HBPC jigsaw, and now strive to define, standardize, and optimize palliative care services delivered to targeted patient populations in the community. Despite the incredible need for palliative care services, and the solutions it offers to the care of seriously ill patients, payment systems lag and often preclude the unfettered development of mission-driven palliative care programs.

The enactment of the Affordable Care Act[26] created opportunities to develop alternative payment models (APMs), where incentive payments are offered for high-quality and cost-efficient care, such as with Accountable Care Organizations.[26] APMs can apply to a specific clinical condition, a care episode (i.e., for a specific illness, condition, or medical event), or a population, and they served as an impetus to expand HBPC programs.[27] Medicare Advantage operates similarly to a managed care organization in that a health plan receives a per member per month payment to provide comprehensive inpatient and outpatient healthcare, and therefore provides further incentive to expand access to HBPC. A value-based payment model combines a basic monthly payment with incentives for reaching pre-specified value targets,[28] a model that works well with HBPC.[29] Many of these payment models include incentives for healthcare providers to improve quality of care while reducing high medical care costs,[30] such as emergency room visits and hospitalizations—an outcome that is strongly associated with provision of HBPC. This creates an opportunity for growth in HBPC, with increasing numbers of these payment systems offering providers flexibility to provide care in response to patient needs.

The growing body of evidence attesting to both improved patient outcomes and significant cost savings has motivated some insurance companies to develop new payment structures for HBPC.[31] This new insurance coverage has also expanded into other managed care payment systems. For example, in 2018, California implemented as law State Bill 1004 requiring Medi-Cal (California's version of Medicaid) managed care plans to provide access to outpatient palliative care for eligible members, thus expanding HBPC services for this population.[1,32]

The Center to Advance Palliative Care has developed a range of creative strategies around payment options for community, including home-based, palliative care programs. Payment structures range from including a specialized fee schedule within a fee-for-service plan to shared savings and/or loss, add-on fees for typically unreimbursed services, lump sum payments, or capitation.[33] These payment structure solutions may be too complicated or risky for smaller community-based HBPC agencies and may be more appropriate for HBPC provided within a larger healthcare system where innovative payment strategies are easier to formulate and implement.[33] For those HBPC programs serving a Medicare fee-for-service population, limited payment options may be available to cover some in-home services, largely provided by physicians and nurse practitioners.[34]

Variability of Home-Based Palliative Care Programs

Although the Joint Commission has developed accreditation standards for community-based palliative care (which includes HBPC) that mirror the research evidence for HBPC (e.g., complete interprofessional team, including physician, nurse, social worker, and chaplain), those paying for HBPC do not consistently require their HBPC providers (whether internal or contracted) to obtain accreditation; thus, oversight and standardization of services are lacking.[35] Some HBPC administrators lack awareness of these standards, leading to inconsistencies in practices. Even among accredited organizations, service patterns and core team members included in care may vary based on payor. And generally, in the absence of palliative care regulations, accreditation organizations merely verify that the HBPC organization under review is following its own palliative care policies. Therefore, current efforts at standardizing care and quality outcomes remain deficient.

The lack of Medicare fee-for-service payment for HBPC services has contributed to a lack of standardization in HBPC, resulting in a broad range of HBPC program aims, structures, and services offered. Some HBPC programs have been developed to identify patients with serious illness, and act as a guide or a path when patients become eligible for hospice care. With this strategy, the HBPC team focuses on building patient rapport, preparing them for reflecting on their condition, and setting the stage for the election of hospice services when patients have a life expectancy of 6 months or less and the end of life is approaching. Other HBPC programs were created to extend the hospice benefit and therefore require some similar eligibility for service, namely stipulating that patients forgo curative care in exchange for HBPC. Table 15.1 contains a comparison of the gold standard (i.e., evidence-based model) model of HBPC and compares elements of these practices with the large range of current HBPC practices.

Some hospice agencies may offer free, limited HBPC with the goal of serving patients in their service area who may not qualify for hospice care but have palliative care needs. Many of these patients eventually enroll in hospice care; however, each organization must also ensure that they separate free palliative care services they provide from cases where there is any expectation of hospice care enrollment in order to avoid fraudulent practices according to the anti-kickback statute.[36] Other programs may fund telephone case management calls, with infrequent and limited nursing visits in the home, while only a few may provide full interprofessional team home visits. These programs may be funded by philanthropy. In effect, payment systems often drive the structure and functions of HBPC programs, with services offered based on the payment or reimbursement available through insurance billing, grants, or monthly self-pay rates.

In addition to being influenced by payment streams, HBPC programs are also designed around a multitude of factors that guide the program structure. The organic growth of HBPC programs occurs as a result of experiences among healthcare personnel caring for seriously ill patients, and a desire to offer services to address unmet needs. Of importance are the characteristics of the healthcare professions, their skills and abilities to design and build a service line to provide the desired service; and further, the relationships among healthcare personnel who facilitate, cheerlead, and refer to fledgling HBPC programs with the goal of providing access to care to enhance the quality of care already provided to their patient populations.

HBPC programs associated with health systems will often identify high utilizers of healthcare services, frequent hospitalizations, and emergency room visits, and offer CBPC, including HBPC services, during periods of transition, to targeted patients who fit specific inclusion criteria. Inclusion criteria generally include patients upstream from hospice-eligible patients to include those with a serious illness and a prognosis of 1–2 years. Eligibility criteria might also clearly define patient populations by diagnosis or diagnosis group and further delineate those who have advanced disease. CBPC programs often control their growth by selecting a payor source and building their program around the payor source's eligibility criteria. An example would be an HBPC program in a rural area designed around a managed Medicaid payor and the criteria designated by the health plan for patients who would benefit from palliative care services.[32]

Currently, the majority of HBPC programs focus on a broad range of advanced illnesses that influence HBPC program goals. Program goals might be to reduce hospitalizations for a patient population, or reduce hospitalization days or ICU days for the targeted group. Other program goals might include patients who qualify for palliative care, who have a singular payor source and seek primary care services in the emergency room. The goal of the HBPC program might be to connect the patient with a primary care provider, other community-based services, and work collaboratively on palliative care needs. Thus, HPBC programs are structured in different and important ways in order to deliver the care needed to meet the requirements of the program goals. For example, an HBPC program may partner with hospital system departments to identify specific triggers for referral such as patient populations with a prognosis of 1–2 years. Healthcare organizations including acute care hospitals have evolved to using tools such as the Rothman Index to identify patients who maybe decompensating in the hospital, and who might benefit from palliative care services in the post-acute-care setting.[37] A set of services are offered by the HBPC program with the goal of decreasing hospitalizations, and stabilizing their disease process in the community.

Without dedicated funding and consistent services, some HBPC agencies struggle to sustain their business operations, particularly those that are not associated with or part of a larger healthcare organization. These HBPC agencies operating outside of a large healthcare organization generally do not have access to electronic medical records, preventing the ability for patient referral based on algorithms or referral alerts.[17] Instead, they rely on primary care and hospital-based physicians for referral.

Lack of Awareness about HBPC

Overall, general understanding and knowledge of palliative care is low among healthcare professionals and the public.[38] For hospital-based palliative care, where referrals are generated through electronic medical record alerts or by physician referral from hospital colleagues familiar with palliative care services, this low level of knowledge does not impede access in the same way as with referrals to HBPC. Studies have documented that both healthcare providers and consumers have limited knowledge of HBPC.[39-41] For providers, this includes lack of understanding of the services provided, clarity about how to refer patients, and confusion between palliative care and hospice care. This knowledge gap impedes patient identification and referral.[40,42,43]

Consumers also have limited knowledge of palliative care, and among those with some knowledge, many confuse palliative care with hospice care.[41] This is particularly true for HBPC, given the similarity to hospice care in location of services provided. This misunderstanding of palliative care also serves as a barrier for patients who may be reluctant to accept services they believe are for terminally ill patients. Moreover, when consumers are unfamiliar with palliative care, many may turn to the internet for information. This, too, is problematic, as internet searches often present palliative care definitions alongside hospice definitions or discussion, further obscuring understanding of HBPC.[44] In some cases, HBPC is a line of business under a hospice agency, and if contacted by a patient or family member, they may be greeted by someone identifying as a hospice agency.

Palliative Care Telehealth

Many early telehealth programs focused on extending the reach of HBPC to rural and isolated communities. The use of HBPC telehealth has continued to increase for these communities while expanding to other populations because of its convenience and effectiveness. Telehealth is defined as "the use of electronic information and telecommunications technologies to support long-distance clinical healthcare, patient and professional health-related education, public health and health administration. Technologies include video conferencing, the internet, store-and-forward imaging, streaming media, and terrestrial and wireless communications."[45(np)] Telehealth and telemedicine are often used interchangeably; however, telemedicine refers specifically to remote clinical services and is defined by the World Health Organization as "the delivery of healthcare services, where distance is a critical factor by all healthcare professionals using information and communication technologies for the exchange of valid information for diagnosis, treatment and prevention of disease and injuries, research and evaluation, and for the continuing education of healthcare providers, all in the interests of advancing the health of individuals and their communities."[46(np)] While telemedicine is provided by a specialist to a patient who is facilitated by a healthcare worker, often in a remote clinic, video visits refers to the type of healthcare that became common as a response to COVID-19 shelter-in-place mandates, where the provider meets with the patient in their own home using secure videoconferencing technology.[47]

Telehealth has resulted in the provision of palliative care services to communities and populations who would otherwise have limited or no access to HBPC services. The provision of palliative care may be delivered in a variety of ways: through technologies that allow for video, or simply by telephone. Further, some telehealth programs rely on technologies available to the patient (telephone or video interfaces), while other programs send a staff member (a nurse, social worker, chaplain, or outreach worker) with telehealth technology to the patient's home to facilitate the consultation by a healthcare provider, or other clinical staff working from an office. Telehealth clinical care is similar to in-person treatment in that it incorporates pain and symptom management, advance care planning, and psychosocial and spiritual support. These virtual programs have been well received by patients and caregivers, with systematic reviews supporting the feasibility and acceptability of telehealth palliative care.[48,49]

With the onset of COVID-19, telehealth expanded under the Coronavirus Aid, Relief, and Economic Security (CARES) Act, and the Centers for Medicare and Medicaid Services (CMS) subsequently increased telehealth payment to include all beneficiaries, not just those in rural areas. Through these regulatory waivers, both hospice and palliative providers were able to provide care via telehealth, including re-certification visits, and to demonstrate the value of tele-palliative care.[50,51] As a result, telehealth services are here to stay, along with emerging mHealth (mobile health) technologies designed to perform remote patient monitoring, and utilize other technologies and applications for remote care that can be used to support HBPC programs and services.[52] Despite these promising developments, systematic research reviews have identified a lack of clear evidence to support HBPC telehealth practice. Specifically, there is little evidence to support effectiveness in addressing patient-level outcomes, including pain, symptoms, and psychosocial management.[48,49]

Future Directions

The ongoing deficit in palliative care trained workforce and anticipated future workforce decline,[53] coupled with the recent sudden onset and expansion of HBPC telehealth visits, will shape the future of HBPC to include additional innovations in remote monitoring, including technologies that track physical activities, vital signs, and social interactions. Currently, the evidence comparing the effectiveness of telehealth to standard in-home visits is not available, although emerging research explores mHealth technology focused on HBPC.[51] Future directions will no doubt expand the reach, efficiency, and effectiveness of HBPC through the implementation of novel technology sensing, monitoring, and alerts.

Conclusion

Significant evidence attests to the effectiveness of HBPC in improving patient outcomes while reducing emergency room visits and hospitalizations, subsequently reducing healthcare costs. Contrary to the criteria for the hospice care benefit, the provision of HBPC does not require patients to forgo curative care and may be offered earlier in the disease trajectory. Unlike hospice care services, HBPC programs are not funded by Medicare, and therefore lack universal access to care and a standardized model of care across all patients and payors. Implementation of policies such as the CHRONIC Act and alternate payment models have expanded access to HBPC; however, CMS funding and standardized services are needed to provide a stronger foundation for HBPC programs. Finally, with expansion of telehealth in HBPC, more research is needed to understand the benefits and limitations of telehealth services in HBPC.

Discussion Questions

1. What outcome measures offer value to guide the development of an HBPC program?
2. Discuss opportunities within HPBC programs that might address the deficits in trained palliative care workforce.
3. What strategies can HBPC programs undertake to overcome challenges in the provision of HBPC?
4. What policy, payment, and practice changes need to be made in order to increase access and to strengthen HBPC services and programs?

Additional Resources

- Center to Advance Palliative Care (2016). Palliative Care in the Home. A guide to program design. Retrieved from https://media.capc.org/filer_public/5e/07/5e070659-e350-4f7e-83a8-096a7e61e7b8/4467_2066_hbcp-final-web.pdf.
- Clinical Practice Guidelines for Quality Palliative Care, 4th edition. Retrieved from https://www.nationalcoalitionhpc.org/ncp/.
- The Palliative Care Quality Collaborative: https://palliativequality.org/.

References

1. California Healthcare Foundation. *Up Close: A Field Guide to Community-Based Palliative Care in California.* Accessed December 9, 2020. https://www.chcf.org/publication/up-close-a-field-guide-to-community-based-palliative-care-in-california/
2. Heaton J, Tadi P. Managed care organization. Updated March 9, 2022. StatPearls. https://www.ncbi.nlm.nih.gov/books/NBK557797/.
3. U.S. Department of Health & Human Services, Centers for Medicare and Medicaid Services. *Medicare and Home Health Care.* 2020. https://www.medicare.gov/Pubs/pdf/10969-medicare-and-home-health-care.pdf.
4. Brumley R, Enguidanos S, Cherin D. Effectiveness of a home-based palliative care program for end-of-life. *J Palliat Med.* 2003;6(5):715–724. doi:10.1089/109662103322515220.
5. Brumley R, Enguidanos S, Jamison P, et al. Increased satisfaction with care and lower costs: results of a randomized trial of in-home palliative care. *J Am Geriatr Soc.* 2007;55(7):993–1000. doi:10.1111/j.1532-5415.2007.01234.x.
6. Periyakoil VS, Neri E, Kraemer H. Common items on a bucket list. *J Palliat Med.* 2018;21(5):652–658. doi:10.1089/jpm.2017.0512.

7. Ornstein K, Wajnberg A, Kaye-Kauderer H, et al. Reduction in symptoms for homebound patients receiving home-based primary and palliative care. *J Palliat Med.* 2013;16(9):1048–1054. doi:10.1089/jpm.2012.0546.

8. Cai J, Zhang L, Guerriere D, Coyte PC. Congruence between preferred and actual place of death for those in receipt of home-based palliative care. *J Palliat Med.* 2020;23(11):1460–1467. doi:10.1089/jpm.2019.0582.

9. Hamel L, Wu B, Brodie M. Views and experiences with end-of-life medical care in the U.S. Kaiser Family Foundation. April 27, 2017. Accessed December 9, 2020. https://www.kff.org/report-section/views-and-experiences-with-end-of-life-medical-care-in-the-us-findings/.

10. Cassel BJ, Kerr KM, McClish DK, et al. Effect of a home-based palliative care program on healthcare use and costs. *J Am Geriatr Soc.* 2016;64(11):2288–2295. doi:10.1111/jgs.14354.

11. Lustbader D, Mudra M, Romano C, et al. The impact of a home-based palliative care program in an accountable care organization. *J Palliat Med.* 2017;20(1):23–28. doi:10.1089/jpm.2016.0265.

12. Enguidanos SM, Cherin D, Brumley R. Home-based palliative care study: site of death, and costs of medical care for patients with congestive heart failure, chronic obstructive pulmonary disease, and cancer. *J Soc Work End Life Palliat Care.* 2005;1(3):37–56. doi:10.1300/J457v01n03_04.

13. Yosick L, Crook RE, Gatto M, et al. Effects of a population health community-based palliative care program on cost and utilization. *J Palliat Med.* 2019;22(9):1075–1081. doi:10.1089/jpm.2018.0489.

14. Enguidanos S, Vesper E, Lorenz K. 30-day readmissions among seriously ill older adults. *J Palliat Med.* 2012;15(12):1356–1361. doi:10.1089/jpm.2012.0259.

15. Ranganathan A, Dougherty M, Waite D, Casarett D. Can palliative home care reduce 30-day readmissions? Results of a propensity score matched cohort study. *J Palliat Med.* 2013;16(10):1290–1293. doi:10.1089/jpm.2013.0213.

16. Kerr CW, Donohue KA, Tangeman JC, et al. Cost savings and enhanced hospice enrollment with a home-based palliative care program implemented as a hospice-private payer partnership. *J Palliat Med.* 2014;17(12):1328–1335. doi:10.1089/jpm.2014.0184.

17. Kerr K. Community-Based Model Programs for the Seriously Ill. Gordon and Betty Moore Foundation website. May 2017. Accessed December 9, 2020. https://www.moore.org/docs/default-source/patient-care-/report-model-programs-for-the-seriously-ill-may-2017-dls.pdf?sfvrsn=529b6c0c_2.

18. Weng K, Shearer J, Grangaard Johnson L. Developing successful palliative care teams in rural communities: a facilitated process. *J Palliat Med.* 2022 May;25(5):734–741. doi:10.1089/jpm.2021.0287. Epub 2021 Nov 11. PMID: 34762493; PMCID: PMC9081037.

19. Finken JS, Clark K, Ryan D, Shea L. The Joint Community Based Palliative Care Certification: lesson learned. (n.d.) Accessed December 9, 2020. https://www.jointcommission.org/-/media/deprecated-unorganized/imported-assets/tjc/system-folders/assetmanager/cbpc_lessons_learned_webinar_final__10_20_16pdf.pdf?db=web&hash=0684ADAB2935649EF547BAFB36932CE8.

20. CAPC. Mapping community palliative care: A snapshot. 2019. https://www.capc.org/documents/download/700/.

21. 115th Congress. Creating High-Quality Results and Outcomes Necessary to Improve Chronic (CHRONIC) Care Act of 2017. https://www.congress.gov/bill/115th-congress/senate-bill/870.

22. Ferrell BR, Twaddle ML, Melnick A, Meier DE. National Consensus Project clinical practice guidelines for quality palliative care guidelines, 4th edition. *J Palliat Med.* 2018;21(12):1684–1689. doi:10.1089/jpm.2018.0431.

23. NHPCO. Palliative Care Certification and Accreditation. 2020. Accessed December 9, 2020. https://www.nhpco.org/palliative-care-overview/palliative-care-accreditation/.

24. Rahman AN, Rahman M. Home-based palliative care: toward a balanced care design. *J Palliat Med.* 2019;22(10):1274–1280. doi:10.1089/jpm.2019.0031.

25. Rahman A, Enguidanos S. Paving pathways on proven ground: the future of home-based palliative care. *J Palliat Med.* 2016;19(4):354–355. doi:10.1089/jpm.2015.0540

26. Affordable Care Act. https://www.healthcare.gov/glossary/affordable-care-act/.

27. APMs Overview. https://qpp.cms.gov/apms/overview.

28. Cattel D, Eijkenaar F, Schut FT. Value-based provider payment: towards a theoretically preferred design. *Health Econ Policy Law.* 2020 Jan;15(1):94–112. doi:10.1017/S1744133118000397. Epub 2018 Sep 27. PMID: 30259825.

29. Bernstein RH, Singh LA. A value-based payment model for palliative care: an analysis of savings and return on investment. *J Ambul Care Manage.* 2019 Jan–Mar;42(1):66–73. doi:10.1097/JAC.0000000000000259. PMID: 30499902.

30. Mandal AK, Tagomori GK, Felix RV, Howell SC. Value-based contracting innovated Medicare Advantage healthcare delivery and improved survival. *Am J Manag Care.* 2017 Feb 1;23(2):e41–e49. PMID: 28245661.

31. California Healthcare Foundation. Five ways to pay: palliative care payment options for plans and providers. September 2015. Accessed December 9, 2020. https://www.chcf.org/wp-content/uploads/2017/12/PDF-FiveWaysPayPalliativeCare.pdf.

32. Kennedy W, Hardin L, Kinderman A, Meier D, Loughnane J, Volandes A. Five strategies to expand palliative care in safety-net populations. *NEJM Catalyst Innovations in Care Delivery,* 2020;1(2): doi:10.1056/CAT.20.0004.

33. Center to Advance Palliative Care. Payment arrangement options for community-based palliative care. (n.d.). Accessed December 9, 2020. https://media.capc.org/filer_public/99/1f/991fb17f-72c0-4cda-b432-4d17cb2728cd/payment_accelerator_payment_arrangement_options.pdf.

34. Acevedo J. Documentation & Coding Handbook: Palliative Care. California Health Care Foundation. 2019. Accessed December 9, 2020. https://www.chcf.org/wp-content/uploads/2019/05/DocumentationCodingHandbookPalliativeCare.pdf.

35. Bowman BA, Twohig JS, Meier DE. Overcoming barriers to growth in home-based palliative care. *J Palliat Med.* 2019;22(4):408–412. doi:10.1089/jpm.2018.0478.

36. Office of Inspector General. Fraud & Abuse Laws. HHS.gov. https://oig.hhs.gov/compliance/physician-education/fraud-abuse-laws/.

37. Chan A, Rout A, Adamo C, Lev I, Yu A, Miller K. Palliative referrals in advanced cancer patients: utilizing the Supportive and Palliative Care Indicators Tool and Rothman Index. *Am J Hosp Palliat Care.* 2022;39(2):164–168. https://doi.org/10.1177/10499091211017873

38. Patel A, Deo S, Bhatnagar S. A survey of medical professionals in an apex tertiary care hospital to assess awareness, interest, practices, and knowledge in palliative care: a descriptive cross-sectional study. *Indian J Palliat Care.* 2019;25(2):172–180. https://doi.org/10.4103/IJPC.IJPC_191_18.

39. Cardenas V, Rahman A, Zhu Y, Enguídanos S. Reluctance to accept palliative care and recommendations for improvement: findings from semi-structured interviews with patients and caregivers. *Am J Hosp Palliat Med.* 2021;39(2):189–195. https://doi.org/10.1177/10499091211012605.

40. Enguidanos S, Cardenas V, Wenceslao M, et al. Health care provider barriers to patient referral to palliative care. *Am J Hosp Palliat Med.* 2021;38(9):1112–1119.

41. Zhu Y, Enguidanos S. When patients say they know about palliative care, how much do they really understand? *J Pain Symptom Manage.* 2019;58(3):460–464.

42. Birch D, Draper J. A critical literature review exploring the challenges of delivering effective palliative care to older people with dementia. *J Clin Nurs.* 2008;17(9):1144–1163. doi:10.1111/j.1365-2702.2007.02220.x.

43. Fadul N, Elsayem A, Palmer JL, et al. Supportive versus palliative care: what's in a name? A survey of medical oncologists and midlevel providers at a comprehensive cancer center. *Cancer.* 2009;115(9):2013–2021. doi:10.1002/cncr.24206.

44. Liu M, Cardenas V, Zhu Y, Enguidanos S. YouTube videos as a source of palliative care education: a review. *J Palliat Med.* 2019;22(12):1568–1573. doi:10.1089/jpm.2019.0047.

45. HealthIT.gov. What is telehealth? How is telehealth different from telemedicine? (n.d.). Accessed December 9, 2020. https://www.healthit.gov/faq/what-telehealth-how-telehealth-different-telemedicine.
46. World Health Organization. Telemedicine: Opportunities and developments in Member States. Report on the second global survey on eHealth. 2010. Accessed December 9, 2020. https://www.who.int/goe/publications/goe_telemedicine_2010.pdf.
47. Leventhal, R. Telehealth and COVID-19: Industry Experts Answer Key Questions. Healthcare Innovations. Accessed December 9, 2020. https://www.hcinnovationgroup.com/covid-19/article/21131066/telehealth-and-covid19-industry-experts-answer-key-questions.
48. Hancock S, Preston N, Jones H, Gadoud A. Telehealth in palliative care is being described but not evaluated: a systematic review. *BMC Palliat Care.* 2019;18(1):114. doi:10.1186/s12904-019-0495-5.
49. Steindal SA, Nes AAG, Godskesen TE, et al. Patients' experiences of telehealth in palliative home care: scoping review. *J Med Internet Res.* 2020;22(5):e16218. doi:10.2196/16218.
50. Center for Medicare & Medicaid Services. Hospice: CMS flexibilities to fight COVID-19. November 4, 2020. Accessed December 9, 2020. https://www.cms.gov/files/document/covid-hospices.pdf.
51. Padmanabhan, P. How the COVID-19 pandemic is reshaping healthcare with technology. *CIO Magazine.* March 27, 2020. Accessed December 9, 2020. https://www.cio.com/article/3534499/how-the-covid-19-pandemic-is-reshaping-healthcare-with-technology.html.
52. Park Y-T. Emerging new era of mobile health technologies. *Healthc Inform Res.* 2016 Oct; 22(4): 253–254.
53. Kamal AH, Wolf SP, Troy J, et al. Policy changes key to promoting sustainability and growth of the specialty palliative care workforce. *Health Aff (Millwood).* 2019;38(6):910–918. doi:10.1377/hlthaff.2019.00018.

16

Interprofessional Palliative Care Philosophy as Standard Care across Settings

Amanda J. Kirkpatrick and Stephanie W. Chow

Key Points

- While there are a number of profession-specific theoretical models that align with palliative care philosophy and practice, there is an absence of theoretical literature providing a holistic interprofessional lens.
- A clear and unified model for interprofessional palliative care would assist in establishing primary palliative care philosophy as standard care across settings.
- The "5C" skill set for quality relationship-centered care delivery requires interprofessional team members who are competent, cognizant, communicative, collaborative, and compassionate.
- The primary expected outcome of interprofessional palliative care is well-being for the patient, family/caregiver, and interprofessional care team, achieved through 5 team attributes: personalized, holistic, harmonious, reciprocal, and versatile care delivery.
- We must mobilize the transition to relationship-centered care as a lifestyle and adopt interprofessional palliative care philosophy as standard care for all patients.

Introduction

What if palliative care was perceived as more than a series of advance care planning conversations and instead adopted as a complete lifestyle? What if palliative care was in our water? What if mindfulness of palliative care was pervasive in everyday life? How would this change current practices in interprofessional palliative care? Current practices in healthcare? As the life span of the human population increases, coupled with the sustaining abilities of advanced and improved modern medical knowledge and technology, individuals are living longer with chronic conditions beyond what was previously possible.

Living with chronic or serious illness presents many challenges, and palliative care is an important and fundamental tenet to living a full and quality life. Palliative care has been advocated as a "human right"[1] and should be embedded into daily practice for individuals living with serious illness to ensure optimal living. In fact, we aspire to expand interprofessional palliative care philosophy and application beyond serious illness care, to care coordination of persons with multiple comorbidities and their families. Suffering can occur in multiple domains, is encountered in any care setting, and may begin as early as diagnosis with a serious or chronic illness. Palliative care should be implemented earlier in illness trajectories, moving beyond symptom management to address suffering encountered with complex physical, psychosocial, spiritual, and cultural issues. In transitioning to this aspirational paradigm, we provide a specific skill set for interprofessional team members and a description of the characteristics inherent to quality interprofessional palliative care delivery.

However, the number of palliative care specialists is not sufficient to meet the demand of this world's changing demographic.[2-4] Additionally, many existing teams are limited by providing only select domains of palliative care, without the benefit of a full interprofessional team. These challenges call for creative solutions to meet the growing demand. This chapter provides a concept analysis of interprofessional palliative care and outlines a theoretical model as a visual framework for implementing palliative care as standard care across settings. *This concept analysis and theoretical model generate further understanding of primary palliative care theory that can be used in the education and expansion of palliative, relationship-centered, care delivery as standard care across professions, settings, trajectories, and the life span.*

Current Palliative Care and an Aspirational Future

Ideally, love and relief of suffering are the very essence of healthcare. By love, we are referring to professional love, or the emotional relationship that the health professional enters into with a patient that promotes quality of care while providing a sense of fulfillment that outweighs the burden of providing care.[5] In traditional training for the healthcare field, goals focus on finding a cure or a "fix" to systematic failures. Rather, the primary goal of each interprofessional team member, regardless of healthcare field or professional role (including the patient and their support system), should be to improve the quality of life of the patient. To achieve this aim, these individuals must agree to enter a relationship where achieving optimal health and function is central.[6] In this relationship the patient works with the healthcare team to define what optimal health and function means to them.

Palliative care is an exemplary model of relationship-centered care that is focused on achieving optimal well-being for the patient, as defined by the patient.[7] In both specialty and primary palliative care, these principles are central, as the focus is on addressing multiple, comorbid sources of suffering, mapping patient values, and establishing goals of care to achieve greater quality of life. Primary palliative care can be delivered at any encounter with a health professional. Primary palliative care, or palliative care delivered by generalist health professionals who have not specialized in palliative care, is the quintessential relationship-centered care delivery model that transcends the boundaries of age, disease, specialty, and even death. It stands to reason, then, that palliative care philosophy should be adopted as a standard interprofessional care model across settings, including and beyond advanced illness, from birth through survivorship or end of life and bereavement, and to address sources of suffering in all domains of care (physical, psychological, social, spiritual, and cultural).

While not all chronic disease is classified as serious or advanced illness, there are many chronic diseases that increase risk of serious illness or trigger sources of suffering in more than one domain as the disease progresses. Once palliative care philosophy and its benefits are understood by generalist health professionals, it can, and should, be easily infused into all primary care of chronically and seriously ill patients early in their illness trajectory. While some primary care providers may think they are already providing palliative care to these populations, evidence suggests that further education is needed to promote this cultural shift.[1] Adoption of primary palliative care as a lifestyle, or as a standard of care, requires demonstrated understanding and abilities in primary palliative care as a baseline competence for all interprofessional team members. Thus, this philosophy must be learned by all clinicians and any discipline[†] that has the potential to impact the quality of life of the patient.[8,9]

The palliative care concept is thought to have originated in religion and nursing care,[8] and has since expanded to other realms of healthcare as specialist palliative care: in the medical specialty itself and integrated into supportive cardiology, oncology, and pediatrics, to name a few.[10,11] The philosophical shift in focus from quantity of years to quality of life has gained prominence with the aging population demographic. "What Matters Most" to a patient is now an important piece of the Institute for Healthcare Improvement–led Age-Friendly Health System's initiative to describe geriatric medicine to non-geriatricians, placing a patient's life values and motivations at the forefront of health discussions.[12] Additionally, catastrophic events such as the pandemic of SARS-CoV-2 has prompted patients and families to further recognize the need for exploring and discussing an individual's end-of-life

---

[†] Although often used interchangeably, "discipline" refers to a branch of knowledge, while "profession" refers to an occupation that requires special education and/or prolonged training and a formal qualification. In this book, we have attempted to standardize the use of the term "profession" when referring to occupations such as chaplaincy, medicine, nursing, and social work, but occasionally the term "discipline" is used, especially when focused on the theory and knowledge development of the professions.

goals of care and life values.[13] Challenging conversations that had previously been pushed off for "another time" now take on greater urgency.

Figure 16.1 displays palliative care models of the past, present, and an aspirational future. The past and present models demonstrate the relationship between life-prolonging care and hospice and palliative care delivery.[14] As modern medicine increasingly embraces the concept of palliative care, this care model should continue to be promoted in the everyday setting. A vision for the future of palliative care illustrates a paradigm shift, where palliative care philosophy becomes standard care for patients with chronic or serious illness and suffering, even during periods of optimal health, to promote continued well-being. Beyond this, however, we propose palliative care as a lifestyle, one that extends beyond the healthcare system and includes both clinician (all members of the healthcare team) and non-clinician team members (described below).

Care is a result of human relationships, and the network of relationships that impact patient care extend beyond obvious relationships directly with the patient.[15,16] Non-clinician team members include individuals with indirect relationships that impact care delivery, like housekeeping and food services, or that influence access to care and social determinants of health, like education, technology, health policy, and community resources. These relationships should be considered as part of the collective whole.[16] Any part of care delivery (i.e., any professional role that involves human life) has a palliative component. Dyess and colleagues refer to this as the "continuum of living and healing,"[7] describing interprofessional palliative care as

PALLIATIVE CARE MODELS

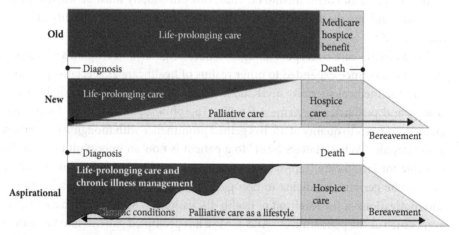

Figure 16.1. "What if palliative care was not a series of advanced care planning conversations, but a complete lifestyle?"

Reprinted from Journal of Pain and Symptom Management, 24/2, Ferris, F.D.; Balfour, H.M.; Bowen, K.; Farley, J.; Hardwick, M.; Lamontagne, C.; Lundy, M.; Syme, A.; West, P.J., A Model to Guide Patient and Family Care Based on Nationally Accepted Principles and Norms of Practice, 106-123, ©2002. Modified with permission from Elsevier. In the aspirational model, the sine wave to demonstrate peaks and troughs in the palliative support required during exacerbation and remission periods of life-prolonging care and chronic illness management.

a synergistic and unified approach where all collaborators put forth shared effort to achieve optimal patient care. These collaborators include unique disciplines and integrative therapies that may at times be overlooked, like music and pet therapy, and non-health professionals like volunteers, lawyers, researchers, law enforcement, and corrections personnel. Everyone has a potential role and should feel empowered to promote palliative care philosophy despite discipline and setting, with contributions flowing freely and synergistically. Palliative care, as an expectation of general healthcare and modern living for persons with chronic or serious illness, would facilitate the seamless flow of conversations between patients, families, and healthcare personnel in discussions of life goals and values, allowing for a natural centering of a person's care at all times.

Philosophical Exploration

Palliative care as a philosophy of care delivery is an intuitive and humanistic approach that results in enhanced and efficient care delivery and improves quality of life for all. In today's healthcare system, high-quality care is an expectation, not just an objective. To achieve commitment to quality, one must begin with sufficient knowledge.[15] Adequate knowledge in a profession is derived from theory, so identifying and articulating an interprofessional framework for primary palliative care practice is important. Having a guiding model promotes standardized and systematic care and enhances each profession. While there are a number of profession-specific theoretical models that align with palliative care philosophy and practice—including many in nursing (Desbiens's Shared Theory of Palliative Care, Kirkpatrick's CHAARM Concept Model, and Watson's Human Caring Theory)—there is an absence of theoretical literature providing a holistic interprofessional lens.[7, 9,15,17-20] However, these profession-specific models share the fundamental principle that promotion of health, dignity, and harmony are achieved through human-to-human interactions.[15,18] While patient-centered care is a non-discipline-specific model that closely aligns with palliative care, it focuses on the patient-provider dyad and excludes the network of relationships existing among the rest of the care team.[16] Relationship-centered care, however, is a patient-centric model that includes both the interconnectedness of the care team and care of the patient in its theoretical framework.[21]

A clear and unified model for interprofessional palliative care would assist in establishing primary palliative care philosophy as standard care across settings.[7,9,17] We believe that aligning the frameworks of profession-specific palliative care and relationship-centered care theories into a unified model would assist in clarifying the shared principles of interprofessional team members and would provide a guide for educators, researchers, and all team members who implement primary palliative care. Thus, a concept analysis of interprofessional palliative care was undertaken.

Concept Analysis

Literature detailing various profession-specific palliative, interprofessional, and relationship-centered care philosophies were reviewed to determine the mutual threads present in primary palliative care delivery.[7,9,15-21] This concept analysis of interprofessional palliative care was conducted using Walker and Avant's method.[22] Walker and Avant's approach to concept analysis includes: (1) identifying the necessary antecedents that precede a concept, (2) defining its central attributes, and (3) revealing the consequences or expected outcomes of the concept occurring. Walker and Avant also describe borderline cases, or cases that contain most, but not all defining attributes of a concept, and model cases, which depict all of a concept's defining attributes. Our concept analysis of interprofessional palliative care revealed 5 common antecedents, 5 shared attributes, and several outcomes that can be expected for the patient, family, and team member when palliative care philosophy is effectively employed. These results were used to build a conceptual model depicting our interprofessional palliative care framework (see Figure 16.2).

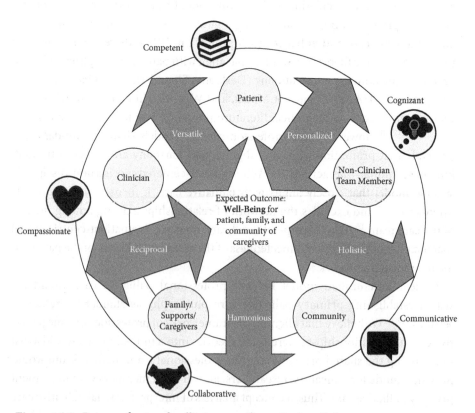

Figure 16.2. Interprofessional palliative care theoretical model.

Antecedents

Antecedents are those characteristics that are proposed as necessary for a concept to occur and to achieve a desired outcome. In the case of interprofessional palliative care, high-quality relationship-centered care delivery requires clinicians who are *competent, cognizant, communicative, collaborative,* and *compassionate.* These 5Cs comprise the knowledge, skills, attitudes, and values that are essential for every interprofessional team member for delivery of optimal palliative care.

While individual clinician team members may have strengths in one or more of these antecedents, interprofessional teams achieve balance through the blended unique strengths of its clinician team members.[23] This is an inherent quality of being an interprofessional team member—balanced membership with varied strengths to achieve a shared goal. It is the role of team leadership to ensure that the skill sets of each clinician contribute to balance on the team, and to evaluate when the team membership is unbalanced and restructuring is needed.

In this chapter, we refer to these antecedents as the "5C Skill Set" and have placed them in the outer circle of our theoretical model (Figure 16.2). These skills envelope all other elements of interprofessional palliative care, representing the prerequisite traits of clinician and non-clinician team members for delivery of quality relationship-centered care. We will now describe each trait in the 5C Skill Set.

Competent

Competence is the aptitude to deliver high-quality interprofessional palliative care and is comprised of the knowledge, skill, experience, and confidence that all interprofessional team members must possess.[19,23] These qualities of competence are interrelated; for example, increased knowledge and experience may foster greater self-efficacy, and with greater confidence, improved skill demonstration.[19] For healthcare clinicians involved in direct care delivery, foundational knowledge includes all dimensions of interprofessional and palliative care as set forth by the National Consensus Project for Quality Palliative Care and the Interprofessional Education Collaborative.[23,24] This includes understanding of the roles of others on the care team.[23] For those team members with non-clinical roles, such as volunteers, community members, teachers, public agency employees, law enforcement, non-profit service providers, and administrators, competence includes the core skills necessary to adequately perform job functions and positively impact palliative care delivery to individuals with chronic or serious illness and suffering.[16]

Cognizant

Cognizance is the caring consciousness and self-awareness achieved in the process of competence development and through intentional reflection on the significance and meaning behind illness, health, and care.[15,19,20] It requires recognition that one's own values, beliefs, feelings, and experiences contribute to the formation of worldviews and inclinations that should not be imposed on others or may interfere with the development of deep and effective relationships.[21] This self-reflection fosters the development of empathy and the recognition of prejudgments, and assists in overcoming prejudices while accepting and valuing patients, caregivers, and colleagues for who they are.[16,19] Clinicians are often required to attend to the simultaneous needs of the patient, the care environment, the interprofessional team, and their own subjective experience. This sort of multi-awareness is another aspect of cognizance that is promoted through self-awareness strategies like reflection and mindfulness.[25] This mindfulness assists team members in identifying disagreements among team members, conflicts with overlapping scope or professional role, and reflection on whether one is meeting expectations of their role on the team.[23]

Communicative

Communicative refers to the skills of conveying and receiving (listening to) a message, which are key in the assessment, planning, and treatment of patients.[23,24] These skills are necessary to develop a therapeutic rapport, ascertain and relay the patient's unique life experiences and personal values, and to survey and appreciate the unique perspectives of all team members.[9,17] Strong communication is fundamental to sharing feedback, ideas, experiences, and knowledge, and is a critical step in shared decision-making and conflict resolution.[19] Communication surrounding chronic and serious illness can often be difficult, sometimes requiring the delivery of bad news or diffusing tension when patients, families, or team members disagree. Communication in these cases calls for empathy, clarity, and honesty.[19,23,24]

Collaborative

Collaborative refers to the capacity of a clinician to form healing and cooperative relationships with colleagues, patients, families, and communities through positive team dynamics.[21] Collaboration requires effective communication and a concerted effort to seek feedback from others and promotes transparency in coordination and accomplishment of shared goals.[9,16,17] Recognizing the strengths, roles, and responsibilities of team members supports collaboration and reduces leadership hierarchy and power differentials.[23] Collaboration includes coordination of care, assisting all team members, including patients, family caregivers, and professionals in the community such as public agency employees, law enforcement, and non-profit service providers, in developing a collective and unified approach to goal setting, sharing information, decision-making, and advocating for optimal patient outcomes.[7]

Compassionate

Compassion is the conscious awareness of and compulsion to serve others, especially those impacted by suffering.[7] It is linked to intention, honor, respect, and presence. This sense of moral obligation influences the formation of genuine relationships, assisting clinicians in identifying with patients' suffering and driving

Table 16.1 Linking Antecedents and Attributes of Interprofessional Palliative Care

		5C Skill Set				
		Competent	Cognizant	Communicate	Collaborative	Compassionate
Attributes	Personalized		×	×		×
	Holistic	×	×		×	×
	Harmonious			×	×	×
	Reciprocal	×	×	×	×	×
	Versatile	×			×	

them to alleviate it.[21] Compassion has theoretical underpinnings in caring, and as a common professional core value, is a skill that unites interprofessional team members.[7] Team members must also demonstrate compassion for self. Risk of moral distress and burnout highlight the need for respite and effective self-care by caregivers and team members.[25,26]

Attributes

Attributes are the defining characteristics of a concept. In the case of interprofessional primary palliative care, as a philosophy of aspirational care for chronic and serious illness and suffering, 5 key attributes describe the shared principles or tenets of this relationship-centered care approach. We propose a synthesis of disciplinary philosophies of caring as guiding theory for interprofessional palliative care practice because one does not currently exist.[7,16,19,20] In Figure 16.2, these attributes are represented as bi-directional arrows that link the antecedents in our theoretical model to the expected outcome of interprofessional palliative care delivery. Table 16.1 also displays how the 5C Skill Set is linked to each of these attributes, contributing to more effective care delivery.

Personalized
Interprofessional palliative care can be characterized as a personalized approach to caring that respects diversity and dignity, and as relationship-centered care that honors human uniqueness.[7,15] Interprofessional practice assists in personalizing care through identification of a person's suffering, whether it be physical, psychological, social, spiritual, or cultural, and drawing on the strengths of those team members best suited to address their individualized needs. For example, culture, religion, and spirituality are unique and intrinsic factors that may impact how a patient adapts to, accepts, or recovers from disease.[7,15] Involving chaplain team members may be crucial to addressing suffering in these patients.

Personalized care demands sensitivity, attentiveness, intentionality, and active listening (*compassionate* and *communicative*) to attend to these factors and build meaningful connections.[7,21] This unbiased and nonjudgmental approach (cognizant) assists the team in honoring the patient's voice, advocating for their wishes, and adhering to the ethical principles of free choice, autonomy, consent, and assent for pediatric patients.[19] Supporting patients in completing advance directives and discussing their decisions with their family and caregivers is a powerful tool in achieving these aims. Sometimes, personalizing care also means supporting grounded hope, which is hope that is founded in a realistic understanding of the patient's illness trajectory, prognosis, and treatment—assisting the patient and family in transitioning from the goal of cure to a more realistic goal of optimized well-being.[19] Legacy work and self-actualization are also often supported through personalized care by interventions to promote a patient's life review, assist them in their journey to recognize their potential, find meaning in their illness experience, and preserve their dignity and embrace life before they die.[7,19] These interventions are often facilitated by social workers, chaplains, and child life therapists to strengthen bonds and ensure that adults and children receiving palliative care are able to contribute to how they will be remembered.[27]

Holistic
Careful attention must also be paid to holistic aspects of a person and their illness through comprehensive assessment (*competent*) of the patient's needs and suffering—physically, psychologically, socially, and otherwise.[19] While *personalized care* recognizes the uniqueness and autonomy of individuals, *holistic care* attends to their wholeness.[7] Holistic needs encompass not only those of the patient, but also those of the family, support system, or caregiver.[19] Illness experiences are emotionally charged and must be met with genuine empathy, mindfulness, and emotional presence (*cognizant* and *compassionate*). A multifaceted approach is also needed to alleviate suffering. Roles of all interprofessional team members should be maximized (*collaborative*), employing multimodal management of suffering by combining medications and integrative therapies like music, yoga, and aromatherapy, among others.[17,19,21] Additionally, interprofessional teams should address the holistic needs of each other and themselves to prevent burnout, by employing similar strategies that promote reflection and self-care.[26]

Harmonious
Harmony represents the balanced relationship and interconnectedness of the patient, family/caregivers, community, and interprofessional team achieved by working toward a shared goal.[7] Communication, love, and compassion are instruments in this harmonious relationship (*communicative* and *compassionate*), and in achieving balance. Mutual trust, understanding, and support are foundational in creating a safe space where patients and family members can be open and honest about their wishes, and where clinicians can collaborate (*collaborative*) and engage in shared decision-making to promote patient needs being met.[15] Psychological safety among interprofessional teams is fostered through collegiality, civility, and

shared governance.[28] Leaders who role-model openness by creating opportunities for thoughtful dialogue assist in making team members feel supported in sharing their concerns without fear of reprisal. This ultimately promotes cohesion, a positive work environment, and results in improved patient care.

While each team member brings the same "skill set" from their profession to the metaphorical table, their strengths may vary. Each team member or caregiver may possess more of one skill than another, but the collective whole within an ideal contained system may be greater than the sum of its parts. The varied strengths of team members should complement each other to achieve harmony. This dynamic is also represented in Figure 16.2 with equivalent circles representing the patient, family/caregivers/support system, community, non-clinicians, and clinicians as collaborating members of the interprofessional team. The patient and caregivers are equal team members and thus should be empowered participants in care, achieving equilibrium on the interprofessional team. Ideally, all members should take an active role at their meetings by preparing for visits with talking points and questions. They also need to speak up when there is something they do not understand, letting the team know when they feel unheard or misunderstood, and expressing appreciation when they feel heard and/or supported.[16]

Reciprocal

Reciprocity refers to the idea that care is not unidirectional but mutually transformative, offering opportunities for growth for team members as people and professionals.[21] Clinicians should be open to the idea that patient and colleague encounters might influence their personal attitudes and personal practice, often as a result of contemplation about the human experience of healing, living, and dying.[7] Table 16.1 highlights the reciprocal and cyclical relationship between the 5C Skills Set and the attributes of interprofessional palliative care, particularly reciprocity. Clinician transformation can occur as subtle shifts or powerful breakthroughs, strengthening both the clinicians' moral commitment to serve (*compassionate*) and their personal awareness (*cognizant*), and thus setting in motion a cycle of further skill development (*competent* and *communicative*) while simultaneously delivering higher-quality care.[21] Reciprocity deepens connections and role appreciation resulting from these caring encounters that occur for and with patients, families, caregivers, and team members (*collaborative*), touching the hearts and providing intangible rewards to all parties in the process.[7]

Versatile

Versatility describes the way in which the interprofessional team and the care they deliver is flexible and adjusts to the changing needs of the patient, team, and institution, and the changing realities of the disease.[19] Versatility also refers to the integration of palliative care as a continuum of care that spans settings, populations, and all levels of care, focused not only on the end of life and bereavement, but on disease prevention, early diagnosis, treatment of chronic and serious illness, and suffering (*competent*).[7] Interprofessional palliative care follows the patient across care transitions. The composition of the team may be adjusted (*collaborative*), from primarily clinician team members in the acute-care setting to non-clinician team members when the patient transitions back home and into the community.[21] The interprofessional team in primary palliative care is fluid, with not all team members present at every meeting and varied levels of engagement depending on the care setting. For example, community members will not regularly attend inpatient hospital rounds, but will be called upon as a patient is approaching time for discharge.

The interprofessional team must also pivot from a patient- to family-centered approach during certain developmental or transitional phases of care, or when patient goals change.[20] An example of this adaptability occurs during the end of life and bereavement phase, when a focus on cure shifts to that of preserving comfort and dignity and building meaningful memories.[19]

Expected Outcomes

According to Walker and Avant, expected outcomes are the consequence of a concept occurring. While the optimal outcome of effective interprofessional palliative care is patient well-being, our literature review revealed that well-being is often achieved for the family/caregiver and interprofessional care team as well.[9,17,19] Thus, we have identified "well-being" as the primary expected outcome of interprofessional palliative care and have placed it at the center of our theoretical model (see Figure 16.2). Development of the 5C Skill Set by team members addresses their well-being by ensuring they are adequately prepared for quality relationship-centered care delivery, promoting self-efficacy, effective self-care, and satisfaction of the team and team members. Well-being for the patient and interprofessional team are promoted through personalized, holistic, harmonious, reciprocal, and versatile care delivery. Well-being can be equated to quality of life, and the qualifications for achieving maximized well-being (such as relief of suffering, optimal living, dignity, satisfaction, etc.) should be personalized and defined by the target individual(s) or population(s) for whom this shared goal is intended.

Well-being should be viewed holistically, and patient and family outcome aims should be grounded in a realistic understanding of the patient's prognosis. Dependent on patient prognosis and illness trajectory, outcomes that we can reasonably expect to impact through effective interprofessional palliative care include: current and future living status, relationships, optimized function, prolonged life, advance care planning, improved symptoms, relief of suffering, comfort, dignity, self-esteem, coping, effective closure, acceptance, discovering meaning, bereavement support, and relief from financial burden.[9,17,19] Reciprocal team member well-being outcomes of interprofessional palliative care may include: positive and therapeutic relationships, job satisfaction, and enhancement of their 5C Skill Set (greater self-awareness [*cognizant*], improved listening and verbal skills [*communicative*], enhanced understanding and appreciation for interprofessional roles and skills in shared decision-making [*collaborative*], increased knowledge and self-confidence [*competent*], and deepened empathy and moral imperative [*compassionate*].[19,23,24]

Model of Care Adoption

Health policy requires transformation of the healthcare system to be cross-functional and collaborative, and to build partnerships with patients.[21] The National Academies of Practice (formerly the Institute of Medicine) is also calling for a shift of focus from technical skill mastery to teaching human dimensions of care and interpersonal skills.[21] These key stakeholders have realized that the efficiency and quality of technical work are determined by the quality of the provider-patient relationship. Trust and mutual commitment are necessary to affect behavioral change and achieve optimal health outcomes.[21]

In a world where healthcare spending is a glaring issue for patients and policymakers alike, cost is a consideration in adopting a model of care. While health system administrators emphasize *efficiency* with time and money, *efficacy* with care is equally important, and both can be achieved by mindfully addressing care encounters in a humane and caring way.[29] Efficacy and efficiency require a personalized approach to assist clinicians in understanding patient values and meeting their care needs. Palliative care is an ideal model for a value-based health system, as it leverages clinician strengths to deliver optimal healthcare through a relationship-centered approach, improving the patient's experience *and* fully considering their healthcare goals. All of these outcomes are exalted by stakeholders—patients, interprofessional teams, administrators, and politicians.[29] The vision, then, should be for all patients to receive care that is congruent with their values, where their symptoms are managed, their humanity is recognized, and all members of the team are mutually committed to achieving optimal health and quality of life for the patient. We understand that while expanding the palliative care workforce or providing interprofessional primary palliative care education to existing clinicians may be a resource challenge, evidence shows that such care simultaneously boosts improvement in life quality as well as cost savings.[30] While expansion of the palliative care workforce is the necessary first step, the aspirational vision would be for communities to simultaneously begin introducing and implementing palliative care principles into all industries, mobilizing the transition to relationship-centered care as a lifestyle for all and adopting palliative care philosophy as a standard of care for all patients.

Hirschmann and Schlair[21] identify four primary areas where investment in relationship-centeredness must occur: interprofessional teamwork, education, administration, and patient care. Our concept analysis explores the ways in which interprofessional team members must invest in teamwork to achieve relationship-centered care. This section will further explore methods of education, models of primary palliative care administration, and exploration of usual care compared with aspirational, interprofessional patient care that demonstrate investment in a relationship-centered palliative care approach.

Interprofessional Palliative Care Education

Interprofessional team members require abilities in patient-centeredness and collaboration to promote communication, reduce medical errors, and build long-term relationships with patients, families, colleagues, and communities.[31] Uni-professional training models, though common, are inadequate in meeting the learning needs of clinician team members because every team member—clinical or non-clinical—should partake in this palliative care experience.[32] Weiss and Swede[31] argue that education should be transformed, beginning at the pre-professional level, to better prepare learners for relationship-centered care. The deeper that learners get into disciplinary siloes, the more challenging it becomes for these learners to develop empathy, overcome negative stereotypes about other disciplines, and ultimately prepare for shared decision-making.

To achieve this cultural shift, care teams must be simultaneously transformed and transformative. Care teams must deliberately transition away from the historical perspective of the physician as an omniscient provider to a more balanced view of their role as collaborator and member of an interprofessional team. We must enhance the delivery of care and address specialty workforce shortages by developing current practicing generalists as primary palliative care providers. Experienced palliative care champions would be needed to teach and promote a palliative care perspective and work-life culture that establishes this introductory foundation. Thoughtful interprofessional curriculum development for new trainees of this ubiquitous palliative care training model will involve an "upstream" approach, teaching fundamentals and core competencies while simultaneously fostering changes in learner attitude and behavior.[16,21]

We propose that the 5C Skill Set in our theoretical model should be developed by integrating interprofessional and palliative care competencies established by the Interprofessional Education Collaborative and the National Consensus Project for Quality Palliative Care (see Table 16.2),[23,24] applying educational theory, and weaving key concepts of collaboration into pre-professional team member curricula.[32] The development of relational skills, as they align with the 5C Skill Set, have been described as attending to four dimensions: (1) relationship with self, (2) relationship with patient, (3) relationship with peers, and (4) relationship with the community.[31] *Relationship with self* is the dimension that addresses development of *competence* and *cognizance*. Promoting meditation, reflection, and contemplation, and teaching students about the importance of self-care, assist in developing this dimension. Attending to the dimension of *relationship with*

Table 16.2 Clinician Competence Requirements for Interprofessional Palliative Care

Clinical Practice Guidelines for Quality Palliative Care	Interprofessional Education Collaborative Core Competencies
Domain 1: Structure & Process of Care Includes interdisciplinary team education and support, comprehensive planning and assessment, and continuity, stability, sustainability, coordination, and quality across care transitions and settings.	Competency 1: Value & Ethics for Interprofessional Practice Includes climate of mutual respect and shared values.
Domain 2: Physical Aspects of Care Includes screening, assessment, treatment, and ongoing care.	Competency 2: Roles & Responsibilities Includes knowledge of one's own role and that of others to assess and address patient needs.
Domain 3: Psychological and Psychiatric Aspects Inclusions same as Domain 2	Competency 3: Interprofessional Communication Includes responsive and responsible communication that supports a team approach to treatment.
Domain 4: Social Aspects of Care Inclusions same as Domain 2	
Domain 5: Spiritual, Religious, Existential Aspects Inclusions same as Domain 2	Competency 4: Teams & Teamwork Includes relationship-building values and team principles to deliver safe, timely, efficient, effective, and equitable care.
Domain 6: Culture Aspects of Care Inclusions same as Domain 2	
Domain 7: Care of the Patient Near End of Life Inclusions same as Domain 2 & Bereavement care	
Domain 8: Ethical & Legal Aspects of Care Includes ongoing decision-making	

the patient is crucial in the development of *compassion* and empathy, requiring learners to focus on the subjective illness experience of the patient. To attend to *relationships with peers* and the interprofessional care team, a culture of *collaboration*, mutual respect, and shared-decision making is required. The individual and team-based qualities of humility and kindness, and establishment of psychological safety among teams, assist in effective *communication*, conflict resolution, and prevention of errors. Service-learning is the application of theory through experiential learning and civic engagement in community-based settings. This educational approach fosters assessment skills to identify community needs, the impacts of programs, and inspires advocacy for population health—all crucial in attending to the *relationship with community domain*.[31]

Narrative medicine is 1 of 2 pedagogical paradigms that center around the development of relational skills in each of the 5Cs, and thus should be widely adopted to facilitate a pervasive palliative approach. Narrative medicine leverages the core curricula of clinician (health professionals) and non-clinician team members (housekeeping and food services, caregivers, education and technology supports, public health servants, etc.) by maximizing modalities of expression like the arts and humanities, which are common among many pre-professional programs.[31,32] Techniques in narrative medicine are compatible with relationship-centered care, sensitizing students to human suffering.[31] Incorporation of narrative approaches in general education courses, such as creative writing, slow viewing, or careful reading, instill a pervasive "understanding of other's perspectives." These strategies foster a natural desire to be mindful and bring meaning to the lives of others, which are inherent principles in achieving a palliative lifestyle. Educators should collaborate with English, visual arts, and film faculty to develop effective narrative strategies that can be blended within pre-professional courses.[31]

A second pedagogical paradigm is interprofessional education. Hall and colleagues[32] advocate 3 key concepts in interprofessional education to foster collaboration and integrate multiple perspectives: idea dominance, knot-working, and situational awareness. Idea dominance requires learners to focus on common goals and use shared language, often through case-based problems, to shift focus from one's own professional goals to the unified ideal of holistic care. This approach is effective in building partnerships by directing attention away from team member behaviors and toward patient concerns.[32] Likewise, knot-working requires active group work and the incorporation of multiple perspectives (through role-play or simulation) to appropriately address evolving situations while involving patients and families as equal contributors on the care team. Narrative medicine can be blended with this approach through interactive theater or exploring patient and family voices within written scripts or audio/video clips. Finally, situational awareness is the skill of knowing when, why, and how to access appropriate resources and get others involved who could provide a valuable contribution, and can also be fostered through role-play or simulation, or can be developed in various care settings.[32]

Models of Interprofessional Palliative Care Administration

During a time of particular healthcare system scrutiny, we need to re-examine both the framework and platform for palliative care. Increasing calls for thoughtful integration of palliative care into broader domains is welcomed and sensible.[33] Models of care that include a palliative care provider, for example, working alongside a heart failure specialist, or oncologist, or other chronic disease provider, are being considered and adopted in health systems throughout the country. Such collaborations are found to promote Berwick's triple aim, or rather to improve the health system through improved patient care experience, improved population health, and reduced costs.[34]

Mahmood-Yousuf and colleagues found that the best-performing palliative care teams in the United Kingdom were those in which the diverse team members developed a clear shared purpose,[35] had a non-hierarchical team structure, and had a combination of formal meetings for regular patient management, as well as a mechanism for informal meetings for urgent patient care issues. Although the authors observed that different disciplines may prefer different styles of workflow and communication (for example, the nurses valued formal meetings while general practitioners preferred ad hoc informal dialogue), the overall alignment of palliative care philosophy centered the team in a meaningful way. Current literature provides extensive examples of healthcare-related interprofessional collaboration demonstrating this cohesion.

Cohesion of interprofessional teammates may also be modeled in various forms. For example, Fendler and team[36] identified a multilayered approach to care, in which the patient, caregiver, and loved ones are at the center of a concentric circular arrangement. In this model, an inner ring consists of the heart failure specialist team, palliative service, and primary care team, and an enveloping outer ring of further support includes social work teams, pharmacy, nursing, therapists, art therapists, geriatricians, psychiatrist, and other specialists. This circular diagram suggests a more balanced 2-tier arrangement of support, but professionals within each tier are of equal influence.

Another style of care to consider would be more chronological in nature, known as the "time-based model."[37] In this model, palliative team members and the intensity of their involvement may change over time as the individual's disease course progresses. This may be represented as overlapping care teams, who may substitute or "swap out" team members based on palliative need. Regardless of the delivery model (cohesive, multilayered, or chronological), we should expand our platform for palliative care beyond a singular field of palliative care or its cohort of enlightened champions. Palliative care as a standard of care extends the platform to the greater community.

As patients are not simply composed of the medical ailments that affect them, palliative care should not simply belong to the medical or healthcare domain. For example, industries in arts and music, exercise and sports, retail and manufacturing would benefit from better understanding the increasingly longer life trajectories and challenges of chronic conditions of their patrons and customers. Industries in finance, business, and information technology would benefit from adjusting their models and algorithms to consider the spending and needs of an older, increasingly comorbid population of clients who may prioritize quality of life over quantity of years. Better understanding people's perceptions in life quality may allow industries in food, retail, and manufacturing to reshape their practices in product distribution and delivery.

Each industry would likely benefit from greater empowerment and better quality of care for their target clientele when looking through the lens of palliation and symptom management. Take, for example, a clothing company whose chief executive officer (CEO) has a granddaughter with ulcerative colitis. This granddaughter just had a colectomy and is self-conscious about her clothing choices. The CEO now invites her company's creative design team to research, design, and produce a line of new clothing items for ostomy covers and belts that allow children and adults alike to live comfortably and feel supported with their chronic conditions. Upon completion of this project and buoyed by the positive publicity and humanitarian ideals, this same design team begins investing resources in designing clothing for accommodation of other chronic disease conditions, such as insulin pumps, hearing aids, and prosthetic limbs.

Societal change is key. The complexity and interdependence of patient care delivery call for increased personal accountability, because when human beings are not valued and treated with dignity, "everyone suffers."[21] With limited resources and high costs of healthcare, the community needs to step in and contribute, sharing the workload (see Scenario 2). This societal movement aims to create a "ripple effect" for positive palliative change. The more diverse the collective community, the richer the experience. When thinking of ways that we can maximize health and quality of life, we should ask questions like: Who else possesses the background or skill set that is currently underutilized but could be beneficial to this patient? How can we help them feel empowered? How can they advocate? What is their role or within their scope?

Most jobs require some form of human-to-human interaction and betterment of our lives. Increased understanding of palliative care could impact the way we approach our interactions with others regardless of role, that is, becoming more compassionate human beings, and linking the understanding that quality of health is the new goal (quality vs. quantity). The common denominator is a palliative philosophy and if as a society we can think about the day-to-day improvement of life (symptom appeasement), then it is easier to understand how palliative care philosophy spans all domains and thus should be adopted as standard care. Adopting a broad public health strategy to translate the skills and knowledge into actionable cultural changes in the community is important to reach everyone in the population.[38]

Interprofessional Palliative Care Case Examples

Placing this chapter's philosophies and practices in context, we present 2 theoretical case examples to demonstrate how our proposed interprofessional palliative care model can be employed by each discipline/team member's practice. One "current world" or usual care example illustrates system failures that are commonplace in today's healthcare system, termed a "borderline case" by Walker and Avant's classification.[22] The second example proposes what an ideal world—or what Walker and Avant call a "model case," and our idea of "palliative care as a lifestyle"—would look like.[22]

Following these examples, we provide a table to display the effective and ineffective demonstration of interprofessional palliative care characteristics (see Table 16.3).

Table 16.3 Demonstration of Interprofessional Palliative Care Characteristics

Skills/Traits	"Current World Example" (Borderline Case)	"Aspirational Future Example" (Model Case)
	Clinician Level – 5C Skill Set (Antecedents)	
Competent	Physician is competent.	Physician, parent, family members, nurses, social worker, occupational therapist, school administration, daycare providers, and church leaders are competent.
Cognizant	Physician is not cognizant (busy parent does not share concerns).	Physician, social worker, and parent are both cognizant and anticipatory of Mariam's needs and potential hardship.
Communicative	Lack of communication between parent, teachers, community support	Frequent
Collaborative	Very little	Mariam participates in support groups, diabetes education, and occupational therapy beginning early in childhood and morphing into other support as she matures
Compassionate	Yes	Yes
	Team Level – Care Delivery Traits For Interprofessional Relationship-Centered Practice (Attributes)	
Personalized	No	Yes
Holistic	No; community resources are siloed	Yes; entire community is supportive
Harmonious	No culture of balanced support	Part of community culture
Reciprocal	Untested as Mariam never engages her community	Supportive and harmonious community culture leads to positive relationships and reinforcing rewards.
Versatile	Untested as Mariam never engages her community	Community able to adapt to Mariam's changing needs (childhood, pre-adolescence, teenager)
	Interprofessional Palliative Care Outcomes (Expected Outcomes)	
Well-Being • Patient	No, not until she reached college when she was independent, autonomous, and secured her own resources	Yes; Mariam was able to thrive in a supportive community.
• Family/Caregiver	No, Mariam's mother did not have an understanding of Mariam's emotional state and its impact on her physical and social well-being.	Yes; resources were readily available in the community from birth and significantly unburdened the mother.
• Team	No, the non-clinicians in Mariam's life did not have the 5C Skill Set and thus did not operate as a team.	Yes; the team was dynamic and collaborative, working together to address Mariam's holistic needs.

Scenario 1: Current World

Mariam S. is a lovely child born with type 1 diabetes mellitus and mild persistent asthma. She lives in a small rural town with one hospital and a handful of family physicians. Her parents are divorced and she is cared for by a single parent who needs to work long hours to pay the bills. Her parent is unable to spend much time with Mariam, and does not have the resources or health system literacy to understand how best to support Mariam through her challenging chronic conditions. Mariam spends her early childhood in a local daycare program where she is the only child required to bring snacks and meals from home because of her diabetic dietary restriction. She often cries when not allowed to eat shared foods from her classmates and is not allowed to eat any birthday treats when other classmates celebrate. Because she had a few asthmatic exacerbations during gym class, as she was struggling to learn how to use her inhaler, her gym teacher excluded Mariam from subsequent intensive activities, causing Mariam to feel excluded and a burden on her classmates. Her teachers feel sad that they cannot help, and while they understand the general medical concept of diabetes to keep Mariam safe, they do not know how to support Mariam's emotional suffering and isolation, although as attentive and caring teachers they recognize it. While Mariam's school does have a school nurse, because Mariam's blood glucose is generally closely monitored and tightly controlled, she does not often need medical attention, and her emotional needs are overlooked; consequently, her school team does not communicate these concerns to each other.

As Mariam grows, she develops an instinct to hide her diabetes and her asthma, for fear of being singled out and embarrassed. Because of her busy single parent, she has not attended any support groups as a child, and always feels that she is alone in her battle with her chronic conditions. She becomes resentful of her glucometer and the need to frequently worry about her blood glucose levels. She tries her best to assimilate into life as a teenager, and with her growing independence tries to ignore her diabetes to the point where she fights frequently with her parent over her diabetes management and poor glucose control. Her parent and family doctor are both frustrated at her rebelliousness and refusal to follow the plan of care. Her teachers are also concerned about her poor academic performance, likely resulting from missed class periods due to illness or spending time in the school nurse's office, which has become a regular occurrence when her glucose levels are out of range or when she needs to use her asthma inhaler. She often lies about her adherence to her insulin, and refuses to answer telephone calls from her hospital's endocrine clinic who try to check in on her regularly. Mariam has had several emergency room visits for episodes of hyperglycemia, after which she remains increasingly resentful of her health and of the health system. It is not until college, when she finds herself in a community of newly independent individuals and joins a diabetes support group, that she learns how it might have been to live a life supported by those who understand her chronic illness and suffering.

Scenario 2: Aspirational Interprofessional Palliative Care

Mariam S. is a lovely child born with type 1 diabetes mellitus and mild persistent asthma. She lives in a small rural town with one hospital and a handful of family physicians. Her parents are divorced and she is cared for by a single parent, who needs to work long hours to pay the bills. Her parent is unable to spend much time with Mariam, but having lived in the same town for 35 years, fortunately appreciates the community's inclusive culture and empathic approach to recognizing a person's individual needs. Her parent anticipates and recognizes that Mariam's diabetes will be a significant challenge. Her parent quickly engages her primary care physician, who connects her from birth with a diabetes nurse educator and social worker within the community and establishes a regular pattern of care conferences throughout pivotal points of Mariam's childhood. In addition to childhood vaccinations and regular childhood visits, Mariam also attends the recommended endocrinology appointments for her diabetes care. When her parent is not available, transportation is provided as a benefit of her health insurance plan. As insulin management and diabetes surveillance is overwhelming for a child, Mariam's nurse educator and social worker recommend engaging in social supportive groups at her local church, daycare, and weekend play groups, in which the childcare providers often inquire about her well-being and emotional health with regard to her physiological symptoms. She is also referred to an outpatient occupational therapist who assists Mariam with integrating her medical management seamlessly into her activities of daily living that promote both her physical and emotional well-being. Her parent and family members, as well as school administration and church leaders, follow the lead of the occupational therapist by trying their best not to medicalize her life, and encourage her to feel comfortable discussing her feelings and life with respect to what she understands to be most important to her living at her current age. Her teachers feel comforted that while they cannot cure Mariam's diabetes and asthma, they do know how to support Mariam's emotional suffering and isolation, and feel supported by the school system and local community. Her teachers, gym teacher, and school nurse collaborate to keep Mariam included in all activities. Mariam's school nurse communicates often with the teachers, primary care provider, and parent about Mariam's diabetes and asthma plan of care, and while surveilling Mariam's compliance the school nurse supports Mariam's independence in managing glucose abnormalities in class to ensure active attendance and engagement, without risk of isolating her.

As Mariam grows, she is able to engage in thoughtful discussion about a "palliative lifestyle" without needing to share the unnecessary details of her medical history with teachers and friends in school. While there are no other young people living with type 1 diabetes in her small rural town, she knows other classmates living with chronic conditions who are also experiencing challenges and health concerns. She learns to focus her energy on reducing and alleviating her symptoms and emotional burdens. She has an appreciation for her parent, medical care team, and community in providing a holistic yet individualized and versatile support structure. She finds a part-time job as a volunteer at a local nursing home and enjoys spending time with the older members of her community, as they remind her of what is important and valuable with her life. As she enters college, she realizes that her new support system has similar characteristics to her hometown, because she is able to identify and assess what she needs to maintain a palliative lifestyle for herself and to share this with her college friends who also understand her chronic illness and potential suffering.

Conclusion

Our concept analysis of interprofessional palliative care was a necessary first step in mobilizing palliative care as standard care across disciplines, settings, trajectories, and the life span. The theoretical model in Figure 16.2 is a feasible product and synthesis of existing philosophies. While the aspirational vision we propose may seem idyllic, this model is founded in present-day perspectives. We have demonstrated how this model is both visionary and practical, with usefulness for educators, administrators, politicians, researchers, and as a complement to other care-delivery models already in practice.

Movement toward an aspirational future of interprofessional palliative care requires health-system adaptation, a societal awareness of relationship-centered care principles, and recognition that quality of life and well-being across the life span are as important as the current healthcare system's focus on attempting to cure all ailments. This integrated care model could meet the current demands of a changing population demographic by supporting and expanding the healthcare workforce beyond clinicians to non-clinician team members. As palliative care becomes a more natural and pervasive phenomenon in communities, society may find itself transformed, with patients, families, and team members achieving optimal well-being through healing relationships.

Problem-Based Learning Scenario

Mr. P is a 72-year-old retired farmer and grandfather, who lives on his own farm with his wife in a small rural town in the Midwest United States. He greatly appreciates and values his independence and self-sufficiency. His past medical history includes hypertension, benign prostatic hypertrophy, and osteoarthritis. Recently Mr. P suffered a traumatic fall from a 16-foot ladder, leaving him with a traumatic brain injury, paraplegia, and significant limitations to his daily function and quality of life.

Questions for the Reader

1. What challenges do you anticipate would result from this catastrophic injury?
2. What interprofessional team members might be engaged to provide palliative care support to Mr. P and his family?

After 6 months of acute care and skilled nursing and rehabilitation, Mr. P laments being unable to use his bicycle for his emotional release—previously riding 20–30 miles daily to enjoy the countryside. Yet, both he and his wife remain active in their local church, regularly attending services, weekly Bible study, and potluck events. While Mr. P's cognitive function is sufficient to recognize and enjoy his friends and family and remember details of daily living, his mood and executive functions are limited, resulting in angry outbursts and poor emotional control, especially when recognizing that he cannot organize his activities as he could previously. His wife of 60 years has also developed mild cognitive impairment, causing the couple to bicker increasingly as they are unable to compensate for each other's faltering memories, executive functions, and mood shifts. These verbal altercations escalate more frequently, causing neighbors to grow concerned and at times call for law enforcement to provide transport to the local emergency room for evaluation of Mr. P's mental status.

Questions for the Reader

3. What 5C skills would be essential in each team member, and which professions might contribute the most care initially?
4. How might this team composition shift as processes stabilize?
5. What team-level care-delivery traits—or attributes—would be valuable in interprofessional relationship-centered practice?

Mr. P becomes more resistant to receiving care from his wife and caregiver, and frequently calls 911 to report that he is being held against his will or to request transport to the hospital for evaluation. Once in the emergency room, Mr. P becomes more agitated and distressed, unfamiliar with the nurses and doctors who check on him, confused with the hospital environment, and unable to rest comfortably. With each hospitalization, the clinical team increasingly seeks guidance from the palliative care team to provide perspective. Mr. P's daughter and healthcare proxy states repeatedly that she is not yet ready to speak about palliative care. She expresses disappointment that a shared in-patient/community-care plan cannot be devised to support her parents in their home.

Questions for the Reader

6. What appear to be some barriers to accepting palliative care in this case? How might teams shift or activate attributes/5C skills to accommodate?
7. Where might more upstream approaches have changed outcomes, if implemented earlier in Mr. P's life trajectory?

Finally, one of Mr. P's grandsons brings him to a race track within a couple hours' drive of his home as a surprise gift experience, family reunion, and picnic. When they arrive, Mr. P is happily overwhelmed and spends the day with his grandson "smelling the fumes" of the racecars, something he had often described as a lifelong dream of his. On the following day, Mr. P's daughter contacts his primary care physician and requests to speak to the palliative care team to learn more about its services. Mr. P is ultimately enrolled in home hospice, and dies peacefully in his home 6 weeks later.

Questions for the Reader

8. How might implementing an aspirational model of palliative care as standard care across settings have resulted in different outcomes in well-being at the patient, family/caregiver, and team level?
9. What additional barriers prevent the adoption of palliative care as standard of care in society?
10. How does the view or value we place on persons who are aging or those with disabilities play into this paradigm shift?
11. Consider this from a federal policy, local community, health system, and individual level.

References

1. Rosa WE, Ferrell BR, Mason DJ. Integration of palliative care into all serious illness care as a human right. *JAMA Health Forum.* 2021 Apr 1;2(4):e211099–e211099.
2. Lapu D, Quigley L, Mehfoud N, Salsberg ES. The growing demand for hospice and palliative medicine physicians: will the supply keep up? *J Pain Symptom Manage.* 2018;55(4):1216–1223.
3. Lapu D. Estimate of current hospice and palliative medicine physician workforce shortage. *J Pain Symptom Manage.* 2010;40(6):899–911.
4. Etkind SN, Bone AE, Gomes B, et al. How many people will need palliative care in 2040? Past trends, future projections and implications for services. *BMC Medicine.* 2017;15(1):102.
5. Rollings JC. Professional love in palliative nursing: an exceptional quality or an occupational burden? *Int J Human Caring.* 2008 Apr 1;12(3):53–56.
6. Ferris FD, Balfour HM, Bowen K, et al. A model to guide patient and family care: based on nationally accepted principles and norms of practice. *J Pain Symptom Manage.* 2002;24(2):106–123.
7. Desbiens JF, Gagnon J, Fillion L. Development of a shared theory in palliative care to enhance nursing competence. *Journal of Advanced Nursing.* 2012;68(9):2113–2124.

8. Clark D. History, gender and culture in the rise of palliative care. Palliative care nursing: Principles and evidence for practice. 2004:39–54.

9. Koloroutis M, Abelson D. Advancing relationship-based cultures. Springer Publishing Company, ed. 2017.

10. Crawford GB, Price SD. Team working: palliative care as a model of interdisciplinary practice. *The medical journal of Australia*. 2003;179(6):S32.

11. Hauptman PJ, Havranek EP. Integrating palliative care into heart failure care. *JAMA Internal Med*. 2005;165(4):374–378.

12. Ferrell B, Paice J, Koczywas M. New standards and implications for improving the quality of supportive oncology practice. *J Clinical Oncol*. 2008;26(23):3824–3831.

13. Tinetti M, Huang A, Molnar F. The geriatrics 5M's: a new way of communicating what we do. *J Am Geriatr Soc*. 2017;65(9):2115.

14. Curtis JR, Kross EK, Stapleton RD. The importance of addressing advance care planning and decisions about do-not-resuscitate orders during novel Coronavirus 2019 (COVID-19). *JAMA*. 2020;323(18):1771–1772.

15. Meghani SH. A concept analysis of palliative care in the United States. *J Adv Nurs*. 2004;46(2):152–161.

16. Dyess SM, Prestia AS, Levene R, Gonzalez F. An interdisciplinary framework for palliative and hospice education and practice. *Journal of Holistic Nursing*. 2020; 38(3):320–30.

17. Aghaei MH, Vanaki Z, Mohammadi E. Watson's human caring theory-based palliative care: a discussion paper. *Int J Cancer Manage*. 2020;13(6):e103027. https://doi.org/10.5812/ijcm.103027.

18. Guo Q, Jacelon CS, Marquard J. An evolutionary concept analysis of palliative care. *J Palliat Care Med*. 2012;2(6):1–6.

19. Dobrina R, Tenze M, Palese A. An overview of hospice and palliative care nursing models and theories. *Int J Palliat Nurs*. 2014;20(2):75–81.

20. Kirkpatrick AJ, Cantrell M, Smeltzer SC. A concept analysis of palliative care nursing. *Adv Nurs Sci*. 2017;40(4):356–369.

21. Hirschmann K, Schlair S. *Relationship-Centered Care*. The Patient and Health Care System: Perspectives on High-Quality Care. 2020:173–84.

22. Walker LO, Avant KC. *Strategies for Theory Construction in Nursing*. 5th ed. Pearson/Prentice Hall; 2011.

23. Interprofessional Education Collaborative (IPEC). IPEC core competencies. 2016. https://www.ipecollaborative.org/ipec-core-competencies.

24. National Consensus Project for Quality Palliative Care. Clinical practice guidelines for quality palliative care. 4th ed. 2018. https://www.nationalcoalitionhpc.org/ncp/.

25. Rabow MW. Meaning and relationship-centered care: recommendations for clinicians attending to the spiritual distress of patients at the end of life. *Ethics Med Public Health*. 2019; 9:57–62.

26. Maffoni M, Argentero P, Giorgi I, Hynes J, Giardini A. Healthcare professionals' moral distress in adult palliative care: a systematic review. *BMJ Support Palliat Care*. 2019 Sep 1;9(3):245–254.

27. Boles JC, Jones MT. Legacy perceptions and interventions for adults and children receiving palliative care: A systematic review. *Palliat Med*. 2021 Mar;35(3):529–551.

28. Pfeifer LE, Vessey JA. Psychological safety on the healthcare team. *Nurs Manage*. 2019 Aug 1;50(8):32–38.

29. Dunsford J, Reimer LE. Relationship-centered health care as a Lean intervention. *Int J Qual Health Care*. 2017;29(8):1020–1024 doi: 10.1093/intqhc/mzx156. PMID: 29190380.

30. Morrison RS, Penrod JD, Cassel JB, et al. Cost savings associated with US hospital palliative care consultation programs. *Arch Internal Med*. 2008;168(16):1783–1790.

31. Weiss T, Swede MJ M. Transforming preprofessional health education through relationship-centered care and narrative medicine. *Teach Learn Med*. 2019;31(2):222–233.

32. Hall P, Weaver L, Grassau PA. Theories, relationships and interprofessionalism: learning to weave. *J Interprof Care*. 2013;27(1):73–80.

33. Casarett D, Teno J. Why population health and palliative care need each other. *JAMA*. 2016;316(1):27–28.

34. Berwick DM, Nolan TW, Whittington J. The triple aim: care, health, and cost. *Health Affairs*. 2008; 27(3):759–769.

35. Mahmood-Yousuf K, Munday D, King N, Dale J. Interprofessional relationships and communication in primary palliative care: impact of the Gold Standards Framework. *Br J Gen Pract*. 2008 Apr 1;58(549):256–263.

36. Fendler TJ, Swetz KM, Allen LA. Team-based palliative and end-of-life care for heart failure. *Heart Failure Clin*. 2015 Jul 1;11(3):479–498.

37. Hui D, Bruera E. Models of integration of oncology and palliative care. *Ann Palliat Med*. 2015;4(3):89–98.

38. Stjernsward J, Foley KM, Ferris FD. The public health strategy for palliative care. *J Pain Symptom Manage*. 2007;33(5):486–493.

17

Looking Forward in Interprofessional Palliative Care

Cara L. Wallace, Naomi Tzril Saks, DorAnne Donesky, and Michelle M. Milic

Key Points

- Intentionally interprofessional palliative care is an invitation to assure that the palliative care we offer benefits from the expertise of all core palliative care professions, practicing at the top of their scope of practice and interacting in a transdisciplinary fashion.
- Intentionally interprofessional palliative care encompasses all aspects of the field (i.e., practice, education, administration, research, and sustainability and well-being), and incorporates advocacy, attention to diversity and equity, and deliberate implementation of research to practice.
- When professions are working in close proximity to one another, this does not necessarily mean that interprofessional education and collaboration are occurring.
- We must actively question assumptions and strive to correct systemic barriers to interprofessional collaboration (e.g., payment structures, ideals of professional behavior, protected time, staffing norms).
- For interprofessional palliative care education to result in intentionally collaborative care, palliative care systems and leaders must prioritize advocacy in overcoming barriers; diversity, equity, and access for both aspiring palliative care professionals and patients; and ongoing implementation of evidence-based practice and education.
- Workforce development and unpaid caregivers represent 2 ongoing and vexing challenges within palliative care that could benefit from an intentionally interprofessional approach.

Introduction

This textbook presents an aspirational vision of the practice and education of interprofessional palliative care that is holistic and ethically sustainable for practitioners and patients. However, many challenges remain. In our work, each of us should consider: What is my role in the future of hospice and palliative care? How am I already contributing to this future in my current roles (as a student, educator, clinician, researcher, or administrator)? What is the role of the interprofessional team in addressing each challenge? How can palliative care leadership and institutions catalyze current teams and potential allies to further this vision? This chapter considers the application of *intentionally* interprofessional palliative care and examines current challenges in the field, along with the role of effective interprofessional teams in working to solve them.

Interprofessional Palliative Care—Assumed or Intentional?

By definition, palliative care is interprofessional, as it is "provided by a specially trained team"[1] and "involves a range of services delivered by a range of professionals that all have equally important roles to play."[2(np)] Chapter 1 of this text demonstrates the centrality of interprofessional teamwork across all 8 domains of palliative care, while highlighting the lack of robust, empirical evidence linking teamwork to specific outcomes. Much of current research focuses on specific team members or interventions, rather than considering full palliative care team collaboration (see Chapter 1). Additionally, clinicians remain trained heavily in professional silos (see Chapter 3), with limited opportunities for single-profession or interprofessional palliative care residencies or fellowships outside of medicine (see Chapter 9). While effective interprofessional teams are the signature of and central to the practice of palliative care, working well together cannot be assumed and is not simple in application—as seen in the challenges and interprofessional tensions presented in Chapter 4—without deliberate *intention*.

Intentionally Interprofessional Palliative Care

While this text highlights the role of interprofessional *education* and *practice* in palliative care, the authors cannot underscore enough that intentionally interprofessional palliative care extends beyond education and practice alone—it encompasses research,[3] leadership and administration,[4,5] advocacy,[6] well-being/sustainability in the field,[7,8] and extends to our national organizations.[9] The framework of transdisciplinary team collaboration allows teams to transcend traditional challenges of interprofessional practice through a shared vision and development of common policies and practices (see Chapter 3). This framework requires that teams and their leaders develop processes with equal participation of each team member. If this same approach were extended to our research, our leadership teams, or our advocacy efforts, new, innovative approaches could emerge. How often, though, are we considering diverse perspectives of other professions to inform our research questions or clinical best practices? While many peer-reviewed publications or national organizations invite diverse professionals to disseminate their work through their venue, how many employ varied representation within their leadership teams? In review of research, are investigators intentional in seeking knowledge across professions, or do they review research within familiar outlets in their own occupations?

Intentionally interprofessional palliative care requires building outcome-based evidence for fully staffed interprofessional collaborative team practice. This necessitates advances in both research outcomes and educational competencies. It is especially important for studies to link transdisciplinary practice directly to improvements in social equity among teams and institutions,[10] access to domestic and global palliative care,[11] patient experience, population health, finances, and personal and professional well-being.[12] The field also needs training and research validating the National Consensus Project (NCP) Clinical Practice Guidelines'[13] recommendations for screening across all domains for all professions using evidence-based screening tools to identify urgent and ongoing patient and caregiver needs. If we hope to seed sustainable and systemic improvements beyond an honorable but unrealized ideal, we also must conceptualize interprofessional collaboration as an essential intervention in palliative care, similar to serious illness communication or pain and symptom management. Just as no palliative care provider is born knowing how to facilitate a family meeting,[14] the same is true for how to collaborate effectively with a team.

Authorities in the study of group-based learning and success have illustrated for decades that simply putting smart and well-meaning experts together does not automatically create cooperative practice or mitigate individual and systemic power dynamics and conflicts.[15-17] Yet, across the country, most teams are formed randomly, with members and leadership lacking vision and training in the art of collaboration. Interprofessional education in collaboration should be a required component of pre- and post-licensure education for all team members. Standardized pre- and post-licensure programs should be designed using the 6 characteristics of excellence for interprofessional palliative care education (competencies, content, educational strategies, evaluation, interprofessional focus, and systems integration).[18]

In a recent integrative review of interprofessional teamwork in specialty palliative care from patients and professionals' perspectives, 13 potential competency categories emerged across 4 areas: knowledge, skills, attitudes, and values (see Figure 17.1, reprinted with permission).[19] These 13 competencies provide a high-level focus on valuable characteristics and objectives of all interprofessional team members,[19] which closely align with Interprofessional Education Collaborative (IPEC) competencies.[20,21] What needs further

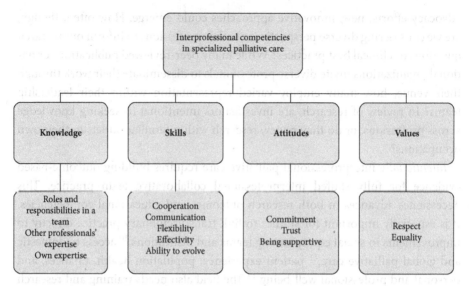

Figure 17.1. Interprofessional competencies in specialized palliative care.

Reprinted from SAGE under CC BY 4.0 license. Kesonen P, Salminen L, Kero J, Aappola J, Haavisto E. An integrative review of interprofessional teamwork and required competence in specialized palliative care. *OMEGA.* 2022; https://journals.sagepub.com/doi/epub/10.1177/00302228221085468

development are the key tasks or skills that might be measurable for implementation and improvement. In another model, Fink and colleagues[22] base their proposed interprofessional palliative care competencies on adapted NCP guidelines and provide a measurement tool to assess learners on these competencies. However, the tool includes many profession-specific skills that are less applicable to the scope of the full team, such as detailed pharmacological symptom management. Beyond the consideration of competencies, which define a minimum level of knowledge for practice, Wu and colleagues[23(p1)] call for an "evidence-based definition of clinical excellence for palliative care specialists," which could provide an aspirational target for elevated care, improved outcomes, and individual development.

New and veteran team members need training to become familiar with the expertise and functions of others' roles, and educators and curriculum developers need to help facilitate the development of a clear dual-identity formation—an interprofessional identity in addition to the learners' existing professional-role identity.[24] For collaborative education to result in collaborative care, palliative care systems must also prioritize the following: (a) role of advocacy in overcoming barriers; (b) diversity, equity, and access; and (c) ongoing implementation of evidence-based practice and education. The field must rally advocates who join with others to create ethical, sustainable practice environments and help transform interactional, organizational, cultural, and financial barriers that influence individual behavior and systems that obstruct teamwork.[25] Programs must address issues of interprofessional and systemic power and conflict requiring particular attention to efforts of diversity and equity. Finally, education and practice must create systems for implementation of new, cutting-edge evidence from the palliative care field.

Advocacy

Though palliative care is *assumed* to be interprofessional, the National Palliative Care Registry 2018 survey data revealed that only 41% of the surveyed adult practices had the full complement of funded core[*] team members (up from 25% in 2016) as defined by the Joint Commission's Advanced Certification Program, providing in-person weekday care and telephone availability 7 days a week.[26] Programs with higher clinical volume were more likely to have the full complement of team members, and those of the interprofessional team most likely to be underrepresented were chaplains at 54% and social workers at 69%.[26] Although this represents an increase from prior years, the identification of specialty trained and Hospice and Palliative Care–certified staff members is surprisingly low at 8% for certified chaplains and 24% for certified social workers.[26] Eighty-two percent (82%) of the surveyed programs included physicians, which is an increase from just two-thirds of the programs in 2016.[27] To overcome barriers to the use of a full interprofessional team, intentionally interprofessional palliative care requires *advocacy*, from the Latin origin "to call" or "to call to one's aid," in our teams, systems, communities, and public policy.

On a comprehensive level, the National Hospice and Palliative Care Organization (NHPCO)[28] and the Hospice Action Network (HAN)[29] promote reforms to improve access, delivery, healthcare equity, and support for patients and families. Top national priorities include access to care for the seriously ill, a focus on quality improvement, and financing care, along with reimbursement for services.[28,29] Resources and an advocacy toolkit for individuals and institutions are available online.[28,29] In another example of national advocacy, the Improving Access to Advance Care Planning Act (S.4873)[30] has been introduced in Congress, which if enacted would permit certified social workers to provide advance care planning services to patients, thereby increasing access to this vitally important component of healthcare delivery. In addition, after 7 years of national collective advocacy, in 2022 the Centers for Medicare and Medicaid Services (CMS) approved chaplaincy codes for recording the work of chaplains through the Healthcare Common Procedure Coding System (HCPCS) for all healthcare settings.[31]

On healthcare teams, some members of the team may garner individual and systemic influence but do not generally hold institutional power. Power, which is typically unequally distributed, is often dynamic and is based on positional authority, while influence may be more evenly distributed and is based on the development of relationships.[32] Advocacy must be prioritized by all members of the team, not

---

[*] In this book, we use the term "core" to refer to chaplains, nurses, physicians, and social workers, who are all named as part of the interprofessional team for both the Medicare hospice guidelines and the NCP guidelines. This designation does not minimize the importance of other team members who contribute to the palliative care of patients

just the groups or team member most impacted by a particular issue. For example, it is common for the least-often represented member of the interprofessional palliative care team, the chaplain or social worker, to advocate for inclusion of a full complement of team members to optimize intentionally interprofessional palliative care. When these team members are already not represented, as shown in the statistics above, are other professions advocating for their inclusion? Another example is when historically marginalized team members are asked to be the main, visible, and outspoken champions of diversity and equity issues, instead of the team and institution acknowledging the role of all members and the larger, organizational role in examining and dismantling unjust practices and systems. Though many strides have been made in centering the patient and family in the provision of care, power imbalances remain that restrict patient and family voices in creating systemic change.[33]

Increasing demands for leadership action, advocacy for the team, and adequate staffing may resonate across the team, yet many team members feel powerless to effect these changes. In addition to staffing and workforce challenges, profession-specific practices may dictate structured roles within teams. For example, while physicians often have their time divided between clinical roles, research, and teaching, particularly within large academic or university settings, these positions are rare or nonexistent within social work and chaplain positions. Social workers and chaplains are generally considered either clinical or academic, with little crossover between them. Anecdotally, when physician or nurse scientists invite clinical social workers or chaplains to partner with them on research or education projects where they themselves have protected time, they do not realize that social workers or chaplains must participate without protected time from their 100% clinical roles. Conversely, few research-intensive nurse faculty positions include clinical roles, so nurse scientists who value maintenance of clinical skills must self-advocate for a clinical role to be included in their job description.

With this division often follows the assumption that one role or profession has all or most of the influence and power. For example, in writing this section, we discussed the unconscious bias that arises when the physician, who is more often the team lead, may be viewed by others as having the most power with a particular decision-making capacity on the palliative care team and within the healthcare system. Shedding light on this example of the physician seemingly "in charge" highlights that they may have no legitimate power over decisions such as hiring staff or budgeting. Leadership literature describes the use of "soft power," referred to from this point forward as "power of influence" to avoid downplaying the significance of this form of impact, which is often inaccurately associated with gender. Power of influence is a leadership style that is based on motivation and engagement, exhibiting expertise and role-modeling behaviors rather than direct authority over others. This stylistic approach increases intrinsic motivation, trust, and value of the individuals involved in teamwork.[34] The power of influence can be used by all team members, and this role can be viewed as a privilege and duty within a team, group, or system.

At times, advocacy can be compared to a Sisyphean task. The McKinsey 7-S business model's framework for change employs 6 components interconnected to the shared company values and culture (7th component), including (1) change strategy, (2) structure of the company, (3) business systems and process, (4) style or manner of work, (5) staffing, and (6) skills of the staff.[35] These pathways along with the power of influence and advocacy from all team members may address the challenges of interprofessional advocacy by allowing for change through "gentle pressure, relentlessly applied" (Ray Elliot), see Table 17.1.

Diversity, Equity, and Access

Authors of this chapter embody diversity in professions (each from a different core profession in palliative care), in age, geographical location, political, and religious/spiritual perspectives. However, we all identify as heterosexual, white, and cisgender female—with shared privilege as we consider our interactions as actors, advocates, and disrupters within the healthcare system. We acknowledge this shared privilege as a limitation of our perspectives. We are committed to our own learning and growing as allies and disruptors of systems of oppression and stigmatization in palliative care, interprofessional education and practice, and healthcare. Throughout this text, we have purposely included and celebrated—through contributions, literature, and research—the voices of esteemed colleagues who identify as members of historically marginalized groups. Intentionally interprofessional palliative care involves attention to both the deeply rooted disparities in palliative and end-of-life care,[36-38] and to the experiences and inherent wholeness and systemic well-being of clinicians, staff, and all team members. Though under-researched, clinicians experience patient bias and discrimination with little support or institutional response.[39,40] Healthcare systems rarely address the structural forces (historical, economic, political, social, cultural) that produce, and often uphold, ongoing inequities and disparities.[41] While this chapter is not meant to detail an exhaustive list of activities or action steps for interprofessional teams and workplaces, we hope it highlights the necessity and integral role of *action* related to acknowledging and addressing systemic oppression—"the [structurally] imposed discrimination and inequality that emerge from societal and institutional power [systems]."[42(np)]

Creating spaces and opportunities for individuals to deepen their own understanding and learning about equity and diversity efforts and terminology is an important starting place for teams and systems.[43,44] Public discussion around terms without common understanding of their meaning can be particularly divisive. Providing opportunities for groups to come to shared understanding about terminology and language can help bridge some of these gaps. In one example within the *Oxford Textbook of Palliative Social Work*, Borden and colleagues[45] present theoretical frameworks and terminology for palliative care social workers to center a lens of social justice in their work. Beyond creating time, space, and/or incentives

Table 17.1 Advocacy for Intentionally Interprofessional Palliative Care

7-S Model Components[35]	Change Strategy[35]: Advocacy Opportunities	Example
Skills; Systems	Identify and incorporate national benchmarks for measurement of success and strategic advocacy.	It is beneficial to review and quantify the representation of each profession on the team and compare to the census of outside institutions' services; identify markers of success for a particular group, organization, or system.
Shared values and culture; Skills; Style	Cite specific clinical cases and compelling stories of individual team member's and the team's successful intervention and positive outcomes to leadership to advocate for interprofessional collaborative practice and staffing of positions on the team.	Continually collect a library of compelling stories and patient quotations and insert these into business cases and palliative care service introductions and presentations.
Structure; Systems	Leverage data as it relates to benchmarks; collect and present numbers to support inclusion of the full team or a particular role. This may be empirical data, cost savings analysis, or metrics of the populations served.	Include tables showing reason for consults that include all domains of care. Present graphs showing the growth in visit volume for new or existing services and clinics year to date.
Skills; Shared values and culture	Never let a good emergency go to waste. Use industry crises and local or global environmental urgencies as opportunities to advocate for building capacity and resources on the team.	The publicly visible and acknowledged contribution of palliative care chaplains in advanced support of caregivers and healthcare teams during COVID was successfully leveraged by many palliative care teams to advocate and get approval for hiring more chaplains or transitioning existing part-time positions to full-time.
Structure; Staffing	Leverage social and cultural trends, and changes in policy and legislation to advocate for the hiring of the full core palliative care team.	The Improving Access to Advance Care Planning Act[30] further eliminates barriers to ACP by including a provision for social workers to conduct ACP services. If made into law, this legislation will be used by palliative care leaders to advocate for improving social work staffing.
Systems; Style; Shared values and culture	Ensure that your service and division-wide business plan is tied to institutional drivers and quality metrics. Investigate and determine what the priorities are for your institution, community, or healthcare system. Define how the intentional IP team can serve this mission with concrete examples.	Many healthcare organizations are consolidating and working to extend their reach across geographical areas. Palliative care leadership are on the forefront of this expansion by advocating for satellite palliative care clinics and services, staffed by the core team members in more locations.

Table 17.1 Continued

7-S Model Components[35]	Change Strategy[35]: Advocacy Opportunities	Example
Shared values and culture; Style	Identify and connect with leaders in an organization that have been personally touched by palliative care or hospice. The direct link to personal stories can be a powerful force for support.	The chief of a division of palliative medicine learned that the CEO of the organization cared for her mother while she received palliative then hospice care. The chief reached out to the CEO about her experience, started a series of conversations that resulted in increased support and funding for palliative care.
Staffing	Ask for what is needed, especially when it comes to staffing the core interprofessional team with full time employees (FTEs). Often teams make a smaller ask than what is truly needed out of concern for fear of rejection or asking for too much; however, the approving administrators can always negotiate for less if necessary. Increased staffing can also be phased in over a period.	A nurse director of a growing palliative care service missing nurse members, decided to promote a business plan that included 2 FTE nurses to strengthen the case for the RN's effectiveness on the team and for the unmet need and gap in care.
Style; Systems	Build collaborative relationships across the institution that support your cause; acknowledge the connection and support of others in the institution, community, and healthcare system. Some of those connections may have a strong voice of advocacy for your needs or land in other positions of power or authority for example, leadership or philanthropy, etc.	A newly hired palliative care manager at a community hospital partnered with oncology, ICU, social work, spiritual care, nursing, and ethics leaders in advocating for a new outpatient palliative care clinic.

for trainings, employers can provide additional resources for individuals to continue their own learning and provide ongoing in-services on various topics for voluntary attendance and discussion. Leadership should invite participation, rather than requiring employees to complete trainings, beyond the development of common language which benefits from wide participation.[43,46] While many opportunities exist for training, not all training programs are created equally. Important considerations for identifying quality programs include an intersectional approach, diverse leadership, and access to content and learning, balanced with self-reflection.[46]

While education is an important first step, it cannot be the only step that individuals, teams, and agencies take with the expectation that change will occur. True efforts toward issues of justice, equity, diversity, and inclusion require prioritization and commitment. During 2020, amid Black Lives Matter and social justice movements, alongside disproportionate effects of the pandemic in Black and Brown communities, the number of diversity and equity-related job postings increased 123% across corporations, including healthcare.[47] In addition to new positions, however, considerations of power and resources provided to diversity and equity leaders and their efforts must be a priority to enact and support change in structural processes. What happens to grassroots efforts when diversity and equity leadership is formalized with a hired position? Multifaceted *action* and interventions are needed to address systemic barriers, disparities, implicit and explicit bias, and underrepresentation from underserved groups as clinicians, researchers, policymakers, and leaders.[48]

One identified area for action is within our clinical spaces. It is important to have diverse systems that are racially representative of the populations served.[43] Efforts can be taken to create and support recruitment and training initiatives for clinicians and staff from underrepresented groups, along with identifying opportunities for leadership development.[43] Reid and colleagues[44] suggest "getting grounded" for equity and justice work within healthcare teams by (1) creating safe and healing spaces to discuss solutions, (2) examining local history of inequities, and (3) assessing the current state of health equity within their system. For example, Drs. Curseen and Bullock[49] discuss experiences as Black palliative care clinicians where there is an expectation that they must demonstrate they "know and understand what matters to White patients, families, and colleagues to be deemed competent" amidst a culture emphasizing humility to "absolve us of accountability for competency in knowing and demonstrating skills and behaviors that create equity in the way we care for patients."[49(pp 345-346)] Assessing our own implicit biases is paramount to addressing health equity and should be embedded into clinical training and education, along with use of objective systems for screening and assessing various symptoms.[42,50,51]

In addition to diversity in the workforce, researchers must prioritize representation in palliative care research.[43] In a 2022 review of race and ethnicity in hospice and palliative care research,[52] findings suggest that more than half of included studies did not include race and/or ethnicity in the analysis, few included a rationale for the collection of this data, and a total of 78 unique race and ethnic group labels were used, with the majority including non-standardized designations. Along with improvements in representation, changes in the landscape of academic publishing by establishing new structures (i.e., mentorship of underrepresented scholars in peer review, clear anti-racist guidelines) and processes (i.e., use of equity checklist, focused solicitation of equity-focused content, and self-assessment) across the publishing timeline (peer-review, submission and solicitation, and publication) might lead to more equitable publishing outcomes (i.e., increased diversity among reviewers and submissions).[53]

Finally, examining utilization or outcome differences based on race and other individual characteristics must be implemented so that disparities can be remediated.[43] One example of this is the Association of Social Work Boards' recent release of pass rate analysis, which showed large disparities on the clinical licensure exam for Black test takers, in addition to disparities for older social workers.[54] However, this release only happened after decades-long efforts of advocacy,[55] and advocacy for meaningful action as a result continues. The role of advocacy in addressing diversity and equity efforts cannot be overstated, demonstrating the interconnectedness in the presented priorities in intentionally interprofessional palliative care. One example for advocating at the institutional level is for leaders and clinicians to push their agency to address the 4 "planks" in providing inclusive care, including (1) a nondiscrimination statement; (2) employee benefits, orientation, and training; (3) intake forms and processes; and (4) marketing and community engagement.[56]

Implementation of Research in Practice and Education

A third priority for intentionally interprofessional palliative care is the focus on implementing cutting-edge research that explicitly incorporates the interprofessional team into clinical practice. For this to occur, research funding and growth driven from an interprofessional perspective, designed and conducted by interprofessional investigators, are needed, along with processes within interprofessional teams for integration of the evidence base. One important acknowledgment is that different professions have different models for evidence-based practice, and considerations for a transdisciplinary model of implementation in healthcare settings is important.[3] Understanding the state of palliative care research, particularly related to interprofessional teams, is a starting point for translating knowledge into practice and education.

The research base is growing exponentially in support of palliative care, but very little of that research is intentionally interprofessional. As shown in our own PubMed title search, palliative care mentioned in article titles has expanded from 16 articles in the 1970s to 2846 articles in 2021, of which 80 articles were randomized control trials (RCTs), meta-analyses, or clinical trials. In a separate, CAPC-led PubMed search, excluding 2 main palliative care journals (*Journal of Palliative Medicine* and *Journal of Pain & Symptom Management*), palliative care publications have grown across healthcare literature from several hundred in the year 2000 to 1500+ in the year 2022.[57] However, when considering knowledge translation and research implementation outside of specialized palliative care services, one 2022 scoping review found that the majority of studies were focused on cancer and/or in hospital systems, with only 7% of the identified articles focused on early palliative care.[58] Identified implementation barriers to the early integration of palliative care include an inadequate number of clinicians trained in palliative care, challenges in identifying appropriate patients for palliative care referral, and the overarching need for culture change across settings.[59] Similarly, identified barriers to high-quality research by interprofessional palliative care researchers included lack of funding, institutional capacity to support research, researcher workforce, population challenges (i.e., attrition, human subject protections), and ongoing misunderstanding and aversion to palliative care topics.[60]

Demiris and colleagues[61] provide an overview of implementation science in the context of hospice and palliative care, outlining several theories and frameworks along with 2 case studies of hospice clinical trials incorporating implementation considerations in their designs. Though the 2022 review on palliative knowledge translation and research implementation found multiple strategies in use with varying success, no single strategy was identified as outstanding, resulting in the continued call for how implementation science theories can be applied in palliative care, alongside consideration of combining strategies and connecting them to specific outcomes.[58] In the 553 clinical trials, RCTs, or meta-analyses published between 1990 and September 2022 from our search, only 5 articles included the terms "interprofessional" or "interdisciplinary" in the title. Topics in palliative care research mostly focus on disease-specific outcomes, symptom-specific outcomes, or profession-specific practices. Very little published palliative care research to date is created interprofessionally, focuses on exploring optimal team interaction, is generated in collaboration with interprofessional palliative care teams outside of the academic setting, or documents the effects of palliative care policy or standards on public health.

Research exploring the effects of interprofessional palliative care on the quadruple aim—improving population health, healthcare experience, per-capita cost, and the needs of the healthcare clinician—is dependent on development of consensus in 3 areas: shared language, outcomes that matter, and theoretical models for interprofessional palliative care education and collaborative practice.[62] In the area of shared language, there remains little consensus on key terms, such as the definition of an interprofessional palliative care team. Are 2 professions working together sufficient to meet this definition? What collaborative team characteristics are necessary? Or is presence of various professions alone sufficient? When considering interprofessional palliative care outcomes that matter, what successful clinical outcomes might be responsive to the synergy of transdisciplinary practice? What outcomes are affected by the absence of various team members? What educational outcomes might be responsive to differences between interprofessional and profession-specific education? Finally, many theoretical models have been presented and explored in this book, including the NCP Guidelines, IPEC competencies (see Chapter 5), the Generalist-Specialist Model of Interprofessional Palliative Care (see Chapter 3), and an aspirational model of interprofessional palliative care (see Chapter 16). What evidence is necessary to test the value of these models for interprofessional education and collaborative practice in palliative care in support of the quadruple aim, and how can we meaningfully translate and implement them in our workplaces and learning environments?

Current Opportunities in Palliative Care

Palliative care continues to grow toward goals of changing culture and becoming the standard of medical care, demonstrated in the following ways: representation of palliative care teams in 83.4% of U.S. hospitals with 50+ beds; more than 3000 community-based palliative care programs; new hospice and palliative care subspecialty certificates across specialty areas; increased perceived value of palliative care among referring clinicians and healthcare leadership; growth in non-palliative care clinicians' education in palliative care; and representation of palliative care leaders within policy and greater healthcare spaces.[57] In looking forward, the Center to Advance Palliative Care (CAPC) reminds us to "[practice] flawless basics," including (1) stakeholder alignment—"to understand their priorities, so you can plan your palliative care strategy accordingly"; (2) program financing—to ensure full representation of the interprofessional team; (3) operational efficiency—"continuously [looking] at issues like team communication, role clarity, and workflow to . . . make sure everyone is operating at the top of their license and skills"; and (4) team health—"to promote resilience [well-being] and prevent burnout."[57,63(np)] The interprofessional team is at the center of each of these areas, reminding us that our own teams and working environments serve as a springboard for continued efforts in effecting change in palliative care and beyond. In this chapter, we propose that *intentionally* interprofessional palliative care is key to seeking solutions to the challenges facing the palliative care landscape, for example, limited workforce or overreliance on familial caregiving with limited resources to provide support.

Palliative Care Workforce

Workforce shortage of clinicians is a key challenge to advancing palliative care identified by leaders in the field.[64] One estimate demonstrates that for every 100,000 older adults, there are only 13.35 hospice/palliative physicians (just shy of 7500/ physician),[65] with another suggesting that this will increase to one physician for every 26,000 patients by 2030 without significant growth in training trajectories.[66] While corresponding estimates for other members of the palliative care team do not exist, shortages across the interprofessional team are well acknowledged.[67,68] An additional factor requiring consideration related to workforce issues is that of the high risk for clinician burnout, as patients in hospice and palliative care are often vulnerable and/or complex in nature.[69,70]

Across professions, the most readily published approach for addressing workforce challenges is to improve and/or increase education and training.[68,71-73] In addition to hopefully recruiting larger numbers to specialize in palliative care,[71,72] training programs can focus on preparing generalist clinicians to incorporate primary palliative care across settings.[73,74] In nursing, the End-of-Life Nursing Education Consortium (ELNEC)[75] was launched in 2000 to improve end-of-life care with a widespread train-the-trainers curriculum to disseminate knowledge about caring for patients and families near the end of life. More recently, the National Association of Social Workers partnered with MJHS Institute for Innovation in Palliative Care and the Social Work Hospice & Palliative Care Network (SWHPN) to begin offering the Educating Social Workers in Palliative and End-of-Life Care (ESPEC) training program to help health social workers integrate primary palliative care in their clinical practice.[76] Few opportunities for interprofessional palliative care trainings currently exist at any level (see Chapter 10). Other efforts have focused on interventions addressing clinician burnout,[77,78] though most currently focus on individuals rather than approaching change systemically, which is needed.[69,79]

Coordinated interprofessional efforts to address workforce shortages are in their infancy, though one approach for overcoming physician shortages includes relying on and expanding use of interprofessional teams.[80] Applying an intentionally interprofessional approach as outlined here, efforts must span all levels (i.e., clinical, leadership, policy, education, research) and include focused efforts for advocacy, equity and diversity, and building interprofessional research for implementation. Opportunities for advocacy in public policy to address workforce shortages and lack of diversity include the Resident Physicians Shortage Act, which would address systemic barriers impacting physicians of color, and the Palliative Care Hospice Education and Training Act, which would help expand the interprofessional workforce through development of career awards, loan forgiveness programs, and provision of funding to health professional programs who teach palliative care.[42] Currently, schools with the highest percentages of Black residents have less access to opportunities for palliative care trainings.[81] At clinical and system levels, advocating for inclusive recruiting and hiring practices, such as use of standardized policies, evaluation of implicit biases, and provision of adequate mentorship and growth opportunities for diverse candidates, is equally important in addressing lack of diversity in the palliative care workforce. Finally, in addition to improving access to trainings and inclusive recruitment and hiring practices, research on expanding the palliative care workforce must be developed and tested interprofessionally. Trainings should also be built using an interprofessional framework and guided by interprofessionally led research.

Burden of Unpaid Caregivers

The family and friends who care for people living with serious illness describe an intense, overwhelming experience, often without acknowledgment or understanding of their role from the healthcare system.[82] Caregivers' experience not only is important to the individual or patient, but also is an essential consideration for the effectiveness of the provision of palliative care because caregivers influence patients' health behaviors, psychological well-being, quality of life, and healthcare utilization.[83] The patchwork of federal, state, and local policies and programs focused on serious illness that currently exist do not address the diverse needs of caregivers. A systematic evaluation of policies and programs with gaps in our understanding of what works, for whom, and under what circumstances still needs to be done.[84] Holistic solutions to the problem of accessible, affordable, skilled caregiving requires a multipronged approach, co-created across professions, agencies, programs, and policy. A kaleidoscope of perspectives is needed, all working together in a transdisciplinary way, to find a solution that provides the care needed by people with chronic, terminal, and serious illness.

With the exception of a few who have invested in very expensive long-term care insurance and those who qualify for Medicaid-funded custodial care in skilled nursing facilities or a few hours per week of caregiving from In-Home Support Services (IHSS), most people living with serious illness must fund their own caregiving needs. Most caregiving at the end of life is unpaid, while these caregivers spend up to 3 times as many hours offering care in the last month of life compared to caregivers at other times of life, especially in the case of spousal involvement.[84] Despite the increased hours and need, older adults at end of life are not more likely than other older adults to receive government, state, or private insurance-funded care.[85] The burden to the unpaid caregiver includes negative effects on employment, health, and well-being, with associated individual and societal costs.[86] One must also note the inequity that exists in the experiences and impacts of caregiver financial burden, reflected by diagnosis (cancer vs. non-cancer), socioeconomic status, gender, cultural and ethnic identity, and employment status influencing access to specialized palliative care.[87] Beyond the considerable financial burden of this responsibility,[87] families struggle with discord related to the amount of care that is necessary for their loved one and balancing autonomy with safety for their loved one with serious illness.

Additional challenges relate to caring for the cognitive and physical needs of the person while still attending to social and cultural aspects of care, and retaining paid and unpaid caregivers with the appropriate expertise. Conflicts among family members and caring communities may arise when responsibilities are not shared equally among caregivers. Maintaining one's own well-being, family, job, and other personal responsibilities adds tension when caring for someone who is seriously ill and aging. A consequence of these challenges is many days of avoidable hospitalization when families are no longer able to care for their loved one and drop them off at the emergency department, or delayed discharges when attempts to find a discharge solution that works for the patient are foiled by so many competing demands and interests.

The Rosalynn Carter Institute for Caregivers (RCI), which recognizes advocacy, equity, and knowledge (i.e., research and data) as 3 of its core values,[88] conducted a national survey of working caregivers and voters which documented these challenges.[89] They found that the biggest challenge facing caregivers was the emotional stress of balancing the caregivers' own career with their caregiving responsibilities. Although the proposed solutions that received the highest level of voter and caregiver support related to finances, primarily in the form of tax credits, caregivers expressed their desire for flexible scheduling, remote work, job sharing or reducing their workload, or availability of specialized caregiver services such as case management, back-up care, or safety modifications in the home. The problem of caregiving is multifaceted and not "owned" by government, employers, or the health system.

Commonly proposed, broad categories of potentially effective interventions to support unpaid caregivers include indirect support (services for the care-recipient), direct support (such as psychological therapies or financial funding), improvement to care conditions, or a combination of these.[86] There are also opportunities within the current healthcare system to engage family and other unpaid caregivers, support end-of-life care, provide long-term supports and services, and better utilize technology.[84] The RCI report recommends some solutions that could be implemented relatively easily, such as tax credits for families or companies that support family caregivers. But those financial solutions are not sufficient to solve the emotional stress experienced by caregivers. A number of interventions for supporting caregivers have been tested with promising results, led by chaplains,[90,91] social workers,[92] nurses,[93-95] or a collaboration of clinical team members,[96] though one systematic review noted the lack of research on supporting caregivers' physical health or health outcomes and the need for long-term efficacy.[97] The solution is not in a biomedical model. It requires the synergy, the alchemy, of an interprofessional and an interdisciplinary[†] team, brainstorming solutions, testing them using community-based participatory research methodologies, and then advocating for implementation of those solutions in support of patients with serious illness and their caregivers.

Conclusion

Informed by what has been learned from the inception of this text, this chapter outlines essential next steps in transforming the abstract ideas of deep-rooted interprofessionalism into practical reality. Here, we offer a platform for intentionally interprofessional palliative care. This starts with a petition to position interprofessional collaboration at the center of palliative care competency. It then moves to include and transcend standard directives for growth in education and practice to embrace additional necessary advances in interprofessional research, leadership, administration, advocacy, and well-being. This essentially egalitarian vision cannot manifest without a sobering examination and disruption of professional and social systems of inequity and inclusivity inherent in teamwork and institutional palliative care. Substantive change will also be energized from funding for robust evidence-based and outcome-focused

---

[†] Although often used interchangeably, "discipline" refers to a branch of knowledge, while "profession" refers to an occupation that requires special education and/or prolonged training and a formal qualification. In this book, we have attempted to standardize the use of the term "profession" when referring to occupations such as chaplaincy, medicine, nursing, and social work, but occasionally the term "discipline" is used, especially when focused on the theory and knowledge development of the professions.

interprofessionally generated research. Intentionally interprofessional palliative care, as imagined here, has the potential to address some of the most concerning issues currently facing the field while transforming the provision of care for patients and caregivers, including sustainability for all who devote themselves to the fierce and loving accompaniment of the seriously ill and dying.

At the start of this book project, authors of this chapter asked themselves: What would the world look like if palliative care education and practice were truly interprofessional? Through energized discourse and creative imagining, our esteemed author-collaborators have helped us respond to this inquiry throughout the chapters in this book. Conceived, written, and edited interprofessionally, both the process and product of this text are a dynamic testament to the power of evolutionary collaboration.

Discussion Questions:

1. Based on your role, name three concrete behaviors you can implement to be more intentionally interprofessional moving forward.
2. Identify three barriers or challenges to intentionally interprofessional palliative care in your setting (this can include learning environments). What suggestions or strategies might be useful in addressing these barriers and/or challenges?

References

1. Center to Advance Palliative Care. About Palliative Care. Accessed November 16, 2022. https://www.capc.org/about/palliative-care/.
2. World Health Organization. Palliative Care. Published 2020. Accessed November 28, 2022. https://www.who.int/news-room/fact-sheets/detail/palliative-care.
3. Satterfield JM, Spring B, Brownson RC, et al. Toward a transdisciplinary model of evidence-based practice. Milbank Q. 2009;87(2):368–390.
4. Klarare A, Lind S, Hansson J, Fossum B, Fürst CJ, Lundh Hagelin C. Leadership in specialist palliative home care teams: a qualitative study. J Nurs Manage. 2020;28(1):102–111.
5. Twaddle M. Teamwork—the new way. Health Prog St Louis. 2012;93(2):12.
6. Otis-Green S, Ferrell B, Spolum M, et al. An overview of the ACE Project—advocating for clinical excellence: transdisciplinary palliative care education. J Cancer Educ. 2009;24(2):120–126.
7. Dréano-Hartz S, Rhondali W, Ledoux M, et al. Burnout among physicians in palliative care: impact of clinical settings. Palliat Support Care. 2016;14(4):402–410.
8. Zanatta F, Maffoni M, Giardini A. Resilience in palliative healthcare professionals: a systematic review. Support Care Cancer. 2020;28(3):971–978.
9. Kwak J, Jamal A, Jones B, Timmerman GM, Hughes B, Fry L. An interprofessional approach to advance care planning. Am J Hosp Palliat Med. 2022;39(3):321–331.
10. Terashita-Tan S. Striving for wholeness and transdisciplinary teamwork at a Pacific Basin's pain and palliative care department. OMEGA. 2013;67(1–2):207–212.
11. Shah MA. Oncologic and palliative care in a global setting in the twenty-first century: the patient, family, and oncologic health care team. J Global Oncol. 2018;4:1–3.
12. Arnetz BB, Goetz CM, Arnetz JE, et al. Enhancing healthcare efficiency to achieve the Quadruple Aim: an exploratory study. BMC Res Notes. 2020;13(1):1–6.
13. National Consensus Project for Quality Palliative Care. Clinical Practice Guidelines for Quality Palliative Care. 4th ed. National Coalition for Hospice and Palliative Care; 2018.

14. VITALtalk. About us. Accessed November 28, 2022. https://www.vitaltalk.org/about-us/.

15. Paolini S, White F, Tropp L, et al. Transforming society with intergroup contact: current debates, state of the science, and pathways to engaging with social cohesion practitioners and policy makers. *J Social Issues*. 2021;77(1):11–37.

16. Rosen MA, DiazGranados D, Dietz AS, et al. Teamwork in healthcare: key discoveries enabling safer, high-quality care. *Am Psychologist*. 2018;73(4):433.

17. Wax A, DeChurch LA, Contractor NS. Self-organizing into winning teams: understanding the mechanisms that drive successful collaborations. *Small Group Res*. 2017;48(6):665–718.

18. Donesky D, De Leon K, Bailey A, et al. Excellence in postlicensure interprofessional palliative care education: consensus through a Delphi survey. *J Hosp Palliat Nurs*. 2020;22(1):17–25.

19. Kesonen P, Salminen L, Kero J, Aappola J, Haavisto E. An integrative review of interprofessional teamwork and required competence in specialized palliative care. *OMEGA*. 2022:00302228221085468.

20. Head BA, Schapmire T, Hermann C, et al. The Interdisciplinary Curriculum for Oncology Palliative Care Education (iCOPE): meeting the challenge of interprofessional education. *J Palliat Med*. 2014;17(10):1107–1114.

21. Schapmire TJ, Head BA, Furman CD, et al. The interprofessional education exchange: the impact of a faculty development program in interprofessional palliative oncology education on trainee competencies, skills, and satisfaction. *Palliat Medicine Rep*. 2021;2(1):296–304.

22. Fink RM, Arora K, Gleason SE, et al. Interprofessional master of science in palliative care: on becoming a palliative care community specialist. *J Palliat Med*. 2020;23(10):1370–1376.

23. Wu DS, Mehta AK, Brewer CB, et al. Defining clinical excellence for palliative care specialists: a concept whose time has come. *Am J Hosp Palliat Med*. 2022;39(12):1377–1382.

24. Khalili H, Orchard C, Laschinger HKS, Farah R. An interprofessional socialization framework for developing an interprofessional identity among health professions students. *J Interprof Care*. 2013;27(6):448–453.

25. Paradis E, Whitehead CR. Beyond the lamppost: a proposal for a fourth wave of education for collaboration. *Acad Med*. 2018;93(10):1457.

26. Rogers M, Meier DE, Heitner R, et al. The national palliative care registry: a decade of supporting growth and sustainability of palliative care programs. *J Palliat Med*. 2019;22(9):1026–1031.

27. Spetz J, Dudley N, Trupin L, Rogers M, Meier DE, Dumanovsky T. Few hospital palliative care programs meet national staffing recommendations. *Health Affairs*. 2016;35(9):1690–1697.

28. National Hospice and Palliative Care Organization. Advocacy. Published 2022. Accessed November 28, 2022. https://www.nhpco.org/advocacy/.

29. Hospice Action Network. National Hospice and Palliative Care Association. Published 2022. Accessed November 28, 2022. https://www.hospiceactionnetwork.org/.

30. S.4873 Improving Access to Advance Care Planning Act. Published 2022. Accessed November 28, 2022. https://www.warner.senate.gov/public/_cache/files/b/3/b3ccfab0-0ed9-4954-9695-2b5ce962ea2f/20382D2A1668A5EE3160BDC143157973.goe22520-1-.pdf.

31. Department of Health & Human Services, Centers for Medicare & Medicaid Services. Centers for Medicare & Medicaid Services' (CMS') Healthcare Common Procedure Coding System (HCPCS) Level II Final Coding, Benefit Category and Payment Determinations. Published 2022. Accessed November 28, 2022. https://www.cms.gov/files/document/2022-hcpcs-application-summary-biannual-1-2022-non-drug-and-non-biological-items-and-services.pdf.

32. McIntosh P, Luecke R. *Increase Your Influence at Work*. American Management Association; 2011.

33. Scholz B, Bocking J, Platania-Phung C, Banfield M, Happell B. "Not an afterthought": power imbalances in systemic partnerships between health service providers and consumers in a hospital setting. *Health Policy*. 2018;122(8):922–928.

34. Kelly D. Soft power and leadership. *Int J Palliat Nurs*. 2021;27(7):331–332.

35. Waterman RH, Peters TJ, Phillips JR. Structure is not organization. *Business Horizons*. 1980;23(3):14–26.

36. Gardner DS, Doherty M, Bates G, Koplow A, Johnson S. Racial and ethnic disparities in palliative care: a systematic scoping review. *Families Soc*. 2018;99(4):301–316.

37. Johnson KS. Racial and ethnic disparities in palliative care. *J Palliat Med.* 2013;16(11):1329–1334.

38. Orlovic M, Smith K, Mossialos E. Racial and ethnic differences in end-of-life care in the United States: evidence from the Health and Retirement Study (HRS). *SSM Population Health.* 2019;7:100331.

39. Chandrashekar P, Jain SH. Addressing patient bias and discrimination against clinicians of diverse backgrounds. *Acad Med.* 2020;95(12S):S33–S43.

40. Paul-Emile K, Critchfield JM, Wheeler M, de Bourmont S, Fernandez A. Addressing patient bias toward health care workers: recommendations for medical centers. *Ann Internal Med.* 2020;173(6):468–473.

41. Paradis E, Nimmon L, Wondimagegn D, Whitehead CR. Critical theory: broadening our thinking to explore the structural factors at play in health professions education. *Acad Med.* 2020;95(6):842–845.

42. Rosa W, Gray T, Chambers B. Palliative care in the face of racism: a call to transform clinical practice, research, policy, and leadership. *Health Affairs Forefront.* 2022.

43. Algu K. Denied the right to comfort: racial inequities in palliative care provision. *EClinicalMed.* 2021;34:1–2.

44. Reid A, Brandes R, Butler-MacKay D, et al. Getting grounded: building a foundation for health equity and racial justice work in health care teams. *NEJM Catalyst Innovations in Care Delivery.* 2022;3(1):1–13.

45. Borden E, Leimena ML, Sumser B. Centering the lens of social justice. In: Altilio T, Otis-Green S, Cagle JG, eds. *The Oxford Textbook of Palliative Social Work.* Oxford University Press; 2022:1.

46. Griffin SR. Where "diversity training" goes wrong, Part I: 10 essential questions to ask before engaging in social justice & DEI work. Justice Leaders Collaborative. Published 2021. Accessed November 28, 2022. https://www.justiceleaderscollaborative.com/blog/where-diversity-training-goes-wrong-10-essential-questions-to-ask-before-engaging-in-social-justice-amp-dei-work.

47. Dong S. The history and growth of the diversity, equity, and inclusion profession. Global Research and Consulting Group Insights. Published 2021. Accessed November 28, 2022. https://insights.grcglobalgroup.com/the-history-and-growth-of-the-diversity-equity-and-inclusion-profession/.

48. Rhodes RL. The ethnogeriatric implications of the COVID-19 pandemic. *J Health Care Poor Underserved.* 2021;32(1):64–67.

49. Curseen KA, Bullock K. Response to Fitzgerald Jones et al., Top Ten Tips Palliative Care Clinicians Should Know about Delivering Antiracist Care to Black Americans (DOI: 10.1089/jpm. 2021.05021). *J Palliat Med.* 2022;25(3):345–346.

50. Rivera-Burciaga AR, Palacios M, Kemery SA. Educating for equity in palliative care: implications of the Future of Nursing 2030 Report. *J Prof Nurs.* 2022;42:134–139.

51. Gazaway SB, Barnett MD, Bowman EH, et al. Health professionals palliative care education for older adults: overcoming ageism, racism, and gender bias. *Curr Geriatr Rep.* 2021;10:148–156.

52. Rhodes RL, Barrett NJ, Ejem DB, et al. A review of race and ethnicity in hospice and palliative medicine research: representation matters. *J Pain Symptom Manage.* 2022;64(5):e289–e299.

53. Sanders JJ, Gray TF, Sihlongonyane B, Durieux BN, Graham L. A framework for anti-racist publication in palliative care: structures, processes, and outcomes. *J Pain Symptom Manage.* 2022;63(3):e337–e343.

54. Association of Social Work Boards. 2022 ASWB Exam Pass Rate Analysis, Final Report. Published 2022. Accessed November 28, 2022. https://www.aswb.org/wp-content/uploads/2022/07/2022-ASWB-Exam-Pass-Rate-Analysis.pdf.

55. National Association of Social Workers. ASWB social work licensing exam pass rate data confirm concern over racial disparities. Published 2022. Accessed November 28, 2022. https://www.socialworkers.org/News/News-Releases/ID/2531/ASWB-social-work-licensing-exam-pass-rate-data-confirm-concern-over-racial-disparities.

56. Acquaviva KD. *LGBTQ-Inclusive Hospice and Palliative Care: A Practical Guide to Transforming Professional Practice*. Columbia University Press; 2017.

57. Bowman BM, Diane E. BRIEFING: Palliative care state of the field 2022. CAPC. Published 2022. Accessed December 1, 2022. https://www.capc.org/events/recorded-webinars/brief ing-palliative-care-state-of-the-field-2022/.

58. Öhlén J, Böling S, HamdanAlshehri H, et al. Strategies for knowledge translation of a palliative approach outside specialized palliative care services: a scoping review. *BMC Palliat Care*. 2022;21(1):1–14.

59. Aldridge MD, Hasselaar J, Garralda E, et al. Education, implementation, and policy barriers to greater integration of palliative care: a literature review. *Palliat Med*. 2016;30(3):224–239.

60. Chen EK, Riffin C, Reid MC, et al. Why is high-quality research on palliative care so hard to do? Barriers to improved research from a survey of palliative care researchers. *J Palliat Med*. 2014;17(7):782–787.

61. Demiris G, Parker Oliver D, Capurro D, Wittenberg-Lyles E. Implementation science: implications for intervention research in hospice and palliative care. *Gerontologist*. 2014;54(2):163–171.

62. Kirkpatrick AJ, Donesky D, Kitko LA. A systematic review of interprofessional palliative care education programs. *J Pain Symptom Manage*. 2023;65(5):e439–e466. doi:10.1016/ j.jpainsymman.2023.01.022. PMID: 36736863.

63. Center to Advance Palliative Care. Practicing flawless basics: palliative care sustainability in the COVID era. Accessed December 6, 2022. https://www.capc.org/practicing-flawless-bas ics-palliative-care-sustainability-covid-era/.

64. Cruz-Oliver DM, Bernacki R, Cooper Z, et al. The Cambia Sojourns Scholars Leadership Program: conversations with emerging leaders in palliative care. *J Palliat Med*. 2017;20(8):804–812.

65. Lupu D, Quigley L, Mehfoud N, Salsberg ES. The growing demand for hospice and palliative medicine physicians: will the supply keep up? *J Pain Symptom Manage*. 2018;55(4):1216–1223.

66. Kamal AH, Bull JH, Swetz KM, Wolf SP, Shanafelt TD, Myers ER. Future of the palliative care workforce: preview to an impending crisis. *Am J Med*. 2017;130(2):113–114.

67. World Health Organization. *State of the World's Nursing 2020: Investing in Education, Jobs and Leadership*. WHO; 2020.

68. Berg-Weger M, Schroepfer T. COVID-19 pandemic: workforce implications for gerontological social work. *J Gerontol Social Work*. 2020;63(6–7):524–529.

69. Harrison KL, Dzeng E, Ritchie CS, et al. Addressing palliative care clinician burnout in organizations: a workforce necessity, an ethical imperative. *J Pain Symptom Manage*. 2017;53(6):1091–1096.

70. Schneider C, Bristol A, Ford A, Lin S-Y, Brody AA, Stimpfel AW. A pilot observational exploratory study of well-being in hospice interdisciplinary team members. *Am J Hosp Palliat Med*. 2022;39(3):264–269.

71. Dingfield LE, Jackson VA, deLima Thomas J, Doyle KP, Ferris F, Radwany SM. Looking back, and ahead: a call to action for increasing the hospice and palliative medicine specialty pipeline. *J Palliat Med*. 2020;23(7):895–899.

72. Levine S, O'Mahony S, Baron A, et al. Training the workforce: description of a longitudinal interdisciplinary education and mentoring program in palliative care. *J Pain Symptom Manage*. 2017;53(4):728–737.

73. Duty SM, Loftus J. Transforming the workforce for primary palliative care through a system-wide educational initiative. *JONA*. 2019;49(10):466–472.

74. Pelleg A, Smith CB, Blackhall L. Cultural diversity and palliative care. In: Breitbart W, Chochinov H, eds. *Handbook of Psychiatry in Palliative Medicine: Psychosocial Care of the Terminally Ill*. Oxford University Press; 2022:237.

75. American Association of Colleges of Nursing. End-of-Life Nursing Education Consortium. Accessed January 4, 2023. https://www.aacnnursing.org/ELNEC.

76. National Association of Social Workers. Educating social workers in palliative and end-of-life care. Accessed January 4, 2023. https://www.socialworkers.org/espec.

77. Heeter C, Allbritton M, Lehto R, Miller P, McDaniel P, Paletta M. Feasibility, acceptability, and outcomes of a yoga-based meditation intervention for hospice professionals to combat burnout. *Int J Environ Res Public Health*. 2021;18(5):2515.

78. Mehta DH, Perez GK, Traeger L, et al. Building resiliency in a palliative care team: a pilot study. *J Pain Symptom Manage*. 2016;51(3):604–608.

79. Mills J, Ramachenderan J, Chapman M, Greenland R, Agar M. Prioritising workforce well-being and resilience: what COVID-19 is reminding us about self-care and staff support. *Palliat Med*. 2020;34(9):1137–1139.

80. Flaherty E, Bartels SJ. Addressing the community-based geriatric healthcare workforce shortage by leveraging the potential of interprofessional teams. *J Am Geriatr Soc*. 2019;67(S2):S400–S408.

81. Bell LF, Livingston J, Arnold RM, et al. Lack of exposure to palliative care training for black residents: a study of schools with highest and lowest percentages of Black enrollment. *J Pain Symptom Manage*. 2021;61(5):1023–1027.

82. Anderson EW, White KM. "It has changed my life": an exploration of caregiver experiences in serious illness. *Am J Hosp Palliat Med*. 2018;35(2):266–274.

83. Dionne-Odom JN, Hooker SA, Bekelman D, et al. Family caregiving for persons with heart failure at the intersection of heart failure and palliative care: a state-of-the-science review. *Heart Failure Rev*. 2017;22(5):543–557.

84. Reyes AM, Thunell J, Zissimopoulos J. Addressing the diverse needs of unpaid caregivers through new health-care policy opportunities. *Public Policy Aging Rep*. 2021;31(1):19–23.

85. Ornstein KA, Kelley AS, Bollens-Lund E, Wolff JL. A national profile of end-of-life caregiving in the United States. *Health Affairs*. 2017;36(7):1184–1192.

86. Brimblecombe N, Fernandez J-L, Knapp M, Rehill A, Wittenberg R. Review of the international evidence on support for unpaid carers. *J Long-Term Care*. 2018(September):25–40.

87. Gardiner C, Robinson J, Connolly M, et al. Equity and the financial costs of informal caregiving in palliative care: a critical debate. *BMC Palliat Care*. 2020;19(1):1–7.

88. Rosalynn Carter Institute for Caregivers. About us. Accessed January 4, 2023. https://www.rosalynncarter.org/about-us/.

89. Rosalynn Carter Institute for Caregivers. Working while caring: a national survey of caregiver stress in the U.S. workforce: key findings. Rosalynn Carter Institute for Caregivers. Published 2021. Accessed January 4, 2023. https://www.rosalynncarter.org/wp-content/uploads/2021/09/210140-RCI-National-Surveys-Executive-Summary-Update-9.22.21.pdf.

90. Perez SEV, Maiko S, Burke ES, et al. Spiritual Care Assessment and Intervention (SCAI) for adult outpatients with advanced cancer and caregivers: a pilot trial to assess feasibility, acceptability, and preliminary effects. *Am J Hosp Palliat Med*. 2022;39(8):895–906.

91. Steinhauser KE, Olsen A, Johnson KS, et al. The feasibility and acceptability of a chaplain-led intervention for caregivers of seriously ill patients: a Caregiver Outlook pilot study. *Palliat Support Care*. 2016;14(5):456–467.

92. Demiris G, Oliver DP, Washington K, Pike K. A problem-solving intervention for hospice family caregivers: a randomized clinical trial. *J Am Geriatr Soc*. 2019;67(7):1345–1352.

93. Becqué YN, Rietjens JA, van Driel AG, van der Heide A, Witkamp E. Nursing interventions to support family caregivers in end-of-life care at home: a systematic narrative review. *Int J Nurs Studies*. 2019;97:28–39.

94. Dionne-Odom JN, Ejem DB, Wells R, et al. Effects of a telehealth early palliative care intervention for family caregivers of persons with advanced heart failure: the ENABLE CHF-PC randomized clinical trial. *JAMA Network Open*. 2020;3(4):1–13.

95. Hendricks BA, Lofton C, Azuero A, et al. The project ENABLE Cornerstone randomized pilot trial: protocol for lay navigator-led early palliative care for African-American and rural advanced cancer family caregivers. *Cont Clin Trials Commun*. 2019;16:100485.

96. Toor H, Barrett R, Myers J, Parry N. Implementing a novel interprofessional caregiver support clinic: a palliative medicine and social work collaboration. *Am J Hosp Palliat Med*. 2022;39(8):913–917.

97. Ahn S, Romo RD, Campbell CL. A systematic review of interventions for family caregivers who care for patients with advanced cancer at home. *Patient Educ Counsel*. 2020;103(8):1518–1530.

Index